COMPLICATIONS AND PROBLEMS IN AESTHETIC PLASTIC SURGERY

COMPLICATIONS AND PROBLEMS IN AESTHETIC PLASTIC SURGERY

Edited by

George C. Peck, MD, FACS
Chief, Department of Plastic
and Reconstructive Surgery
Beth Israel Hospital
Passaic, New Jersey

Gower Medical Publishing
New York • London

Distributed in the USA and Canada by:

Raven Press
1185 Avenue of the Americas
New York, NY 10036
USA

Distributed in Japan by:

Nankodo Company Ltd.
42-6, Hongo 3-Chome
Bunkyo-Ku
Tokyo 113
Japan

Distributed in the rest of the world by:

Gower Medical Publishing
Middlesex House
34-42 Cleveland Street
London W1P 5FB
UK

Library of Congress Cataloging-in-Publication Data:
Complications and problems in aesthetic plastic surgery / edited by George C. Peck
    p. cm.
    Includes bibliographical references and index.
    ISBN 0-397-44613-6
    1. Surgery, Plastic--Complications and sequelae. I. Peck, George C., 1927-
    [DNLM: 1. Postoperative Complications. 2. Surgery, Plastic. WO 600 C737]
RD118.7.C66 1992
617.9'501--dc20
DNLM/DLC   91-42808
for Library of Congress

British Library Cataloguing in Publication Data:
Peck, George C. 1927-t
  Complications and problems in aesthetic plastic surgery.
  I. Title
  617.95

ISBN 0-397-44613-6

Editor: Kim Loretucci
Editorial Director: Jane Hunter
Art Director: Jill Feltham
Designer: Jeff Brown
Illustration Supervisor: Patricia Holtz
Illustrator: Carlyn Iverson

Printed in Hong Kong by Imago

10 9 8 7 6 5 4 3 2 1

PREFACE

Since the days of Jacques Joseph, there have been many books written about aesthetic surgery. However, *Complications and Problems in Aesthetic Surgery* is unique in that it is the first book to concentrate on the complications that may occur after aesthetic surgery and the problems that are associated with various procedures. As plastic surgeons, we go to meetings and hear about the many techniques that always seem to yield beautiful results. This book is an attempt to teach the plastic surgeon about the many traps and pitfalls that are always present and ready to ruin the most meticulous surgical procedure.

What better way to learn about a surgical procedure than to read about its complications and problems. If we can avoid these complications, we can become better aesthetic surgeons.

This book includes chapters covering the most commonly performed aesthetic procedures written by surgeons who have already made their mark in their chosen areas. Each chapter discuses the most common complications and problems, why they occur, how to prevent them, and how to correct them.

The book has been printed as a color atlas and much thanks must be given to the publisher, Gower Medical Publishing, for its ability to produce a book with so many vividly colored photographs of such excellent quality. My thanks also go to Kim Loretucci, our editor, who has spent so many tireless hours reviewing the manuscripts and working with our contributors.

George C. Peck, MD

CONTRIBUTORS

James L. Baker, Jr., MD, FACS
Cosmetic Surgeon
Winter Park, Florida

Eugene H. Courtiss, MD, FACS
Associate Clinical Professor of Surgery
Harvard Medical School
Cambridge, Massachusetts

David W. Furnas, MD, FACS
Chief, Division of Plastic Surgery
Department of Surgery
University of California, Irvine
College of Medicine
Irvine, California

Robert M. Goldwyn, MD, FACS
Clinical Professor of Surgery
Harvard Medical School
Cambridge, Massachusetts
Head, Division of Plastic Surgery
Beth Israel Hospital
Boston, Massachusetts

Frederick M. Grazer, MD, FACS
Associate Clinical Professor of Plastic
  and Reconstructive Surgery
  University of California, Irvine
College of Medicine
Irvine, California
Clinical Professor
Department of Surgery
Milton S. Hershey School of Medicine
Pennsylvania State University
Hershey, Pennsylvania

Ronald Gruber, MD
Clinical Instructor of Plastic Surgery
Stanford University Medical Center
Stanford, California

Elizabeth B. Jelks, MD
Assistant Clinical Professor of
  Ophthalmology
New York University Medical Center
New York, New York

Glenn W. Jelks, MD, FACS
Associate Professor of Surgery
  (Plastic Surgery) and of Ophthalmology
New York University Medical Center
New York, New York

Bernard L. Kaye, MD, DMD, FACS
Clinical Professor of Plastic Surgery
University of Florida
College of Medicine
Gainesville, California

Clyde Litton, MD, DDS, FACS
Private Practice
Washington, D.C.

George C. Peck, MD, FACS
Chief, Department of Plastic and
  Reconstructive Surgery
Beth Israel Hospital
Passaic, New Jersey

George C. Peck, Jr., MD
Attending Surgeon
Department of Plastic and
  Reconstructive Surgery
Beth Israel Hospital
Passaic, New Jersey, and
  Saint Barnabus Hospital
  Livingstone, New Jersey

Edward H. Szachowicz II, MD
Assistant Professor
Department of Otolaryngology
University of Minnesota Medical School
Minneapolis, Minnesota

Edward O. Terino, MD, FACS
Director, Plastic Surgery Institute
Agoura Hills, California

W. Graham Wood, MD
Clinical Instructor of Plastic Surgery
University of Southern California
School of Medicine
Los Angeles, California

CONTENTS

1 Rhinoplasty: Classic Problems and Complications

2 Rhinoplasty and Open Rhinoplasty

3 Facelift Surgery

4 Forehead Lift Surgery

5 Blepharoplasty

6 Chin and Malar Augmentation

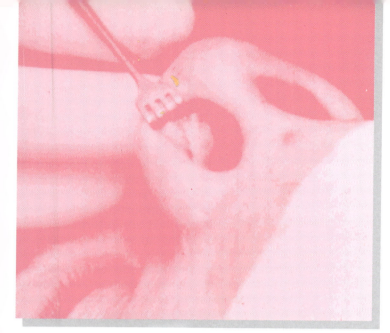

RHINOPLASTY: CLASSIC PROBLEMS AND COMPLICATIONS

George C. Peck
George C. Peck, Jr.

C H A P T E R

1

This chapter on complications in rhinoplasty delineates the most common problems occurring in primary and secondary rhinoplasty. It does not discuss the acute complications after rhinoplasty, such as bleeding or infection, since these problems are comprehensibly discussed in Chapter 2.

The most fundamental problem for the plastic surgeon performing a rhinoplasty is making an accurate diagnosis. The correct preoperative assessment leads to the proper treatment and a predictable aesthetic result. This chapter isolates the most frequently occurring problems in rhinoplasty and discusses their assessment, etiology and treatment.

INADEQUATE TIP PROJECTION

The most common complication after rhinoplasty is inadequate tip protection. This problem usually results after treating a patient with a large dorsal hump and an unsatisfactory nasal tip projection. A simple reduction rhinoplasty will accomplish adequate dorsal hump reduction, but it will not produce adequate tip projection. Furthermore, after sculpturing the lower lateral cartilages, the surgeon can expect further loss of tip projection. All rhinoplasties cannot be simple reductions. The surgery may require reduction, augmentation, or both.

Prevention of inadequate tip projection begins with correct preoperative assessment. The surgeon must evaluate the extent of tip projection as well as septal support. Nasal tip projection is assessed as adequate, inadequate, or excessive. Septal support is determined by simple palpation of the nasal tip. If the nasal tip is well supported by septal cartilage, the surgeon can conclude that the nose has adequate septal support. Once nasal tip projection and septal support are determined, the surgeon can decide on the appropriate surgical course.

The treatment of a patient with inadequate tip projection depends on the adequacy of septal support. A patient with inadequate tip projection and good septal support may only require onlay cartilage grafts to the nasal tip. The same patient with inadequate septal support will require an umbrella graft.

Inadequate Tip Projection with Good Septal Support

An 18-year-old female presented for a primary rhinoplasty. On physical examination, the patient had inadequate tip projection and good septal

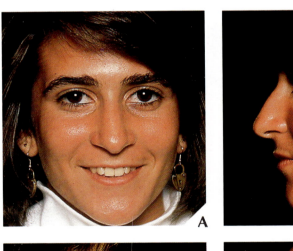
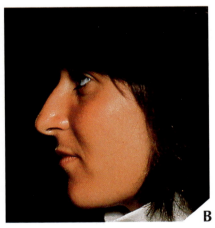
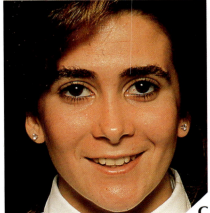
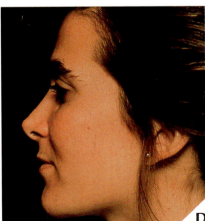

Figure 1.1. (A) Inadequate tip projection with good septal support. (B) Profile shows inadequate tip projection and moderate dorsal hump. (C) Primary rhinoplasty with tip augmentation. (D) Inadequate tip projection treated with onlay grafts.

support. In the lateral view, the patient exhibited a moderate dorsal hump, a long nose, and microgenia (Fig. l.1A,B).

The procedure began as a standard reduction rhinoplasty: sculpturing of the bilateral lower lateral cartilages, shortening and rotation of the tip, rasping of the dorsal nasal bone, lowering of the supratip septal cartilage, and infracturing of the bilateral nasal bones. Since the patient had inadequate tip projection with good septal support, she only required an onlay graft to the nasal tip. In this case, a double onlay graft of lower lateral cartilage was placed in a horizontal pocket over the alar domes. Alar base reduction, using the standard modified Weir's technique, and chin augmentation were also performed.

One year postoperatively, the patient has a nice dorsal line with the nasal tip projecting 2 to 3 mm above the dorsum. The onlay graft accentuates the result by producing a nasal tip that stands out and has good projection (Fig. 1.1C,D).

Inadequate Tip Projection with Inadequate Septal Support

An 18-year-old male presented for a primary rhinoplasty. On examination, the patient had inadequate tip projection with inadequate septal support. The patient also had a moderate dorsal hump with a round and drooping tip. The nose was long and crowded the lip (Fig. 1.2A,B).

The treatment began as a reduction rhinoplasty. The lower lateral cartilages were sculptured to give tip definition. The caudal septum was shortened. The dorsal nasal bone was rasped and the supratip septum was lowered. A V-to-Y advancement of the frenulum was performed to release the hypertrophic band that was causing a crowded lip.

At this point in the procedure, the surgeon has not treated the patient's inadequate tip projection. An umbrella graft was necessary since there was inadequate septal support. The strut for the umbrella graft was harvested from the septal cartilage and placed between the medial crura through a vertical infracartilaginous incision in the columella. The strut is always capped with an onlay graft, usually from conchal cartilage. The conchal cartilage onlay graft is approximately 4 x 9 mm and can be attached to achieve the necessary projection.

Postoperatively, the patient has a nice dorsal line and an appropriate nasolabial angle (Fig. 1.2C,D).

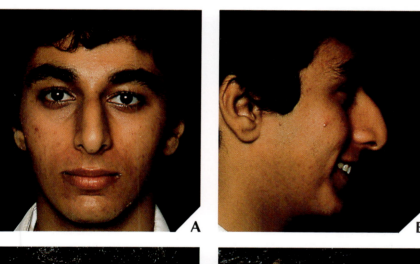
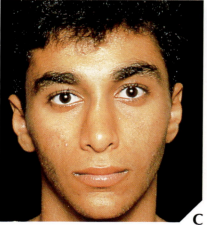
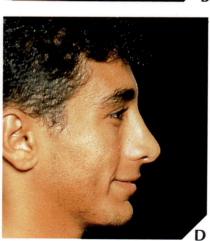

Figure 1.2. (A) Inadequate tip projection and inadequate septal support. (B) Profile shows a long nose, moderate hump, and drooping tip. (C) Primary rhinoplasty and tip augmentation. (D) Inadequate tip projection and drooping tip treated with an umbrella graft.

Inadequate Tip Projection in a Secondary Rhinoplasty

A 40-year-old female with inadequate tip projection presented for a secondary rhinoplasty. On examination, the patient had good septal support, a wide bridge, and a depression in the lateralmost portion of the left lower lateral cartilage (Fig. 1.3A,B).

The procedure for correcting these problems consisted of sculpturing the lower lateral cartilage, rasping the dorsum slightly, and infracturing the nasal bones. A double onlay graft from conchal cartilage was placed in the nasal tip to achieve better nasal tip projection. A filler graft of conchal cartilage was placed in the area of the lateral depression. Alar base reduction and chin augmentation were also done.

In the postoperative photographs, the frontal view shows the resolution of the depressed area in the left lower lateral cartilage. In the lateral view, the patient has satisfactory nasal tip projection (Fig. 1.3C,D).

SADDLE NOSE DEFORMITY

The most common cause of saddle nose deformity is iatrogenic trauma, other causes being accidental trauma and congenital deformity. When the deformity is the result of rhinoplasty, it is caused by over-reduction of the dorsal septal cartilage, nasal bone, or both. Another cause of saddle deformity is the dislocation of the osseo-cartilaginous junction in the dorsal strut following septal surgery.

Surgically produced nasal deformities can be prevented through good surgical technique. For example, the reduction of the nasal bones should always be done with a rasp rather than an osteotome. The rasp offers much better control and reduces the nasal bones more evenly. Also, the sequence of surgery is important. It is much

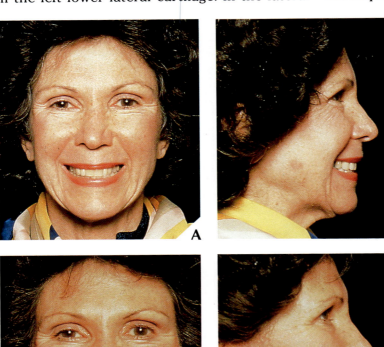
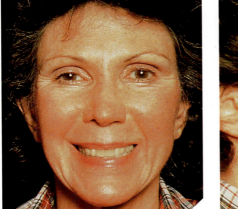
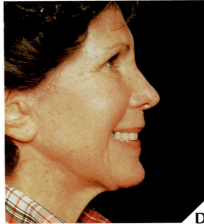

Figure 1.3. (A) Patient presenting for secondary rhinoplasty: depression on left lower lateral cartilage. (B) Profile shows inadequate tip projection. (C) Filler graft to left lower lateral cartilage. (D) Double onlay graft to nasal tip.

safer to do septal surgery after completing rasp reduction of the nasal hump, since a tremendous amount of force is applied to the septum with the rasp.

Correction of a saddle nose deformity involves augmentation with autogenous cartilage or bone. Silastic implants should never be used due to the high rate of complications associated with them.

Moderate saddle deformities can easily be corrected using cartilage grafts. Our preference is a dorsal hull-shaped graft from conchal cartilage because of its great shape and conformity. Septal cartilage is another alternative, although the edges of the graft are more prone to show postoperatively.

A very reliable way of correcting the minimal saddle deformity involves the use of a conchal cartilage graft. This graft is harvested from either ear using a posterior auricular incision. The conchal region just superior to the transverse bar is ideal in shape and length. The shape is similar to the hull of a boat; therefore, the graft is called a dorsal hull-shaped conchal cartilage graft.

The notched alar rims were also treated with conchal cartilage grafts. These rectangular grafts were placed into the involved rim through an intravestibular incision in a pocket as close as possible to the rim's edge.

The postoperative photographs reveal resolution of the saddle deformity and the notched alar rims (Fig. 1.4C,D).

Minimal Saddle Deformity

A 47-year-old female presented with a saddle nose deformity as a result of a previous rhinoplasty. The patient also had notched alar rims that were easily seen in the lateral views (Fig. 1.4A,B).

Moderate Saddle Deformity

A 25-year-old female presented with a moderate saddle deformity and a hanging columella as a result of a previous rhinoplasty. She also had asymmetric alar domes seen in the frontal view

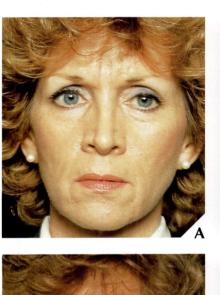
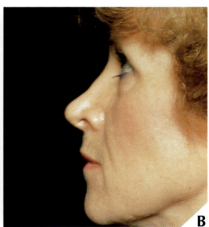
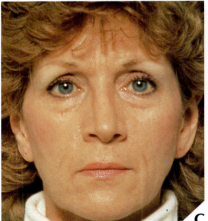
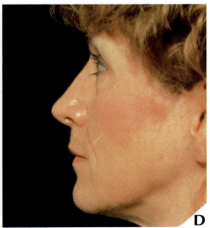

Figure 1.4. **(A)** Patient presenting for secondary rhinoplasty: minimal saddle deformity. **(B)** Saddle nose deformity with notched alar rims. **(C)** Hull-shaped graft from ear to nasal dorsum. **(D)** Rectangular graft to alar rim.

and an abnormal lobule seen in the lateral view (Fig. 1.5A,B).

The patient underwent sculpturing of the lower lateral cartilages, shortening of the caudal septum, and placement of an umbrella graft to the tip, capped with a triple onlay graft. A triple onlay graft from septal cartilage was placed on the dorsum to correct the saddle deformity. A double onlay graft of triangular conchal cartilage was used to reconstruct the underside of the lobule. Suction-assisted lipectomy of the neck was also done.

Postoperatively, the patient has resolution of the saddle deformity and hanging columella. She has good nasal tip projection and an overall good aesthetic result (Fig. 1.5C,D).

THE HANGING COLUMELLA

Another common problem in primary and secondary rhinoplasty is the hanging columella. This deformity is usually a result of excess caudal septum or occasionally due to the medial crural foot plate. Prevention of this problem requires adequate reduction of the caudal septum.

Surgical treatment of the hanging columella involves shortening the caudal end of the septal cartilage and trimming the anterior nasal spine if necessary. The nasal spine should never be completely removed since a recessed nasolabial angle can develop. In shortening the posterior two-thirds of the caudal septum, the surgeon attempts to produce a 90° nasolabial angle. The anterior third of the caudal septum determines tip rotation. The surgeon should trim the anterior third of the caudal septum to produce an obtuse angle.

A patient with a classic case of hanging columella presented for a secondary rhinoplasty. The hanging columella caused by excess caudal septum was prominent and obvious in the lateral preoperative view. The patient also had inadequate tip projection, a short nose, an abnormal lobular angle, microgenia, and malar hypoplasia (Fig. 1.6A,B).

The hanging columella was corrected by shortening the caudal septum, trimming the excess

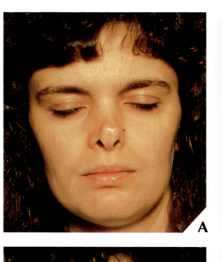
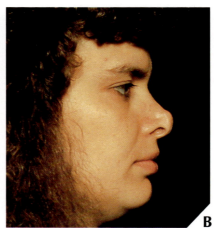
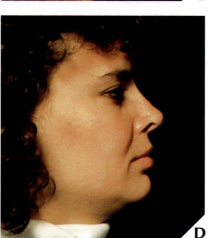

Figure 1.5. (A) Patient presenting for secondary rhinoplasty: asymmetric alar domes. (B) Saddle nose deformity and hanging columella. (C) Umbrella graft with triple onlay to nasal tip. (D) Dorsal graft and double triangular graft to underside of lobule.

A

B

C

D

membranous columella, and partially excising the anterior nasal spine. The patient also underwent lowering of the supratip septum. A double triangular filler graft was placed in the underside of the lobule in order to increase the length of the nose. A double onlay graft from conchal cartilage was placed in the tip. Chin augmentation, malar augmentation, and suction-assisted lipectomy of the neck were also performed. Postoperatively, the patient has an appropriate nasolabial angle, facial symmetry, and balance (Fig. 1.6C,D).

SUPRATIP DEFORMITY (PARROT BEAK DEFORMITY)

The supratip, or parrot beak, deformity is characterized by a high supratip septum and inadequate tip projection. This deformity is caused by inappropriate lowering of the supratip septal cartilage and loss of tip projection.

To avoid this complication during rhinoplasty, the surgeon must lower the supratip septal cartilage appropriately and correct the inadequate tip projection. Treatment requires a reduction and an augmentation rhinoplasty. The augmentation to the nasal tip may only require onlay cartilage grafts, if septal support is adequate. The patient with inadequate septal support requires an umbrella graft.

Supratip Deformity with Adequate Septal Support

A 30-year-old female with a supratip deformity presented for a secondary rhinoplasty. On examination, the patient had a high supratip septum and inadequate tip projection but good septal support. She also had a hanging col-

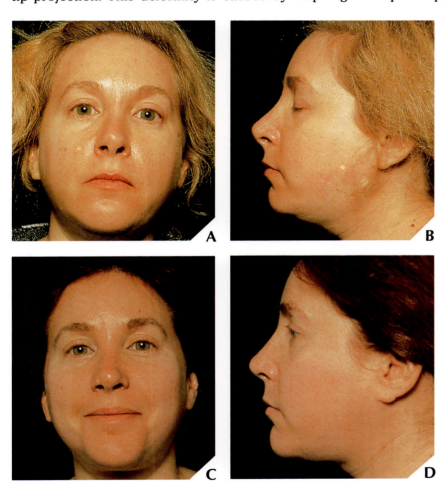

Figure 1.6. (A) Patient presenting for secondary rhinoplasty: hanging columella. (B) Loss of obtuse angle of anterior one-third of columella. (C) Shorter caudal septum and trimmed membranous columella. (D) Partial excision of the nasal spine and triangular graft to underside of lobule.

umella and a cleft of the alar domes at the tip (Fig. 1.7A,B).

The procedure for treating the supratip deformity includes lowering the supratip septum and augmenting nasal tip projection. This patient underwent lowering of the supratip septum, augmentation of the nasal tip projection with a double onlay graft from lower lateral cartilage, sculpturing of the lower lateral cartilages, shortening of the caudal septum with elevation of the tip, and slight rasping of the dorsal nasal bones. A modified lateral rotation of the lower lateral cartilages was done by partially crosscutting the alar domes to make the nasal tip less broad and more defined. An alar base resection using a modified Weir's technique was also performed to narrow the alar base. Postoperatively, the patient has a nice dorsal line and nasolabial angle, as well as good nasal tip projection (Fig. 1.7C,D).

Supratip Deformity with Inadequate Septal Support

A 27-year-old female with a supratip deformity and inadequate tip projection presented for a secondary rhinoplasty. On examination, the patient had inadequate septal support, minimal saddle nose deformity, loss of the obtuse angle on the anterior one-third of the columella, and veiling of the alar rims (Fig. 1.8A,B).

The patient underwent sculpturing of the lower lateral cartilages, lowering of the supratip septum, and placement of a double onlay graft from conchal cartilage to the dorsum. In addition, an umbrella graft was placed in the nasal tip and capped with a quadruple onlay graft. A triangular filler graft was placed to the anterior third of the columella to reconstruct the obtuse angle. A Millard excision of bilateral alar rims was per-

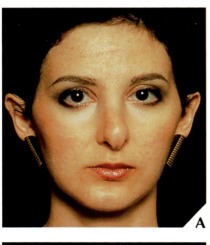
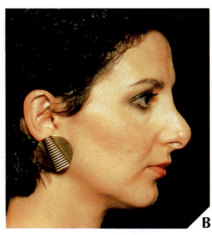
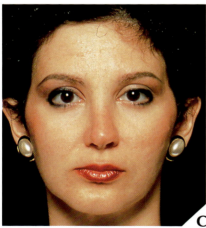
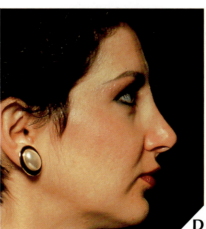

Figure 1.7. (A) Patient presenting for secondary rhinoplasty: supratip deformity. (B) Inadequate tip projection. (C) Shorter caudal septum and lower supratip septum. (D) Double onlay graft to nasal tip from lower lateral cartilage.

formed to correct the veiling of the alar rims. Postoperatively, the patient has a nice dorsal line, good nasal tip projection, and resolution of the veiling alar rims (Fig. 1.8C,D).

THE BROAD NASAL TIP

The complication of a broad nasal tip may result from the inability to refine and narrow the nasal tip during the procedure. After a basic rhinoplasty, the surgeon may find that the nasal tip remains broad. An untreated broad nasal tip will yield an unsatisfactory aesthetic result.

To prevent a broad nasal tip from occurring, the surgeon must first diagnose the problem preoperatively and know how to correct it intraoperatively. The patient may have a minimally broad tip or an extremely broad tip, neither of which resolves by simple sculpturing of the lower lateral cartilages.

The treatment of a *minimally* broad tip requires a crosscutting technique, which achieves narrowing of the dome while preserving the integrity of the lower lateral cartilage. The cartilage is crosscut at the dome, but the incision does not extend from one edge to the other. The integrity of the dome arch is preserved.

The treatment of an *extremely* broad tip requires the same crosscutting technique, as well as excision of a section of the lateral-most portion of the lateral crus. The lateral crus is then repositioned in its bed.

The Broad Nasal Tip and Long Nose

A 16-year-old female with a broad nasal tip presented for a primary rhinoplasty. She also had a broad nasal bridge, a long nose with a crowded

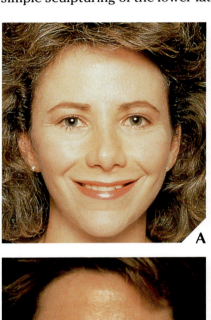
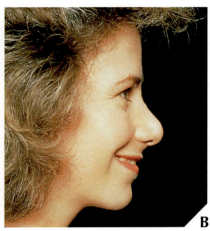
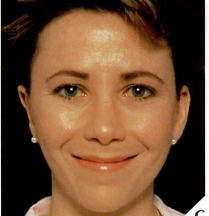
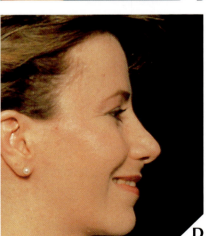

Figure 1.8. **(A)** Supratip deformity and inadequate tip projection. **(B)** Saddle deformity and loss of obtuse angle. **(C)** Lower supratip and double onlay graft to dorsum. **(D)** Umbrella graft and triangular graft to lobule.

lip, and inadequate tip projection with good septal support (Fig. 1.9A,B).

The treatment of this moderately broad nasal tip involved crosscutting of the alar domes. The patient also underwent sculpturing of the lower lateral cartilages, shortening of the caudal septum, slight lowering of the dorsum, raising of the tip, and infracturing of the nasal bones. A double onlay graft from the lower lateral cartilage was placed in the tip. Postoperatively, the patient has a well-defined nasal bridge and nasal tip with good tip projection (Fig. 1.9C,D).

The Broad Nasal Tip and Retracted Columella

A patient with a broad nasal tip and a retracted columella presented for secondary rhinoplasty. On evaluation, she had a minimal saddle deformity, inadequate tip projection with good septal support, a cleft between the alar domes, and a wide alar base (Fig. 1.10A–C).

The treatment of the broad nasal tip began by sculpturing the lower lateral cartilages. The alar domes were partially crosscut and a modified lateral rotation of the lower lateral cartilages was done to give the tip better definition. This patient also underwent placement of a quadruple onlay graft to the nasal tip using ear cartilage, a triangular graft from the septum to the anterior one-third of the columella, and two rectangular grafts to the poste-

rior two-thirds of the columella. An alar base reduction was also performed. Postoperatively, the patient has a defined nasal tip with good projection and resolution of the flared alar rims (Fig. 1.10D–F).

THE LONG NOSE
A long nose is excessively long from the glabella to the nasal tip. This problem results from inappropriate shortening of the caudal septum. The long nose is treated by reduction rhinoplasty and by shortening the posterior two-thirds of the caudal septum.

The Classic Long Nose
A 34-year-old female with a long nose presented for primary rhinoplasty. On examination, she also exhibited a moderate dorsal hump and wide alar base (Fig. 1.11A,B).

In treating the long nose, the surgeon decreases the distance from the root of the nose to the nasal tip by shortening the caudal end of the septum. This patient also underwent sculpturing of the lower lateral cartilages, rotation of the tip, rasping of the dorsal nasal bones, infracturing of the nasal bones, lowering of the supratip septum, and reduction of the alar base. There were no cartilage grafts placed in the nose. Postoperatively, the patient has better symmetry and facial balance (Fig. 1.11C,D).

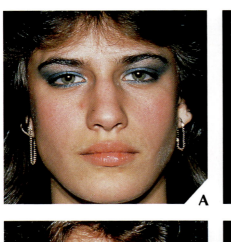
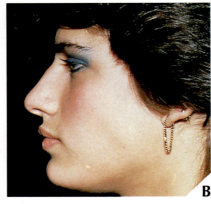
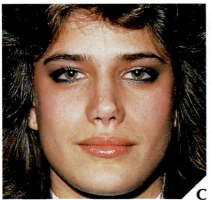
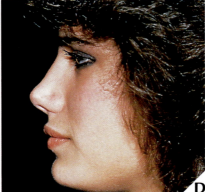

Figure 1.9. (A) Patient presenting for primary rhinoplasty: broad nasal tip and bridge. **(B)** Long nose and inadequate tip projection. **(C)** Crosscut alar domes to narrow nasal tip and infracture. **(D)** Shorter caudal septum and double onlay graft to nasal tip.

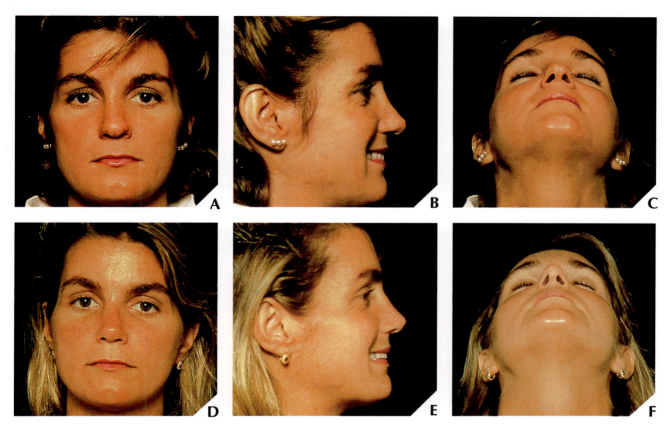

Figure 1.10. (A) Broad nasal tip. **(B)** Inadequate tip projection and retracted columella. **(C)** Cleft between alar domes. **(D)** Crosscut domes and modified lateral rotation of lower lateral cartilages. **(E)** Quadruple graft to nasal tip and rectangular grafts to posterior columella. **(F)** Good tip projection and resolution of cleft.

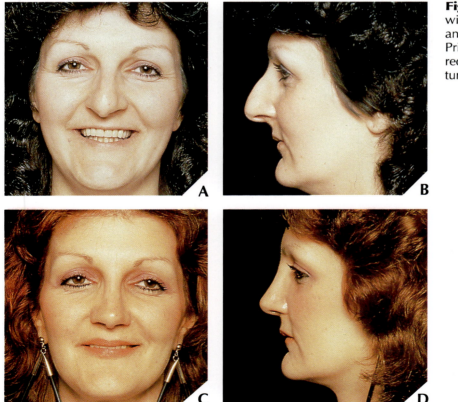

Figure 1.11. (A) Long nose and wide alar base. **(B)** Dorsal hump and adequate tip projection. **(C)** Primary rhinoplasty and alar base reduction. **(D)** Shorter caudal septum and no grafts to nasal tip.

The Long Nose with Saddle Deformity

A 29-year-old female with a long nose, saddle deformity, and hanging columella presented for a secondary rhinoplasty. She also had a collapse of the lateral aspect of the lower lateral cartilage, caused by previous excision of the lateral crus (Fig. 1.12A,B).

The procedure began as a reduction rhinoplasty with sculpturing of the lower lateral cartilages, shortening of the caudal septum, and cephalad rotation of the tip. A dorsal hull-shaped graft was placed to correct the saddle deformity, and alar base reduction was performed. There were no grafts placed in the nasal tip.

In the postoperative photographs, the patient has a nice dorsal line and nasolabial angle. The length of the nose is more appropriate for the face (Fig. 1.12C,D).

THE SHORT NOSE

A short nose is inappropriately short from the glabella to the nasal tip. This problem can result after rhinoplasty from excessive shortening of the posterior two-thirds of the caudal septum and improper tip rotation of the anterior one-third of the caudal septum.

A short nose can be prevented by proper reduction during rhinoplasty. The correction involves nasal reconstruction with autogenous cartilage

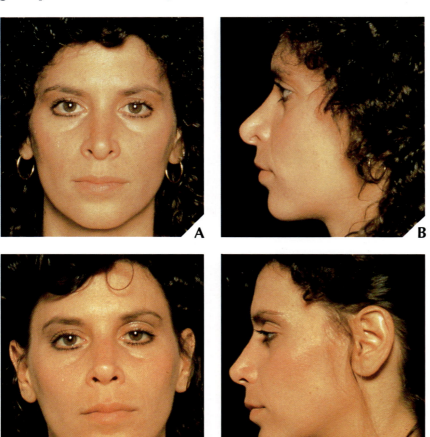

Figure 1.12. (A) Long nose and collapse of lower lateral crus. (B) Saddle deformity and hanging columella. (C) Secondary rhinoplasty. (D) Shorter caudal septum and dorsal hull-shaped graft.

grafts. The posterior two-thirds of the caudal septum is reconstructed with rectangular cartilage grafts. The underside of the lobule (anterior one-third columella) is reconstructed with triangular grafts.

A patient, who had had multiple previous rhinoplasties, presented with a very short nose. On evaluation, she also had inadequate tip projection with inadequate septal support, a saddle deformity, and a wide alar base (Fig. 1.13A,B).

During surgery, a double triangular filler graft was placed in the underside of the lobule on the anterior one-third of the columella and a double rectangular graft was placed in the posterior two-thirds of the columella. A dorsal hull-shaped con-

chal cartilage graft was placed to correct the saddle nose. An umbrella graft capped with a triple onlay graft in the nasal tip increased nasal tip projection. An alar base reduction was also performed. Postoperatively, the patient has a longer nose and a much less noticeable nasal deformity (Fig. 1.13C,D).

OPEN ROOF DEFORMITY

The open roof deformity after rhinoplasty results from improper positioning of the nasal bones. This may be due to inadequate infracturing of the nasal bones or a high-deviated septum preventing proper reduction of the nasal bones.

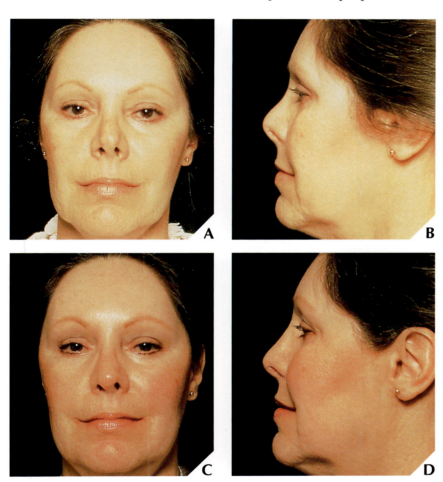

Figure 1.13. (A) Patient presenting for secondary rhinoplasty: very short nose. (B) Saddle deformity and inadequate tip projection. (C) Nasal reconstruction and columellar reconstruction. (D) Dorsal hull-shaped graft and umbrella graft.

Treatment of an open roof deformity requires adequate reduction of the nasal bones. The proper infracture technique and correction of a high-deviated septum assure adequate reduction of the nasal bones.

A 22-year-old female with open roof deformity presented for a secondary rhinoplasty. On examination, the patient was also found to have a wide nasal bridge and inadequate tip projection (Fig. 1.14A,B). In this case, the treatment of the open roof deformity involved infracturing and proper reduction of the nasal bones. The patient also underwent sculpturing of the lower lateral cartilages and placement of an umbrella graft to the nasal tip with a triple onlay graft. The upper lateral cartilages were separated from the septum to narrow the middle vault. Postoperatively, the patient has a narrower nasal bridge and better tip projection (Fig. 1.14C,D).

PINOCCHIO TIP DEFORMITY

The Pinocchio tip deformity is characterized by excessive nasal tip projection. It is one of the most difficult problems to treat in rhinoplasty. The treatment consists of a standard conservative reduction rhinoplasty producing good lines. By sculpturing the lower lateral cartilages and leaving no more than 2 to 3 mm of caudal lower lateral cartilage, the surgeon may achieve an acceptable result. If further reduction is necessary, the surgeon must amputate the alar domes to decrease nasal tip projection. An onlay graft of

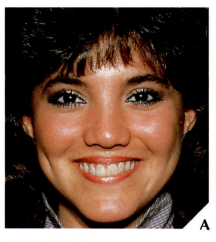
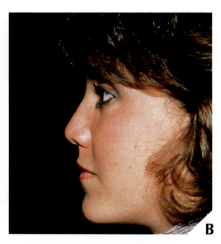
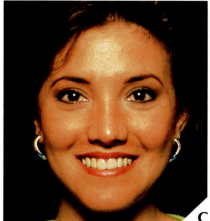
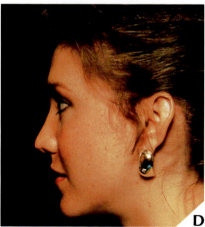

Figure 1.14. (A) Patient presenting for secondary rhinoplasty: open roof deformity. (B) Inadequate tip projection. (C) Infracturing of nasal bones and upper lateral cartilages separated from septum. (D) Umbrella graft to nasal tip with triple onlay graft.

conchal cartilage is added to the tip for permanent tip shaping.

A 47-year-old female with excessive nasal tip projection presented for a primary rhinoplasty. She also had a long nose, a wide nasal bridge, a slightly high dorsum and a wide alar base (Fig. 1.15A,B).

The treatment for this patient with a Pinocchio tip deformity began with a reduction rhinoplasty. However, excessive nasal tip projection persisted. The alar domes were then excised and the nasal tip was reconstructed with cartilage grafts. This patient also underwent sculpturing of the lower lateral cartilages, slight rasping of the dorsum, lowering of the supratip septum, and infracturing of the nasal bones.

Augmentation of the nasal tip was performed by placement of a double onlay graft to the tip. Postoperatively, the patient has a good dorsal line and nasolabial angle, with a resolution of the excessive nasal tip projection (Fig. 1.15C,D).

ALAR RIM DEFORMITIES

Alar rim deformities consist of a wide alar base and notching, veiling, and total collapse of the alar rim. The most common alar rim deformity is a wide alar base. It is caused by flaring of the rims, a wide floor, or both. The treatment consists of reduction of the alar base using the modified Weir's technique.

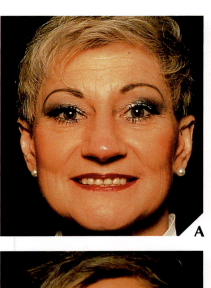
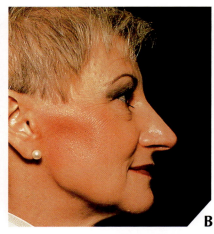
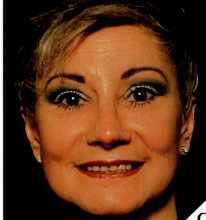
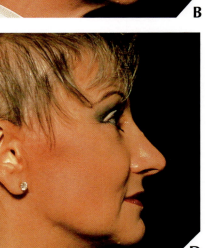

Figure 1.15. (A) Pinocchio tip deformity and wide nasal bridge. **(B)** Excessive tip projection. **(C)** Infracture of nasal bones and alar base reduction. **(D)** Excision alar domes and double onlay to nasal tip.

The Wide Alar Base

A 23-year-old male with alar rim flaring, inadequate tip projection, and a mild saddle deformity presented for primary rhinoplasty (Fig. 1.16A–C). A modified Weir's resection of the alar rims was performed to treat the flared alar rims. The lower lateral cartilages were sculptured, and an umbrella graft was placed in the nasal tip and capped with a double onlay graft. A double onlay graft was also placed in the dorsum of the nose.

Postoperatively, the patient has a narrower alar base and better nasal tip projection (Fig. 1.16D–F).

Alar Rim Veiling

A veiling alar rim is a less common complication; however, the diagnosis and treatment must be understood in order to achieve a good aesthetic result. In the ideal profile, 2 to 3 mm of columella will show. Veiling of the alar rims causes little or no columella to show. Excessive and inappropriate shortening of the caudal septum is the usual cause of veiling of the alar rims.

Surgical correction of the veiling alar rims requires the use of the Millard excision. This procedure involves a wedge excision of the alar rim at the caudal surface of the rim. The incision is closed with interrupted 5-0 nylon sutures and the scar is rarely noticeable.

A 19-year-old female with a veiling alar rim presented for a secondary rhinoplasty. In the patient's lateral view, no columellar show was seen in repose or when smiling (Fig. 1.17A–D).

A wedge excision of the veiling alar rims was performed to correct this problem. The patient also underwent sculpturing of the lower lateral cartilages and lowering of the supratip septum. Her nasal bones were infractured and upper lateral cartilages transected from the midline septum. Her columella was reconstructed with a triangular filler graft to the anterior one-third of the columella, and a double rectangular graft to the posterior two-thirds of the columella. Postoperatively, in both lateral views, the columella is appropriately seen (Fig. 1.17E–H).

CARTILAGE GRAFT COMPLICATIONS

Complications of onlay grafts or umbrella grafts to the nasal tip are not common. Infections and extrusion of the cartilage graft are rarely seen. The most common complication of cartilage graft-

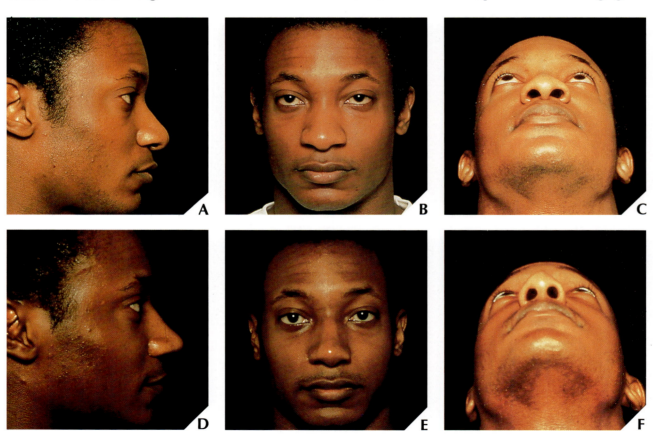

Figure 1.16. (A) Alar rim flaring. **(B)** Inadequate tip projection and mild saddle deformity. **(C)** Wide alar base. **(D)** Alar base reduction. **(E)** Double onlay graft to dorsum. **(F)** Umbrella graft to tip with double onlay graft.

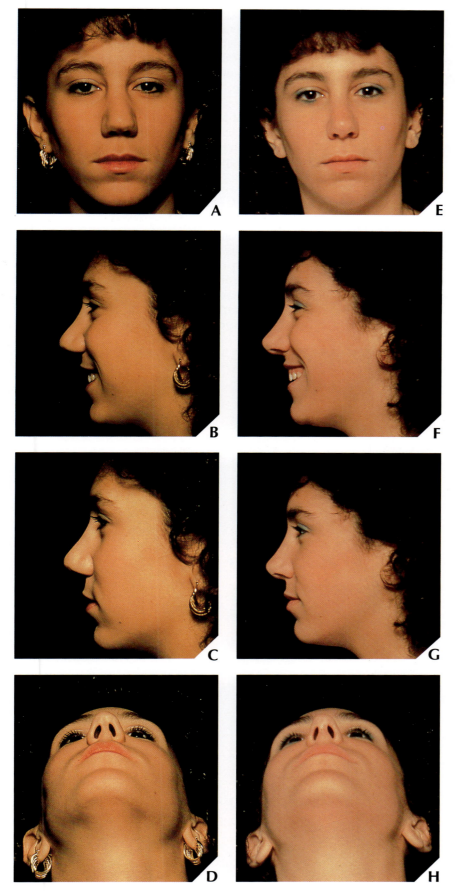

Figure 1.17. (A) Ill-defined nasal tip and wide bridge. (B) Alar rim veiling and no columellar show. (C) Loss of obtuse angle of lobule. (D) Alar rim flaring. (E) Sculpturing of lower lateral cartilages and infracturing of nasal bones. (F) Millard excision of alar rims. (G) Columellar reconstruction. (H) Modified Weir's resection of alar rims.

ing is the visualization of the edge of the cartilage graft through the skin. This complication occurs more often in the patient with very thin skin. In the patient with thick sebaceous skin, the cartilage graft is almost never a problem.

Cartilage Graft Show in the Nasal Tip

A 46-year-old female presented after two previous rhinoplasties with a saddle deformity and a hanging columella (Fig. 1.18A,B). The patient underwent sculpturing of the lower lateral cartilages, shortening of the caudal septum, partial excision of the anterior nasal spine, placement of a hull-shaped graft to the dorsum, and placement of a double onlay graft to the nasal tip from lower lateral cartilage.

Four months postoperatively, the patient has a satisfactory aesthetic result; however, the edge of the cartilage graft is showing through the nasal tip skin and the graft is not well positioned (Fig.

1.18C,D). To correct this complication, the surgeon should remove the graft through an internal incision, morselize the graft, and then reposition it in a horizontal pocket over the alar domes. On occasion, the surgeon may only need to shave the offending edge, rather than morselize the entire graft.

Placement of the Sheen shield graft in the nasal tip is also not without complications. The patient in Figure 1.19 has a shield graft in place, which is showing through the nasal tip skin.

Cartilage Graft Show in the Reconstructed Dorsum

A 31-year-old female presented with a severe saddle deformity as a result of a previous rhinoplasty. She also had a noticeable depression in the area of the left lateral crus from synechia between the left nasal valve and the septum (Fig. 1.20A,B).

Surgery began by harvesting a 1.5 cm x 3 cm elliptical-shaped conchal cartilage graft. An

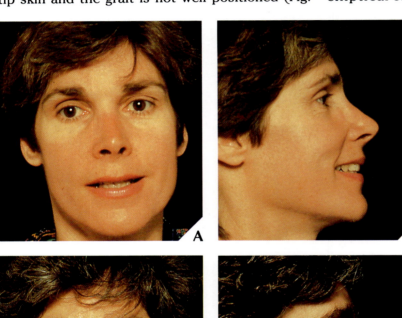
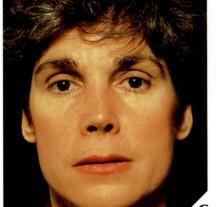
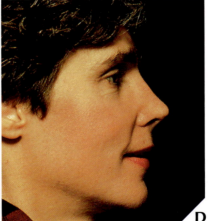

Figure 1.18. (A) Patient presenting for secondary rhinoplasty. (B) Saddle deformity and hanging columella. (C) Onlay cartilage graft showing in nasal tip. (D) Resolution of saddle deformity and hanging columella.

intranasal incision was made at the septal angle and a pocket was developed over the entire dorsum. The cartilage graft was shaped and placed into the pocket. The synechae, causing obstruction of the left intranasal passageway, were released and the raw area was closed with sutures.

Postoperatively, the patient has a good aesthetic result from reconstruction of the dorsum with a hull-shaped conchal cartilage graft. However, the patient has an edge of the cartilage graft showing through the left side of the nasal bridge (Fig. 1.20C,D). This deformity can be easily corrected by shaving the involved cartilage.

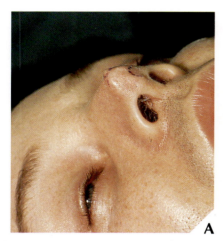

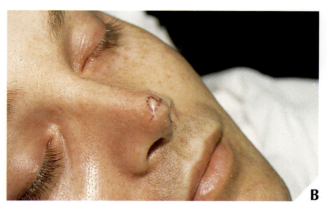

Figure 1.19. (A) Shield graft in the nasal tip. (B) Cartilage edge showing through nasal tip skin.

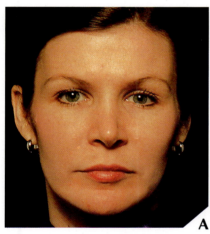

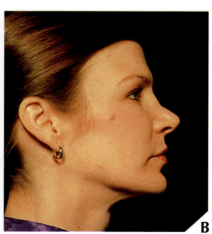

Figure 1.20. (A) Patient presenting for secondary rhinoplasty. (B) Saddle deformity. (C) Cartilage graft showing in left nasal bridge. (D) Resolution of saddle deformity.

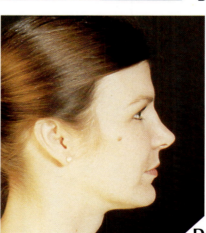

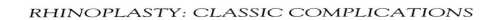

Cartilage Graft Show in the Reconstructed Columella

A 33-year-old female who had multiple previous rhinoplasties presented with an extremely short nose, saddle deformity, and inadequate tip projection (Fig. 1.21A–C). The patient underwent nasal reconstruction with a dorsal hull-shaped graft, an umbrella graft to the nasal tip, and columellar reconstruction. The columellar reconstruction involved placement of a double rectangular graft to the posterior two-thirds of the columella and a double triangular graft to the anterior one-third of the columella.

Five months postoperatively, the patient was re-examined and had a noticeable bump in the middle third of the columella (Fig. 1.21D–F). This deformity is the result of the cartilage graft showing through the reconstructed columella. Even though this deformity will require a revision, the patient has a significantly improved aesthetic result from the nasal reconstruction with autogenous cartilage grafts.

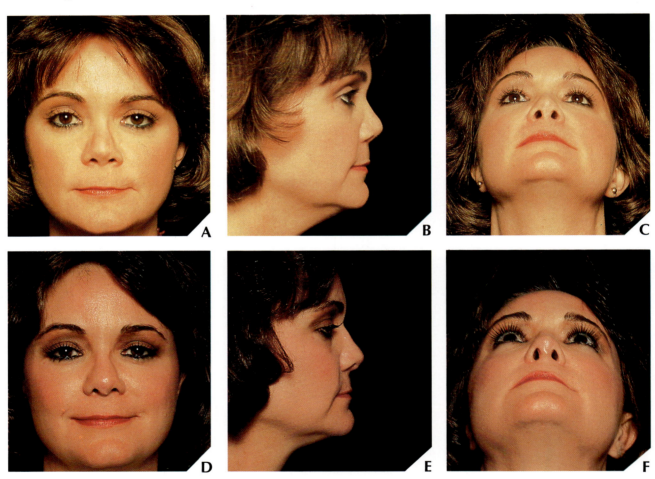

Figure 1.21. (A) Patient presenting for secondary rhinoplasty. (B) Short nose and saddle deformity. (C) Inadequate tip projection and wide alar base. (D) After nasal reconstruction. (E) Resolution of saddle deformity and longer nose. (F) Cartilage graft showing in columella.

Complications of Cartilage Grafts to Lateral Crus Defects

Two patients presented to our office after being treated for defects in the lateral crus area with multi-layered cartilage grafts. The use of multi-layered grafts to fill such a defect does not correct the problem. Since the tensile strength of the external skin is much greater than that of the vestibular skin, the multi-layered graft bulges inwardly rather than outwardly (Fig. 1.22A).

In the second case (Fig. 1.22B), the inferior turbinates had also been trimmed. The inward bulging cartilage grafts, together with the raw surfaces of the inferior turbinate, produced an adhesion with the septum.

CONCLUSION

In practice, most problems and complications in primary and secondary rhinoplasty that are isolated and discussed in this chapter do not occur in their purest form and often are a mixture of multiple problems. Complex problems need comprehensive solutions, while simple problems need subtle solutions. All rhinoplasties are not the same procedure. Our patients are different; their problems are different. The treatment is specific to the needs of the patient. The fundamental process of an accurate preoperative diagnosis, with an understanding of the etiology and treatment, is imperative to achieve a good aesthetic result.

BIBLIOGRAPHY

McCarthy J: Rhinoplasty. In McCarthy J (ed): Plastic Surgery. WB Saunders, Philadelphia, 1989.

Millard DR: Alar margin sculpturing. Plast Reconstr Surg 40:337, 1967.

Peck GC: Techniques in Aesthetic Rhinoplasty, 2nd ed. Gower Medical Publishing, New York, 1990.

Peck GC, Peck GC Jr : Aesthetic rhinoplasty of the nasal tip. In Daniel RK (ed): Aesthetic Plastic Surgery, 2nd ed. Little, Brown, Boston (in press).

Peck GC, Peck GC Jr: Secondary rhinoplasty. In Georgiade NG (ed): Essentials of Plastic, Maxillofacial and Reconstructive Surgery, 2nd ed. Williams & Wilkins, Baltimore (in press).

Peck GC, Peck GC Jr, Michelson L: Secondary rhinoplasty. In Coiffman F (ed): Plastic, Reconstructive and Aesthetic Surgery, 2nd ed. Barcelona, Casa Editora Salvat (in press).

Peck GC: Rhinoplasty. Clinics in Plastic Surgery. WB Saunders, Philadelphia, 1988.

Rees TD (ed): Aesthetic Plastic Surgery. WB Saunders, Philadelphia, 1980.

Sheen JH: Aesthetic Rhinoplasty, 2nd ed. CV Mosby, St. Louis, 1987.

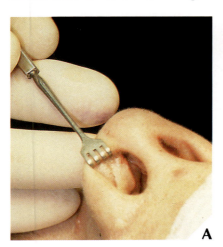 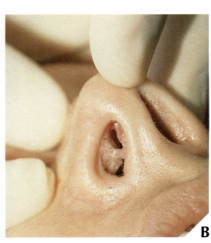

Figure 1.22. **(A)** Multi-layered graft obstructing nasal passageway. **(B)** Adhesion between inferior turbinate and septum.

A

B

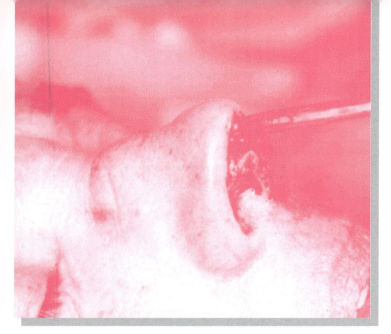

RHINOPLASTY AND OPEN RHINOPLASTY

Ronald Gruber

C H A P T E R 2

This chapter will concern itself with complications of rhinoplasty, with an emphasis on those resulting from the open technique. From the start, it is important to establish what distinguishes a complication from an unfavorable result. Although there is no undisputable distinction between the two, it is generally agreed that a complication is an unexpected postsurgical sequela (and theoretically preventable), while an unfavorable result is an expected sequela (and theoretically unpreventable). In this chapter, only complications, in the sense described above, are discussed and they are divided into those that are common to any rhinoplasty and those that are specific to open rhinoplasty. Within the chapter, the open technique is demonstrated to be a suitable method to treat many of the complications.

INTRAOPERATIVE COMPLICATIONS

Complications following any type of rhinoplasty can begin intraoperatively. Most nasal surgery is done under a local anesthesia with sedation. Numerous cases of hyperventilation have resulted from overdoses of drugs such as Valium and, more recently, Versed. Fortunately, due to the advent of the oximeter, this complication is largely avoidable. In fact, it is fair to say that, because of the oximeter's effectiveness, every patient undergoing heavy sedation should be monitored by one. To minimize the potential for hypoxemia, an oxygen cannula is placed in the corner of the mouth (Fig. 2.1). The risk of fire is avoided by keeping inflammable materials away from the face.

Hypertension, both during and after surgery, is an occasional problem. It is often due to the patient's pre-existing condition; in some cases, it is caused by the adrenaline used with the local anesthetic. It poses a problem during surgery, making it difficult to operate in a blood-filled field, and postoperatively, in terms of epistaxis, swelling, and ecchymosis. Prevention begins by having the patient normotensive prior to the commencement of surgery. Should hypertension occur, 0.5 to 1 cc Indural IV push is given, provided the pulse rate is greater than 70. If needed, an IV push of 2.5 mg of thorazine every 5 minutes is given for a maximum dose of 30 mg, or until the blood pressure has reached a satisfactory level.

EARLY POSTOPERATIVE COMPLICATIONS

Postoperative problems can begin as early as on the first day following surgery. The patient may exhibit an unsatisfactory appearance with the splint in place. In Figure 2.2, an obtuse columella-labial angle caused the patient great anxiety. The possible causes of this problem are threefold: 1) early edema in the upper lip region without any true alteration of the columella-labial angle; 2) malposition of the splint—splints are usually put on when the patient is in a recumbent position—which may be holding the patient's nose in a more cephalic position than desired; or 3) an error in judging the desired columella-labial angle at surgery. Until the cause is known, there exists a need to treat this problem early. Reflection on what transpired at surgery often helps determine which of the three scenarios prevails. If it is simply a matter of readjusting the splint, it is always

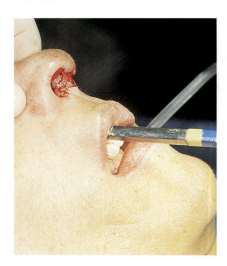
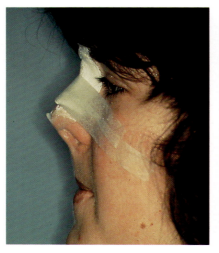
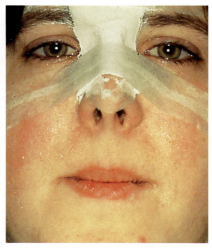

Figure 2.1. To minimize the potential for hypoxemia, an oxygen cannula is placed in the corner of the mouth.

Figure 2.2. If on the first day postoperatively the appearance of the nose is more edematous than expected, the surgeon should consider a cast change, if not a return to surgery. Correcting problems in the early postoperative period is better than waiting for "things to settle down."

worthwhile to apply a new one; it may also help to allay the patient's anxiety. More importantly, if the condition is caused by an error in surgical judgment, it is critical to correct the nasal anatomy early before the problem becomes permanent. Waiting until the swelling subsides and hoping the nose will "settle down" may be an unrealistic expectation. There is no better time than the first few days after surgery to go back and correct these errors.

Epistaxis (Hemorrhage)

Epistaxis (hemorrhage) is usually seen in the first 24 to 48 hours following rhinoplasty. Occasionally it is seen immediately following removal of the packing. The site of bleeding is usually at the caudal edge of the septum. If the patient had a turbinectomy, the bleeding is very likely to emanate from that location. The overall incidence of hemorrhages is approximately 2%. Septal surgery does seem to increase the likelihood of epistaxis, as does turbinectomy. Prevention begins by keeping the patient off aspirin (as well as any of the approximately 300 other products on the market that affect platelet adhesion) for at least 10 days prior to surgery. All patients should be evaluated for a possible family history of bleeding (e.g., von Willebrand's disease).

Good hemostasis during surgery is an obvious factor in outcome. In open rhinoplasty, hemostasis is easier to achieve because there is direct visualization (Fig. 2.3) of the blood vessels along the dorsum of the septum after the hump is removed. Two vessels of the dorsal skin (Fig. 2.4) may be seen in open rhinoplasty and can be coagulated. These vessels often do not bleed until the end of the case when the adrenaline effect has worn off. Even if a closed rhinoplasty is done, these vessels are usually not a problem because pressure from the taping of the nose and the application of a splint provide adequate compression.

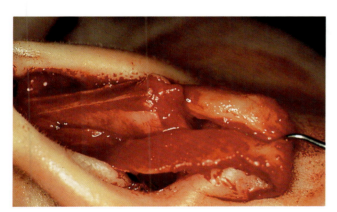

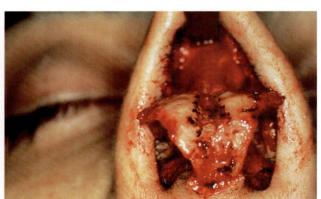

Figure 2.3. One of the causes of epistaxis and hematoma derives from the vessels along the dorsum where the hump has been removed. During an open rhinoplasty these vessels are easily seen and coagulated.

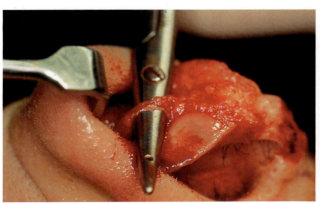

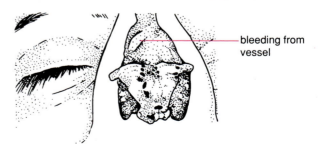

bleeding from vessel

Figure 2.4. Bleeding may come from a vessel on either side of the dorsal nasal skin. It occurs often during open rhinoplasty when the effect of adrenaline has worn off.

The anterior nasal spine is a potential area of bleeding. It is imperative to make every attempt to achieve hemostasis in this region, whether doing an open or a closed rhinoplasty (Fig. 2.5). If the cautery fails, Avitene can be applied. Avitene is also particularly useful in obtaining hemostasis along the cut edge of the inferior turbinates. It is best used here (Fig. 2.6) because, unlike packing, it does not have to be removed postoperatively.

Treatment of epistaxis once it occurs is as follows: under sedation, the patient receives local anesthesia to the base of the nose, columella, and portions of the septum. In addition, cocaine is used for the septum. Often by this time the bleeding will have subsided and nothing further need be done. At this point the bleeding will have diminished to where a specific bleeding site may be seen. If bleeding is from the area of the anterior nasal spine, it may be necessary to remove some of the sutures in the transfixion incision and insert Avitene. If necessary, packing is used. Patients are not happy to have their noses packed

and every means should be used to avoid it. The use of an intranasal balloon serves the same purpose as the packing. Only in rare cases will it be necessary to resort to such a drastic measure as ligation of the internal maxillary artery. Before that point is reached, the patient should be evaluated for the etiology of the epistaxis. That evaluation includes a bleeding panel.

Hematoma

Hematoma is an infrequent complication of rhinoplasty, although it may be more common than appreciated. The actual entrapment of a small quantity of blood, even if it is only 1 to 2 cc under the nasal skin, can cause pain, if not swelling. The patient's discomfort is out of proportion to what is expected with rhinoplasty. Small amounts of hematoma are well tolerated by the skin of the nose but the problem may manifest itself later in an unsatisfactory aesthetic result. Hematoma is a cause of persistent edema and thickening of the subcutaneous tissues for many months; some of

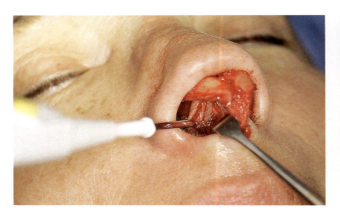

Figure 2.5. Bleeding may be brisk at the anterior nasal spine region, but can be coagulated during either an open or a closed rhinoplasty.

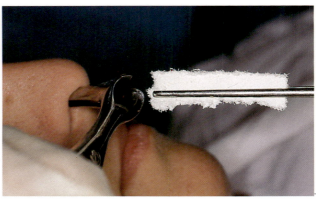

Figure 2.6. Avitene is particularly helpful in obtaining hemostasis. It is especially useful following a turbinectomy, at which time a wafer of Avitene is simply laid along the cut turbinate edge.

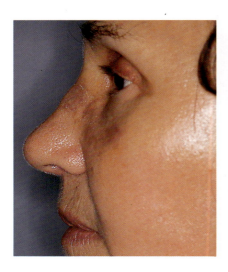

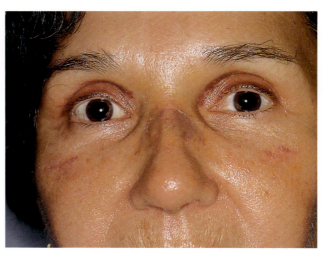

Figure 2.7. On the sixth day postoperatively, at the time of splint removal, a small hematoma was seen near the radix of this patient. Rather than allow it to organize and alter the configuration in this part of the nose, it was aspirated.

this will become permanent. Other sites where small hematomas occur are along the line of the lateral osteotomy and near the radix where the nasal bones are fractured. These hematomas are often not recognized until the splint is removed and some redness and swelling is noted. The symptoms are particularly pronounced in the region of the radix, causing an obliteration of the frontonasal angle.

The causes of hematoma are essentially the same as those enumerated for epistaxis. The patient must be returned to the operating room for evacuation of the hematoma. The subcutaneous space can be irrigated with a thrombin solution. If the swelling is along the lateral nasal bone where the osteotomy was performed, the canal through which the osteotome was passed can be suctioned to evacuate the hematoma. In Figure 2.7, the patient had a small hematoma that was first seen at the time the splint was removed, six days postoperatively. Rather than allow the hematoma to become a source of problems, it was immediately evacuated by suctioning.

Infection and Lacrimal Duct Obstruction

Infection is a rare complication of rhinoplasty (Fig. 2.8). Nonetheless, rhinitis and even sinusitis can result postoperatively. This may be because up to 25% of patients are silent carriers of *Staphylococcus aureus*. In spite of what can be cultured, actual bacteremia resulting from rhinoplasty is rare. Although many feel that antibiotics do not prevent infection, this author strongly favors prophylactic antibiotics, specifically cephalosporin 500 mg IV during surgery and 250 mg potid postoperatively. Treatment involves

drainage and the appropriate choice of antibiotics, as dictated by the culture results.

If packing is left in too long, it can be a potential cause of infection. If nothing else, old packing can produce a foul odor. Therefore, when using a pack, it should be left in place no longer than 3 days postoperatively. Early removal also prevents toxic shock syndrome.

Lacrimal duct obstruction is usually an early, but can be a later, complication of nasal surgery. Upon close scrutiny, many patients do exhibit some form of lacrimal duct obstruction. Most of the obstruction is temporary and disappears quickly. Occasionally, however, a patient will have a persistent problem manifesting itself in swelling in the corner of the eye, with possibly infection. The etiology is usually traced to the lateral osteotomy, which damages the lacrimal sac and drainage system. In these cases, patients will exhibit all the signs and symptoms of dacryocystitis, requiring immediate antibiotics. Once the infection is controlled, the lacrimal drainage will return to normal without further treatment. Prevention of the obstruction mandates careful osteotoma positioning

Edema and Steroid Atrophy

Edema may be the result of overdissection or traumatic surgery. If the edema persists after 6 weeks, it can be treated with judicious use of corticosteroids. Kenalog-10 (Triamcinolone) is injected into such areas as the radix, the supratip, or the lower lateral cartilage region prn. Because some patients are unusually sensitive to corticosteroids, a very small initial dose should be administered (Fig. 2.9). Using a number 27 needle, 0.25 cc (1.25 mg of K-10) and an equal volume of Xylocaine are mixed together.

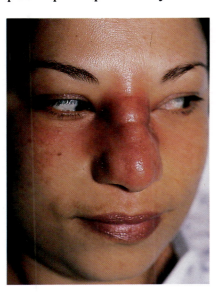

Figure 2.8. Infection is a rare complication of rhinoplasty. Draining the site and the use of appropriate antibiotics are usually all that is required to manage the problem. (Courtesy of Iraj Zandi, M.D.)

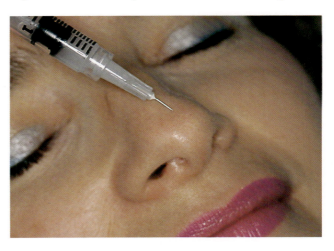

Figure 2.9. Triamcinolone is an effective means of treating persistent postoperative nasal edema.

Initially less than 1 mg of K-10 is injected into the thickened area. Care is taken to avoid a wheal in the skin. This regimen can be repeated at monthly intervals, with the dose steadily increasing.

There is a striking variability of patient response to K-10. Some patients exhibit a significant change in the soft tissues with hardly any K-10, while others exhibit a very slight response to many injections over many months. In Figure 2.10, the patient, following primary rhinoplasty, exhibited significant edema in the region of the lateral crura. The patient was given 2 mg of injectable Triamcinolone and developed a very marked atrophy of the soft tissues, which improved only slightly with the passage of time. The patient in Figure 2.11 underwent an open secondary rhinoplasty to correct some residual problems—an unsatisfactory profile and an abnormal width of the nose. Because there was persistent edema early postoperatively, she received approximately 2 mg of K-10 into the left lateral crural region. Shortly thereafter, she developed a significant depression, which resolved dramatically over the subsequent months and finally disappeared.

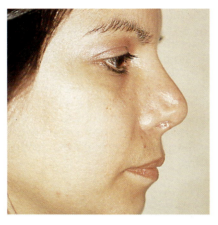
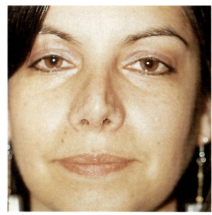

Figure 2.10. Following a primary rhinoplasty, the patient exhibited unusual and persistent edema in a region of the lateral crura. Triamcinolone (2 mg) was given, which caused atrophy of the soft tissues. (Courtesy of Gary Freedman, M.D.)

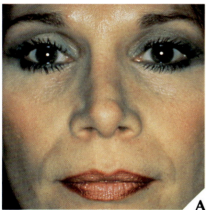
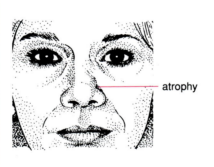

atrophy

A

Figure 2.11. This patient (preoperative, **A**) underwent a secondary rhinoplasty by the open technique. Because of persistent edema and thickening on the left side, 2 mg of Triamcinolone were given. Despite this small dose, the patient developed a small degree of atrophy. Fortunately, it did not mar the overall improved results, as seen 15 months postoperatively (**B**). At 24 months, the atrophy disappeared (**C**).

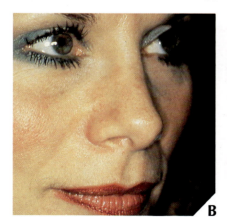
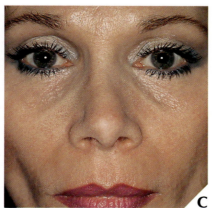

B

C

These problems can be prevented of course by avoiding the use of corticosteroids altogether. Unfortunately that would eliminate the means of treating the many patients who do benefit from the judicious use of corticosteroids. A better approach is to minimize the first dose to less than 1 mg and wait 4 to 6 weeks to observe the response. Most patients who do develop some atrophy will rebound phenomenally—the atrophy will disappear.

Early Skin Problems

Skin problems may be noticed once the splint is removed. Some patients exhibit pustules along the dorsum of the nasal skin. Most of these pustules are due to obstructed sebaceous glands. They are frequently associated with patients who have thick, oily skin and a history of acne. If left untreated, they become frank abscesses and can potentially harm the skin surface (Fig. 2.12). Prevention includes removal of the splint by the fifth or sixth day postoperatively.

On occasion allergic dermatitis due to either the tape and/or Benzoin (Fig. 2.13) can be seen. Prevention involves using a hypoallergenic paper tape for those patients with a strong history of allergies.

Intracranial Complications

Intracranial complications are a very rare cause of early postoperative problems. However, such problems may be lethal; they include pneumocephalus, CSF-rhinorrhea, meningitis, cerebritis, and cavernous sinus thrombosis. Infection can reach the brain via the ophthalmic veins, the bloodstream, or an iatrogenic fracture that extends to the cribriform plate or the anterior cranial fossa. Pneumocephalus (whether seen with or without CSF-rhinorrhea) usually occurs in patients with pre-existing nasal trauma. An even rarer problem is penetration by the osteotome, causing hematoma and/or direct injury to the optic chiasm. This injury causes blindness in one or both eyes.

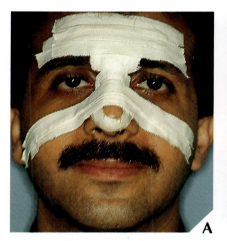
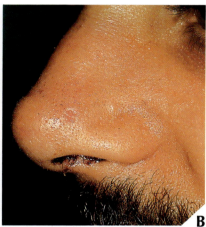
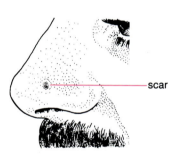

Figure 2.12. Pustules underneath the tape (**A**) can cause permanent skin damage. (**B**) In this case a small, depressed scar resulted.

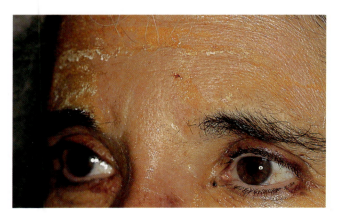

Figure 2.13. Some patients are allergic to the adhesive tape that is used prior to application of a nasal splint, as exhibited here. Nonallergic paper tape is preferable to avoid allergic reaction. However, it may not stick to the skin as well. Removal of the tape and splint by the sixth day postoperatively minimizes these problems should they occur.

LATE POSTOPERATIVE COMPLICATIONS

Saddle Nose Deformity

One of the classic anatomic complications is the saddle nose deformity. If this defect is not recognized at the time of surgery (Fig. 2.14), or if the structural integrity of the septum should fail postoperatively, an evident depression of the nose will result. The problem is usually caused by over-resection of the septum, but in some cases it is due to disruption of the cartilaginous septum (the horizontal component) from the vomer. Still in other cases, it is due to a loss of the integrity of the vertical component of the L-shaped strut remaining after a submucous resection. Prevention is aimed toward cautious and conservative resection of the septum.

Open rhinoplasty lends itself to a relatively easy correction of this problem when it is discovered. When the skin of the dorsum is retracted, the junction of the dorsal septum and bone can be visualized. Direct repair with 4-0 nylon sutures can

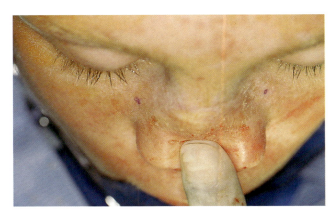

Figure 2.14. During a septoplasty or submucous resection, the support structure may be lost. Failure to recognize this intraoperatively may lead to a saddle nose deformity.

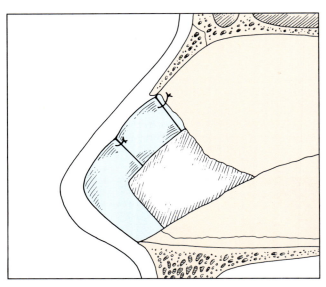

Figure 2.15. After resection of the deformed central cartilage of the septum, an L-shaped strut remains. A saddle nose deformity results if 1) the cartilage becomes disrupted from its attachment to the vomer; 2) too much cartilage is resected from the horizontal component; or 3) there is a loss of structural integrity of the vertical component.

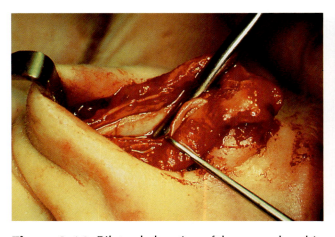
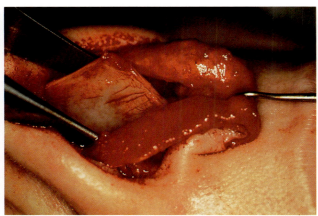

Figure 2.16. Bilateral elevation of the mucochondrium allows good exposure to correct an iatrogenic septal collapse.

restore the integrity of the junction of the dorsal septal cartilage with the nasal bone if that, in fact, is the cause of the potential deformity (Fig. 2.15).

If the problem is due to a collapse of the vertical component of the L-shaped septum following septoplasty, direct exposure of the vertical component can be obtained by elevation of the mucoperiocondrium from both sides of the septum (Fig. 2.16). Reinforcement with cartilage grafts and anchoring the caudal septum to the buccal sulcus will stabilize the vertical component (Fig. 2.17). Late treatment requires grafting cartilage to the dorsum and possibly reconstructing the horizontal or vertical component of the L-shaped strut of the septum with cartilage or bone grafts (Fig. 2.18).

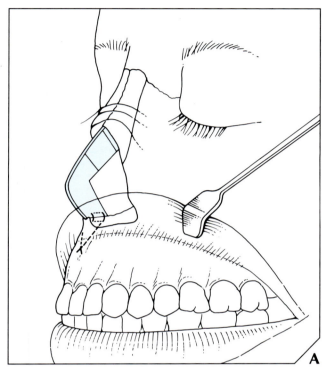

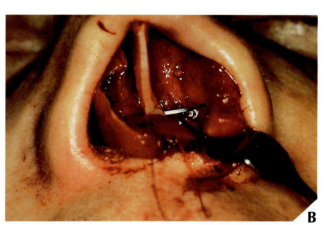

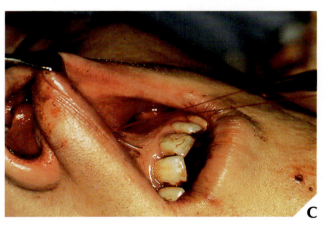

Figure 2.17. The cartilage of the septum, once stabilized, can be held in the proper position by suturing it to the buccal sulcus (**A**). A suture is passed from the buccal sulcus to the caudal edge of the septum (**B**) and back to the buccal sulcus near the frenulum (**C**).

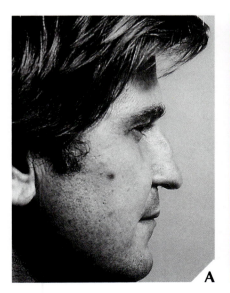

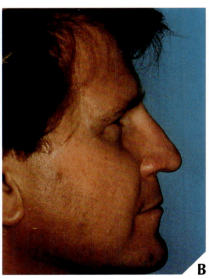

Figure 2.18. (A) This patient sustained a saddle nose deformity following over-resection of the septum. **(B)** Later reconstruction was performed using cranial bone graft for the dorsum and columella. (Courtesy of James Stuzin, M.D.)

Alar Base Over-resection

Alar base over-resection potentially causes inspiratory obstruction and poor aesthetic results. Figure 2.19 illustrates a patient who underwent over-resection of the alar base, which resulted in vestibular stenosis and a severe aesthetic deformity. The problem can be prevented by proper execution of the alar excision. Seldom is it necessary to remove more than 3 or 4 ml of the ala. The stenosis associated with this deformity can be prevented by not extending the Weir excision into the vestibulum. More often than not patients do not require reduction of the perimeter of the vestibulum. Since that is usually the case, the wedge of tissue to be removed should include only the alar skin and not skin from the vestibulum (Fig. 2.20). Treatment for over-resection usually requires a composite graft from the earlobe.

The Unrecognized Crooked Nose

Occasionally, following primary rhinoplasty, the patient will exhibit a crooked nose that was not apparent preoperatively. Sometimes this result is caused by an unrecognized deviation of the dorsal septum camouflaged by the large dorsal hump or lower lateral cartilages, and sometimes it is due to inadvertent scoring or malpositioning of the septum during submucous resection. In Figure 2.21, the patient underwent a primary rhinoplasty. The slight deviation of the nose to the left was not readily apparent preoperatively because it was camouflaged by the overall width of the nose. However, following rhinoplasty when the nose was thinned, the deviation was more apparent.

This problem can be prevented by recognizing the potential for deviation and correcting it intraoperatively by straightening the septum or camouflaging it with cartilage near the dorsal septum. In the case in Figure 2.21, this action was not carried out. To treat the case, the patient was returned to surgery 6 months later to correct the crooked septum. Although camouflaging the deformity with grafts was considered, correcting the deviation of the septum itself was undertaken, rather than risk increasing the width of the nose with a dorsal graft. After elevation of the mucopericondrium bilaterally, the septum was scored vertically on the concave side and was released off the vomerine ridge, allowing it to swing back toward the midline. To secure the sep-

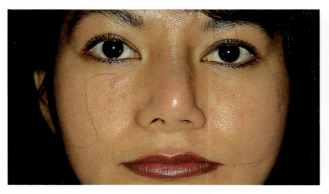 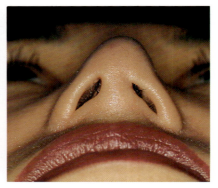

Figure 2.19. This patient underwent over-resection of the ala, producing 1) an unaesthetic result and 2) airway obstruction.

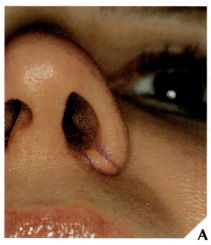 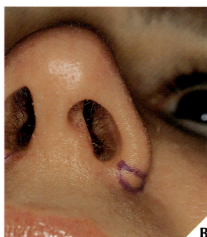

A   B

Figure 2.20. Alar-base resection (Weir excision) is performed by removing usually no more than 3 to 4 mm of the ala (**A**). If the diameter of the vestibule is satisfactory (**B**), there is no need to extend the resection into the vestibulum itself. It is also often not necessary to extend the alar resection to the junction of the ala with the face.

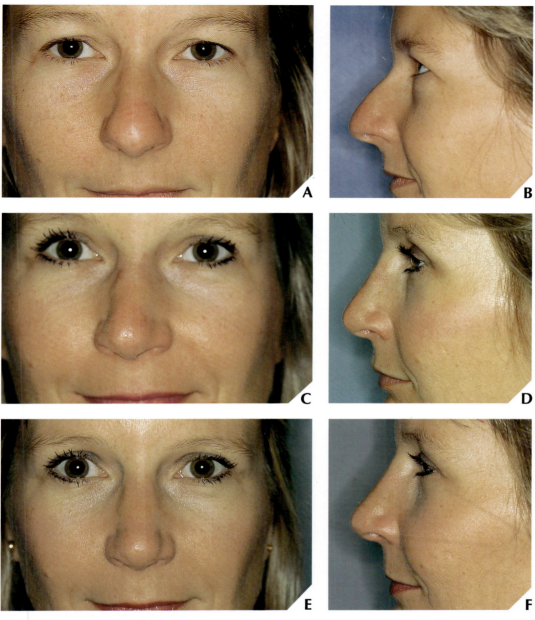

Figure 2.21. Occasionally a patient with a broad nose may have an unrecognized deviation of the nose and/or septum. It is often masked by the thickness and width of the nose. In this patient who underwent an open rhinoplasty, the crookedness of the nose was more apparent following the surgery. In order to correct the deviation, a septoplasty was performed to straighten the nose. Conditions existing before open rhinoplasty (**A, B**) are contrasted with conditions after rhinoplasty (**C, D**) and after secondary septoplasty to straighten the nose (**E, F**). Straightness of the nose is visually verified (**G**) from the perspective at the head of the bed.

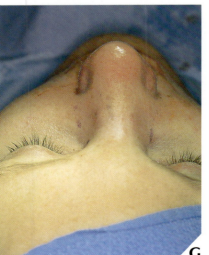

tum in the midline position, a suture was passed from the buccal sulcus to the caudal septum and back to the buccal sulcus.

The Crippled Nose

Each time the patient is returned to the operating room to improve the nose, the chances for success are reduced. The rate of complications increases with each surgery because the skin adapts less and less to the underlying cartilaginous and bony framework and because scar tissue and edema mask the underlying anatomic structure. The patient in Figure 2.22 had multiple operations to improve her appearance. Because of her unrealistic expectations and demands (and because of the willingness of many surgeons to try to meet them), she has ended up with a permanent deformity. The overlying skin is atrophic and irregular and the deformities are numerous. At this point, it is difficult to do anything to improve the nose because the skin surrounding it is no longer resilient and will not conform well to any changes that might be made in the cartilaginous framework.

To avoid producing a crippled nose, the surgeon must know when the risk from further surgery outweighs the gain. Multiple surgeries performed too close together may also increase the likelihood of a crippled nose. Unfortunately, there is no truly satisfactory surgical treatment for the patient with this deformity.

Donor Site Complications

Often the entire concha has to be taken for a graft.

Although no major deformity of the ear occurs, an occasional patient will complain of flattening of the ear as a result of excision of the concha. The patient in Figure 2.23A exhibited considerable flattening of the ear. To prevent this occurrence, a more conservative resection in the cephalic portion can be done (Fig. 2.23B).

Occasionally the scar in the concha can become hypertrophic (Fig. 2.24). Obviously, it is

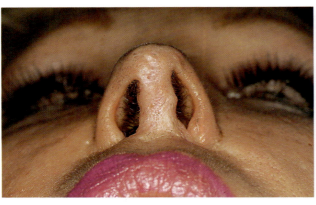

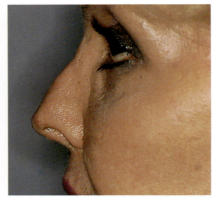

Figure 2.22. Multiple surgeries to achieve perfection often result in a crippled nose. After numerous procedures the skin becomes noncompliant, scarred, and unremediable to further corrections.

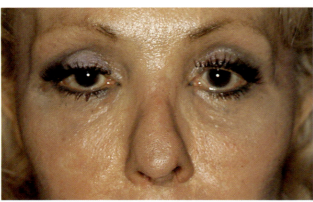

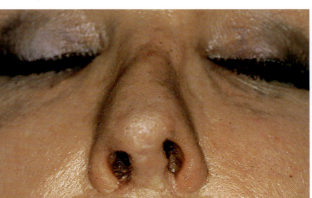

important to do a meticulous closure of the donor site and pack the concha. This type of scar can be prevented by using a posterior approach. However, if the repair is handled with precision, a hypertrophic scar rarely develops. Treatment is the same as that for any unsatisfactory scar.

Implant Exposure

Implant exposure (Fig. 2.25) is a frequent problem with augmentation rhinoplasty; it is the reason most plastic surgeons avoid the use of alloplastic materials. Although prevention of this problem is adequate soft tissue coverage, the best means of

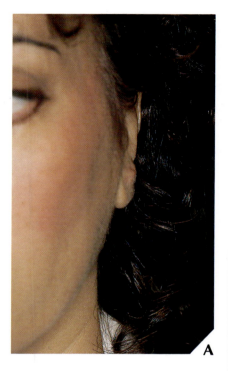

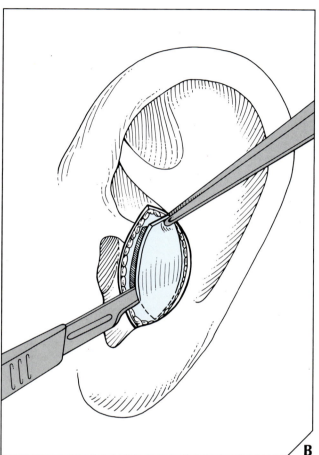

Figure 2.23. In some cases harvesting conchal grafts causes flattening of the ear (**A**). Instead of resecting a crescent of concha (which may cause the concha to collapse), the cephalic portion of the crescent should not be removed.

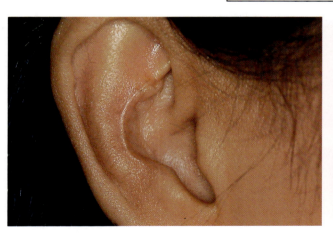

Figure 2.24. Harvesting the conchal graft can in some instances result in a hypertrophic scar.

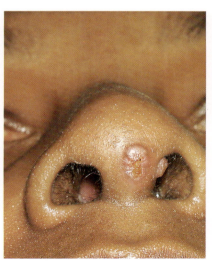

Figure 2.25. Silicone implants may become exposed anywhere on the nose, including the tip.

prevention is simply to avoid using alloplastic materials. If they are to be used at all in the region of the nose, they are probably best confined to the region of the dorsum.

In Figure 2.26, the patient underwent multiple procedures for aesthetic rhinoplasty, the last of which included a silicone implant to the dorsum. In addition to exposure noted within one of the vestibula, the patient developed problems due to a short nose and over-resection of the alae. To treat this condition, the silicone implant was replaced with an autogenous cartilage graft. At the same time, the nose was lengthened by elevating the mucopericondrium bilaterally. The mucopericondrium received staggered, releasing incisions which allowed caudal advancement of the nose. To obtain caudal displacement of the alae, separation between the upper and lower lateral cartilages was done. The columella was main-

tained in its new position with the aid of a baton graft sutured to the septum; and the separation between the upper and lower lateral cartilages was maintained with small cartilage grafts. Postoperatively, the patient exhibits significant improvement.

In Figure 2.27, the patient previously received an L-shaped silicone implant during an aesthetic augmentation rhinoplasty. Unfortunately it too resulted in exposure, as noted from within the vestibulum. Because of the threat of ultimate implant loss and infection, early intervention was undertaken and the implant was replaced with a cartilaginous graft taken from the septum. Because the patient did not want a nose as westernized as she had originally been given with the implant, the vertical height was reduced. To give her a narrow nose, which was the original intention prior to the silicone implant, lateral osteotomies were per-

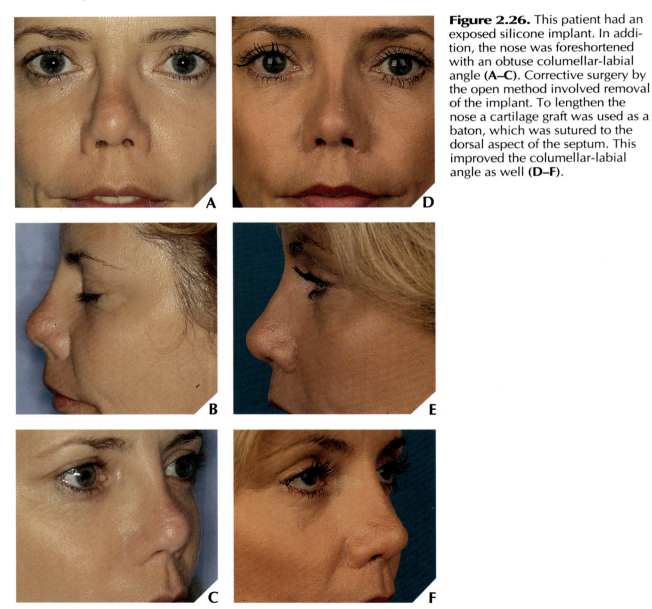

Figure 2.26. This patient had an exposed silicone implant. In addition, the nose was foreshortened with an obtuse columellar-labial angle (**A–C**). Corrective surgery by the open method involved removal of the implant. To lengthen the nose a cartilage graft was used as a baton, which was sutured to the dorsal aspect of the septum. This improved the columellar-labial angle as well (**D–F**).

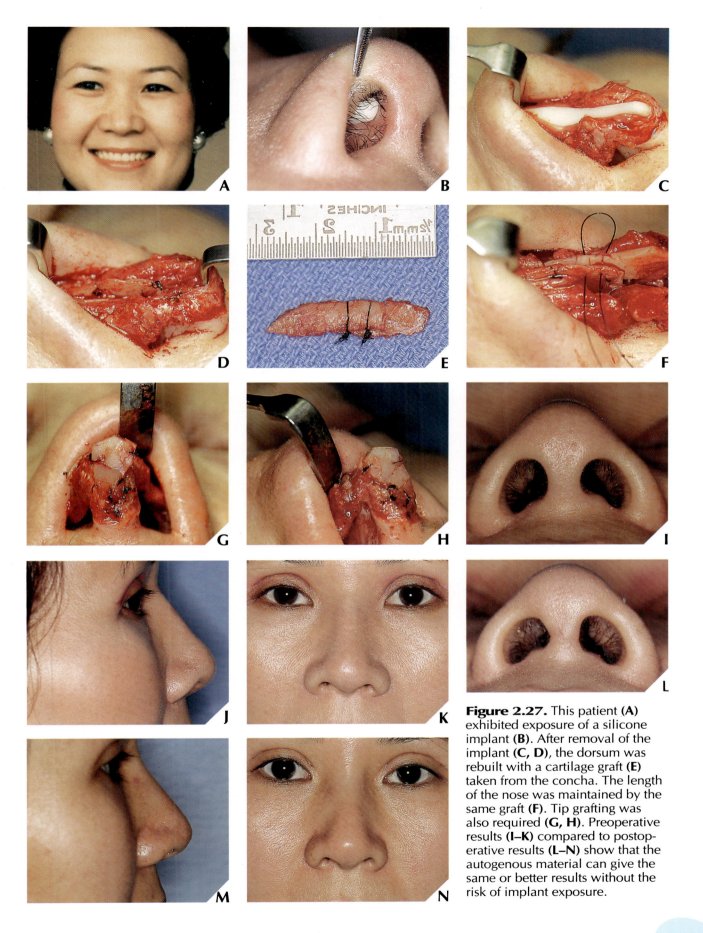

Figure 2.27. This patient (**A**) exhibited exposure of a silicone implant (**B**). After removal of the implant (**C, D**), the dorsum was rebuilt with a cartilage graft (**E**) taken from the concha. The length of the nose was maintained by the same graft (**F**). Tip grafting was also required (**G, H**). Preoperative results (**I–K**) compared to postoperative results (**L–N**) show that the autogenous material can give the same or better results without the risk of implant exposure.

formed. Thus, at 13 months postoperatively, the cartilage graft gives a similar aesthetic result without the risk of silicone exposure.

Occasionally, the silicone implant will not just become exposed, but will become infected and require removal. When this happens, immediate reconstruction with a cartilage graft cannot be undertaken. However, if infection does occur it may be necessary to reconstruct the nose shortly after the infection clears, usually by the sixth week postoperatively. If this is not done, the patient may eventually develop permanent irregularities and distortions of the skin surface. In Figure 2.28, the patient underwent a silicone augmentation rhinoplasty, which resulted in an infection. The implant had to be removed, but early reconstruction was not planned. The skin developed an irregular shape with distortion. Fibrosis

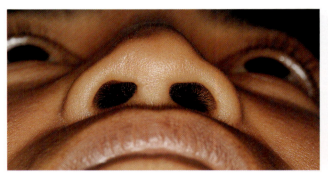
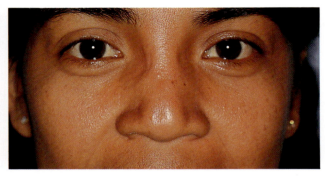

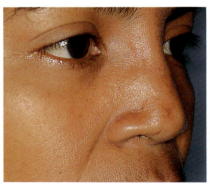
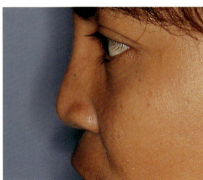

Figure 2.28. This patient underwent removal of a silicone implant that had become exposed and infected. Reconstruction with autogenous material was not done shortly after controlling the infection. Consequently the skin developed irregularities that now become difficult, if not impossible, to correct.

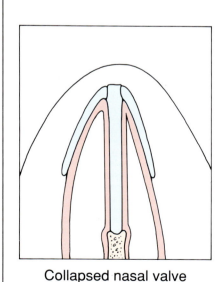
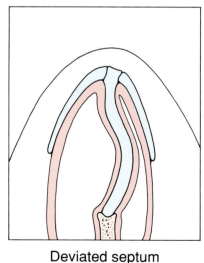
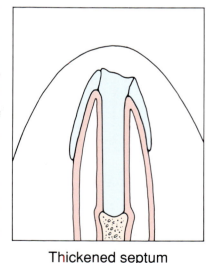

Collapsed nasal valve   Deviated septum   Thickened septum

Figure 2.29. The sources of airway obstruction include: 1) scarring and collapse of the internal valve region, 2) septal deviation, and 3) septal thickening.

developed under the skin and is partly responsible for the distortion. Reconstruction with cartilage grafts is now indicated but may not totally restore the surface contour.

Allograft Rejection

The use of allografts (homografts) carries with it the potential for rejection. Although cartilaginous allografts are generally thought to be immunologically privileged, the fact remains that some of these allografts are absorbed and some will even become infected. Avoiding the use of banked cartilage will prevent this complication. The use of allografts should be confined to small noncritical areas, such as the radix. Treatment mandates removal of the allograft material, should it become exposed or infected, and replacement with autogenous tissues after the infection is cleared.

Breathing Difficulties

Breathing difficulties take the form of either inspiratory obstruction, with collapse of the lower lateral cartilages, or expiratory obstruction. On examination, a variety of problems may present themselves: 1) the internal valve may be narrow as a result of surgery in this area, 2) the external valve (vestibulum) may be narrow, or 3) the septum may be deviated, thickened, or both (Fig. 2.29).

Most problems can be prevented. Inspiratory obstruction can be prevented by maintaining the integrity of the lateral crus. If after resection of the cephalic crus only a very thin rim remains, that rim may not be sufficient to withstand the weight of the overlying skin. Transection of the mid-portion of the lateral crus is not necessarily a cause of collapse (Fig. 2.30). In fact, if properly done, it is an excellent method of correcting the

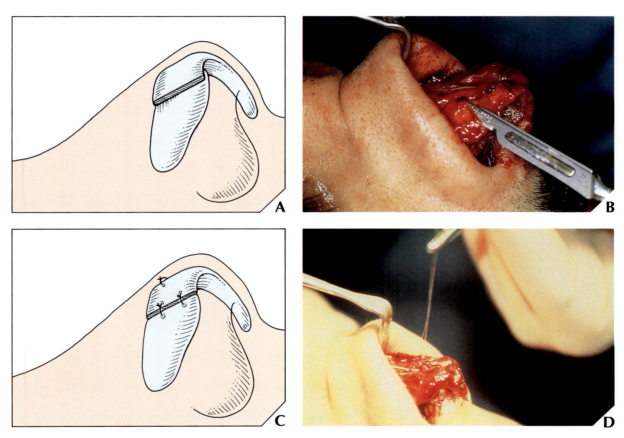

Figure 2.30. Transection of the lateral crus is not necessarily a cause of airway obstruction. By making an incision at the most convex portion of the lateral crus and resecting 1 or 2 mm of cartilage, the convexity can be corrected withoutcausing collapse **(A, B)**. Suturing may be necessary, however **(C, D)**.

bulbous tip. Although the integrity of the dome is important, transection of it alone does not necessarily cause collapse of the lateral crus. Oftentimes when the dome is scored to narrow the tip of the nose, it is completely transected. Yet most of these patients do not develop collapse of the lateral crus and inspiratory obstruction. If, at the time of surgery, weakness or collapse of the lateral crus is noted, a small, thin graft should be applied to the existing lateral crus.

Obstruction of the internal valve is prevented in part by extramucosal surgery (mucosal tunneling). Most plastic surgeons feel that by maintaining the integrity of the mucopericondrium in the vicinity of the valve that there will be less chance of the formation of scar tissue and constriction of the valve. Extramucosal surgery of the nasal valve is not always easily performed, and there is some question as to whether or not it is necessary. It is the author's opinion that extramucosal dissection is not necessary if a good approximation of the tissues joining the upper lateral cartilage to the septum happens to occur. If not, approximation can be done by sutures. However, this is only possible in open rhinoplasty since the structures can be visualized. During the open approach (Fig. 2.31), the mucous membrane of the upper lateral cartilage can be carefully approximated to the mucous membrane of the septum and held there with sutures. If needed, a splinter graft can be sutured directly in place.

Another means of preventing airway obstruction is to avoid overtrimming the caudal edge of the upper lateral cartilage. It should be allowed to overlap the cephalic edge of the lower lateral cartilage and thus recreate normal valve function. Preservation of the mucous membrane in the region of the nasal valve also helps. Thus, the intercartilaginous incision should be in the sulcus between the upper lateral and lower lateral cartilage, not at the edge of the upper lateral cartilage (Fig. 2.32). Finally, meticulous closure of internal incisions that gap is helpful in preventing formation of a scar band.

Recently, Guyoron recommended the use of nasal packing to prevent airway obstruction and even nasal deviation. In a controlled study, improved airway flow was noted in 96% of the group that was packed versus 64% in the nonpacked group. Also, residual septal deviation was seen in 41% of the group that was not packed compared to 13% of the packed group. Thus, packing is a reasonable means of minimizing breathing difficulties. Unfortunately, it is responsible for some patient discomfort.

Another alternative is to place small, plastic catheter breathing tubes along the floor of the nose and pack above them. Also to consider are the splints with attached breathing tubes, available now through several companies. An alternative this author uses is silicone splints. The septum is sandwiched between the silicone splints (Fig. 2.33) and held there with two 4-0 nylon mat-

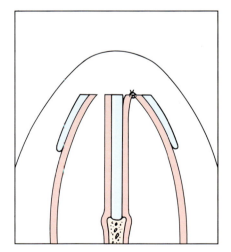

Figure 2.31. If the mucosal tunneling technique is not used and the mucoperichondrium at the junction of the upper lateral cartilage with the septum is transected, it is important that the tissues approximate each other. If necessary, this can be done by sutures. If needed, a splinter graft can be sutured directly into place.

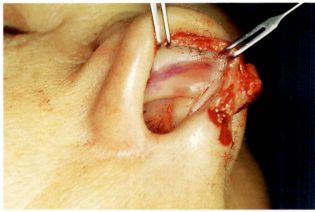

Figure 2.32. To minimize scarring of the internal valve, the intercartilaginous incision must be placed in the sulcus between the upper and lower lateral cartilages, not at the edge of the upper lateral cartilage.

tress sutures. The silicone splints are removed approximately 3 to 5 days later.

Treatment of breathing difficulties is beyond the scope of this chapter and will not be discussed in detail. In general when lateral crural integrity is destroyed, an overlay cartilage graft will provide support. If the internal valve collapses, a spreader graft will improve the constriction. If the ala has been over-resected, composite grafts, using material such as the earlobe, may be necessary. If the septum is deviated or thickened, a formal septoplasty is often required. If the pre-existing enlarged turbinate hypertrophy is a factor in the amount of air flowing through the nose, a turbinectomy may be indicated.

Late Skin Problems

Late skin problems include erythema and telangiectasia (Fig. 2.34). The cause of these conditions is undoubtedly related to interference of skin circulation and is very likely exacerbated by extensive surgery, undermining the skin over the dorsum. Prevention therefore should be aimed at minimizing the amount of dissection. Unfortunately such undermining is frequently necessary to accomplish the goals of the rhinoplasty.

Sometimes the telangiectasia seen postoperatively is a mere exacerbation of what existed preoperatively. Therefore it behooves the surgeon to

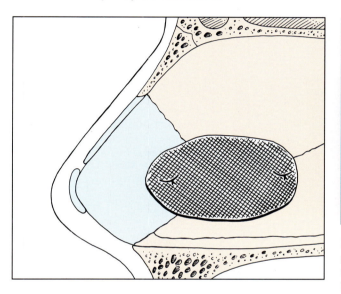

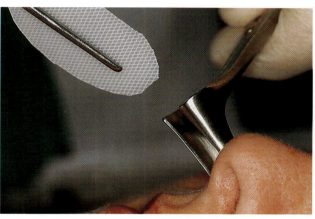

Figure 2.33. The silicone splints applied to either side of the septum following a septoplasty or submucous resection help stabilize the mucoperichondrium to the septal cartilage. These splints reduce postoperative bleeding and reduce problems with airway obstruction.

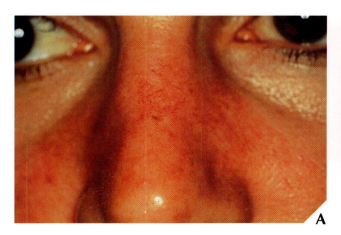

A

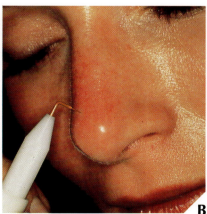

B

Figure 2.34. (A) Telangiectasia to the dorsal skin may follow an open or a closed rhinoplasty. (B) Treatment necessitates the use of an electrocautery or the argon laser.

notice the extent of telangiectasia before surgery, point it out to the patient during the consultation, and let the patient know that this problem may be aggravated by the surgery. To manage the problem, the patient can avoid alcohol and spicy foods, which tend to make the condition flare up. A more definitive treatment is the use of cautery or the argon laser to obliterate the vessels. If the problem is diffuse erythema, such treatment will not be effective, but if it happens to be mostly telangiectasia, then one or more sessions with a cautery should suffice.

Actual nasal skin scarring can be due to rough handling of the tissues, multiple surgeries, or both. Better surgical technique and avoidance of multiple procedures may prevent this complication from occurring. Once the scar occurs it may be difficult to eradicate. Surgical excision of the scar only leaves another scar that may not be any

slighter than the first. Should the scar be quite severe, however (Fig. 2.35), it may be necessary to perform major skin resection with advancement from the cephalic portions of skin to cover the defect. In the case in Figure 2.35, a small skin expander was used to perform immediate skin expansion. Without skin expansion, closure might not be possible. On the other hand, it must be recognized that following skin expansion there is a tendency for scar widening.

Nasal Cysts

Rarely, benign growths in and around the nose may be seen postoperatively. One such problem is the formation of mucocysts, either at the dorsum of the nose or along the area of the lateral nasal bone (Fig. 2.36). This problem is caused by the invagination of the mucous membrane, which

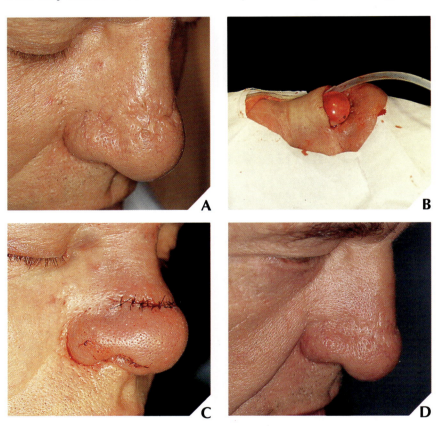

Figure 2.35. If skin damage from a rhinoplasty is extensive (**A**), correction can be achieved by resecting the scar and performing an immediate skin expansion cephalic to the area of the scar (**B, C**). The postoperative result (**D**) can be significantly improved.

eventually forms a cystlike structure. The patient will complain of a persistent swelling and sometimes redness. This problem can be prevented, in the area of the dorsal resection, by careful resection of the exposed mucopericondrium avoiding a large residual that might fall into the subcutaneous space. In the region of the lateral osteotomy, however, there is no adequate means for avoiding the problem. Treatment involves the use of antibiotics if the cyst is inflamed. Frequently a surgical resection of the cyst is necessary.

The Painful Nose

Although infrequently seen, a painful nose can be one of the most disabling complications following a rhinoplasty. The mechanism is unclear, although it is most apt to occur in the patient who has had other neurological and/or psychological problems and who may also have an altered pain threshold. Physical examination usually reveals no signs; yet the patient complains of persistent pain. Prevention is best accomplished by eliciting a his-

tory of psychological and/or neurological problems, such as trigeminal neuralgia, during the interview process. Treatment is similar to the management of other types of pain disorders.

The Difficult or Confused Patient

As is well known by surgeons performing all types of aesthetic surgery, there is a group of patients who are difficult to please. They may have pre-existing psychological problems and their expectations often exceed that of the surgeon's abilities. In McKinney's findings of 200 patients he noted that female patients seem to be more dissatisfied with their postoperative results than males. Other investigators have found just the reverse. Patients over 50 years old and patients not referred by another physician were more likely to be dissatisfied. It is best to avoid surgery in this type of patient. Careful preoperative consultation is the best way to detect this disposition. At the very least, providing informed consent and obtaining a signed statement are imperative.

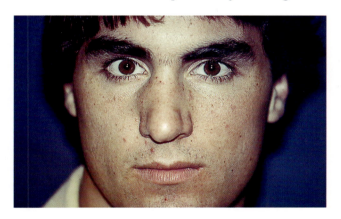

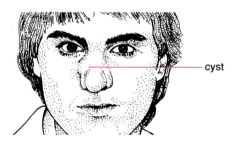

cyst

Figure 2.36. Rarely, a cyst of the nose will occur early in the postoperative period. In this case, a cyst is seen along the right lateral side of the nose where the

osteotomy was performed. It is due to an invagination of the mucous membrane at the osteotomy site.

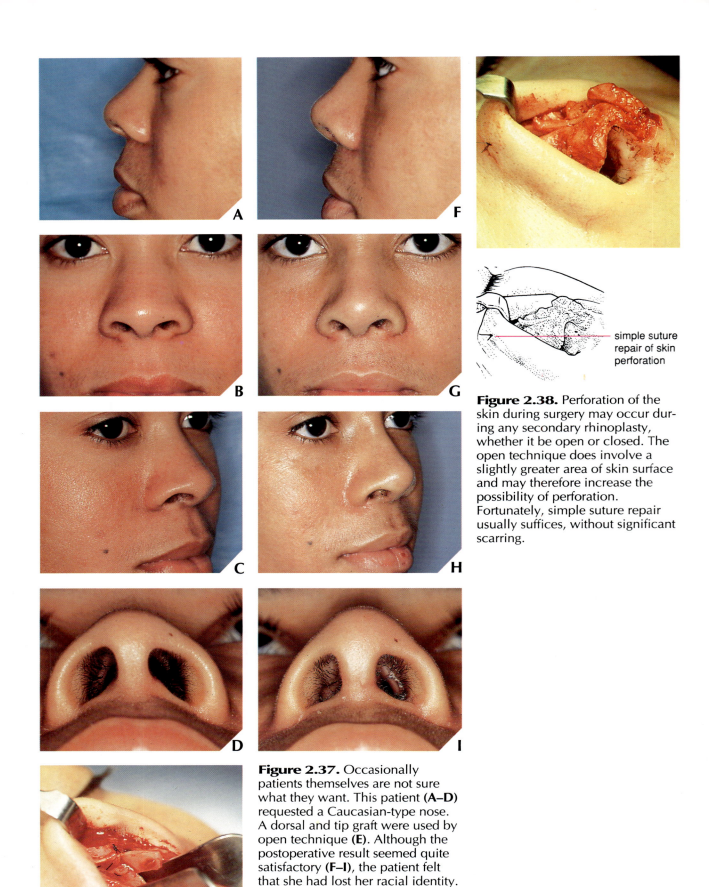

Figure 2.38. Perforation of the skin during surgery may occur during any secondary rhinoplasty, whether it be open or closed. The open technique does involve a slightly greater area of skin surface and may therefore increase the possibility of perforation. Fortunately, simple suture repair usually suffices, without significant scarring.

simple suture repair of skin perforation

Figure 2.37. Occasionally patients themselves are not sure what they want. This patient (**A–D**) requested a Caucasian-type nose. A dorsal and tip graft were used by open technique (**E**). Although the postoperative result seemed quite satisfactory (**F–I**), the patient felt that she had lost her racial identity. Consequently, the cartilage grafts were removed.

Sometimes the patient does not know what he or she really wants. In Figure 2.37, the patient is a black female who requested a Caucasian-type nose. Preoperative photographs were taken on which drawings of the anticipated postoperative result were made. The patient seemed satisfied with the drawings, and it seemed as if there was no problem with communication. At surgery (by open technique) a cartilage graft was applied to the dorsum, the tip cartilages were narrowed, and lateral osteotomies were performed. Early after surgery the patient was quite satisfied, but later her friends and family said she did not look as "black" as she did originally. She promptly requested removal of the cartilaginous graft which was done at her request.

COMPLICATIONS SPECIFIC TO THE OPEN TECHNIQUE

During open rhinoplasty (especially secondary ones), the additional skin that is undermined is approximately 0.5 cm² more than is ordinarily undermined during the course of a traditional technique, such as cartilage evisceration. Nonetheless, the fact that there is an increase in the surface area undermined increases the chance of perforation or buttonholing the skin

(Fig. 2.38). Fortunately these perforations are usually small and can be easily repaired at the time they are discovered.

The Columellar Scar

The complication that most concerns surgeons doing open rhinoplasty is the scar of the columella. The nature of the scar of course depends on the type of incision. Four types of incisions (Fig. 2.39) have been used for open rhinoplasty: 1) a chevron incision at the waist (smallest portion of the columella); 2) a slightly curved incision at the waist of the columella; 3) a stair-step incision at the waist of the columella; and 4) an incision at the junction of the columella and lip in patients with short columellas. In all of these incisions, the potential for scarring exists although it is not great. In the author's experience, approximately 1 out of 100 patients will sustain a scar that is not satisfactory to the patient and will require some form of treatment. Usually the scar will be a retraction. The tissue immediately anterior or cephalic to the scar is often thickened, creating the effect of a hanging columella. Occasionally a patient will even exhibit a small degree of hyperpigmentation within the scar (Fig. 2.40). Sometimes the scar will be notched at the lateral

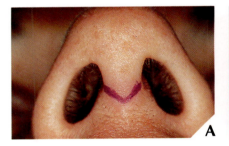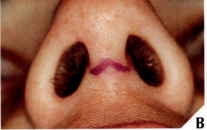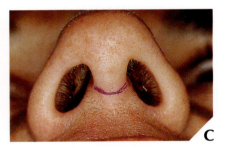

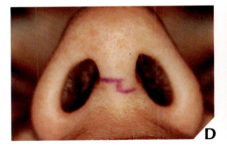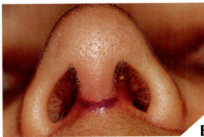

Figure 2.39. There are several possible incisions for the open rhinoplasty: (**A,B**) the chevron incisions; (**C**) the slightly curvilinear incision; (**D**) the stair-step incision ; and (**E**) an incision located near the columella-lip junction when the patient has no "waist" of the columella. The latter two are the best.

Figure 2.40. Rarely, following an open rhinoplasty, a patient will exhibit permanent hyperpigmentation in the area of the scar.

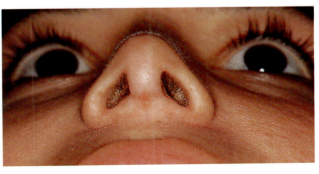

aspect of the columella (Fig. 2.41) or on the profile view (Fig. 2.42). Most problematic scars are isolated, correctable complications. When seen with other unsatisfactory aspects of the rhinoplasty, the scar can appear particularly ominous (Fig. 2.43).

Prevention of scars and patient dissatisfaction experienced from scars can be minimized in the following way. A careful discussion of the nature of the incision and the likelihood of a scar should take place with the patient during the consultation period. Most patients will agree to an open rhinoplasty and accept the scar associated with it once they understand that the open approach allows the surgeon to produce the best aesthetic result. However, there will always be a few

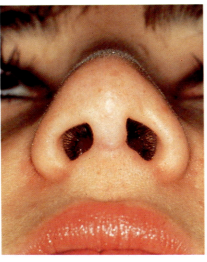

Figure 2.41. Notching following open rhinoplasty is occasionally seen. In this patient it is seen on the lateral aspect of the columella. The patient also exhibits nostril asymmetry, which can occur with either the open or closed technique.

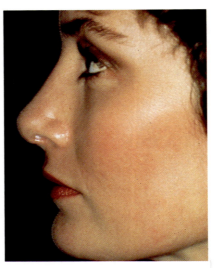

Figure 2.42. Occasionally the notch of the columellar scar can be seen on a profile view. For this reason the stair-step incision is preferred. The stair-step incision tends to camouflage notching seen on the profile view.

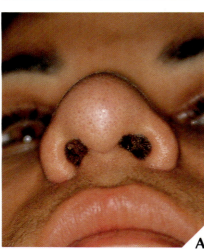

A

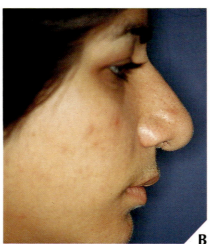

B

Figure 2.43. In this case of an unsatisfactory rhinoplasty result, the patient also exhibited columellar scar retraction and subcutaneous thickening of the columella (**A, B**). If over-resection of the alae compounds a poor scar, the result can appear disastrous (**C, D**).

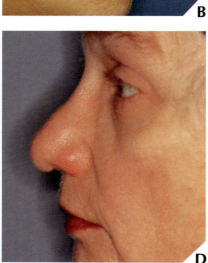

C

D

patients who are not willing to accept that risk, particularly those who point out that others they know with rhinoplasties do not have scars. These patients should be given the option of having a closed rhinoplasty. Doing an open rhinoplasty on such a patient is a setup for a potential problem if the scar is not all but invisible.

The scar can be minimized by the correct choice of incision. When open rhinoplasty was first introduced, the chevron or slightly curved incision at the waist of the columella was popular. With the advent of the stair-step incision, better results were obtained. If there is a significant depression on the profile view, the depressed scar on one side of the columella is camouflaged by the non-scar portion on the other side of the columella, i.e., the stair-step incision breaks up the scar and makes it less apparent on profile. If the patient has a short columella with its waist at the columella-lip junction, an incision here is ideal; the columella-lip junction is a very natural breaking point. In addition, meticulous technique (with magnification) in the repair will greatly facilitate the final result. A deep layer of absorbable sutures is not necessary.

Should a scar of significance occur despite the best attempts to prevent it, correction depends on the type of incision employed. In the case of a chevron or curvilinear incision, a small Z-plasty will effectively break up the depression and improve the results dramatically (Fig. 2.44). The hanging columella effect (convexity of the columella) is due to a small degree of fibrosis and/or edema and is aggravated by the depressed scar. Treatment of it per se is greatly facilitated by revising the depressed scar. Additional measures to treat the convexity within the columella itself can be exceptionally difficult. However, should convexity occur, one can treat the problem much like a hanging columella. A resection of a portion of the membranous septum will be beneficial.

Secondary Open Rhinoplasty Scar

The most difficult scar of the columella is that created from a secondary open rhinoplasty. If a patient already has a scar of the columella, it would seem only reasonable to re-enter the nose through the scar. However, experience has shown that re-entering the columellar scar can aggravate any mild depression that already exists, if not create a depression that did not follow the first open procedure.

The patient in Figure 2.45 had a chevron incision made at the waist of the columella during her

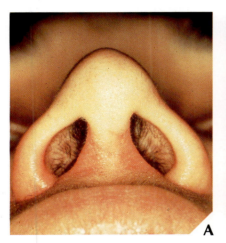
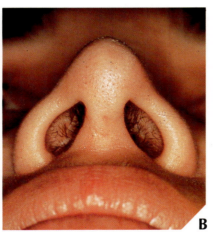

A   **B**

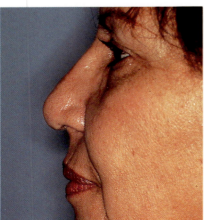
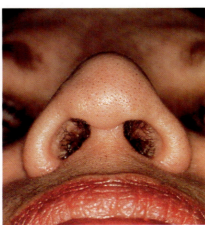

Figure 2.44. Treatment for the columellar scar usually involves a local rotation flap. In this case a Z-plasty was used. Although there was some temporary hyperpigmentation near the lip junction (**A**), that subsided in time and the overall result after scar revision was excellent (**B**).

Figure 2.45. A retracted scar of the columella is most likely to occur in the patient undergoing a secondary open rhinoplasty. When redoing an open rhinoplasty, therefore, the open approach should be avoided unless necessary. If the open approach is used again, plans should be made for a small rotation flap.

first open rhinoplasty. She required a secondary revision of the tip and therefore the old incision was reopened. The actual scar itself was even resected. In spite of this effort, the depression of the eventual columellar scar following the second procedure was significantly more pronounced than·that following the first procedure (which was relatively unnoticeable). Prevention of this problem is twofold: 1) avoid using the open rhinoplasty in those patients who already have a columellar scar, unless it is absolutely necessary to obtain control over the cartilage of the tip. This is especially true if the tissues are not soft; 2) in the event that the open approach is deemed necessary to obtain the maximum result, a Z-plasty or other local flap rotation should be planned at the time that closure of the columella is undertaken. Treatment of the depressed scar and convex columella is similar to that following primary open rhinoplasty.

Persistent Edema

In the early years after open rhinoplasty was introduced, it was thought that edema would be a greater postoperative problem that it is in closed rhinoplasty because the circulation along the columella was disrupted. After reviewing many cases, it appears now that the edema is not necessarily more severe. Although an increase in swelling results from an interference in circulation at the nasal tip, at the same time swelling is reduced by the excellent hemostasis that can be obtained prior to final closure. The small amount of blood that collects under the skin of a closed rhinoplasty when the adrenaline wears off can be as much a cause of postoperative nasal swelling as the interference to the lymphatics and venous return at the columella.

Just as in a closed rhinoplasty, however, loss of facetting can be seen. A small amount of edema

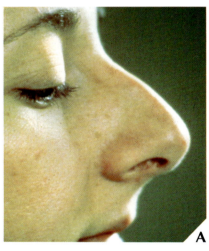 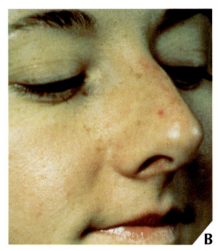

Figure 2.46. Because the surgery in open rhinoplasty is more extensive in the region of the lobule, there may be a greater loss of facetting. This is true of any cartilage-delivering technique, but may be a greater problem in the open approach. Preoperative (**A,B**) and postoperative (**C–E**) results are· shown.

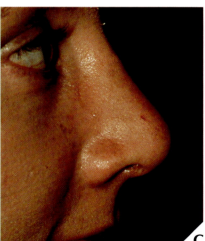 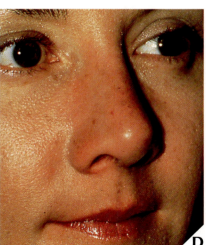 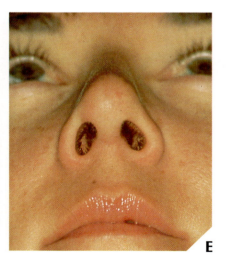

and/or fibrosis in the area of the facets can obliterate the fine structure. Since dissection is undoubtedly more extensive in this area with the open technique, it is not surprising that there should be a tendency for attenuation of the facet surfaces. The patient in Figure 2.46 underwent primary open rhinoplasty. In spite of the overall improvement and patient satisfaction, the result was complicated by a loss of the sculpturing effect, particularly around the area of the facets. Treatment for this condition has not been satisfactory to date.

Flap Necrosis

A major, but extremely rare potential complication in open rhinoplasty is flap necrosis. Seen occasionally intraoperatively or on the first day postoperatively is a slight bluish or other discoloration of the columellar portion of the nasal flap (Fig. 2.47). This discoloration is usually due to tight tape placed around the nasal tip. For this reason patients should be seen on the first day following surgery to evaluate the extent of the circulation in and around the region of the columella and to release the tape if necessary. Fortunately, actual flap necrosis is rare and probably due to poor handling of tissue. To minimize trauma to the columellar flap, it is suggested that the flap not be folded on itself for long periods of time. It is also helpful to uncurl the columellar flap when rasping the dorsum or when using scissors to resect the dorsum (Fig. 2.48).

Although an alar base excision would theoretically carry a great risk for flap necrosis, no problems have been seen with it in the author's experience. Certainly there is the potential for disruption of circulation, particularly if the alar excision is extended into the vestibulum and if the ala is completely detached from the face. To avoid such a problem, the alar base excision should be a conservative one. If an extensive

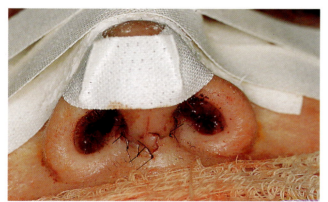

Figure 2.47. Discoloration of the columellar flap may be seen intraoperatively or on the first day postoperatively. When it is seen on the first postoperative day, it is usually due to taping the nose too tightly. Releasing the tape will improve the color. Actual flap necrosis is extremely rare.

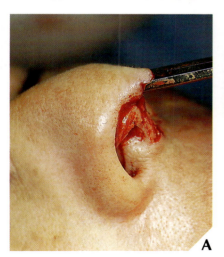
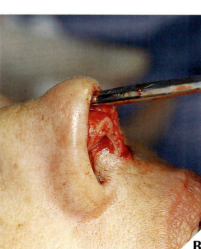

A   B

Figure 2.48. To protect the columellar flap, it should be unfurled when rasping the dorsum or when using a pair of scissors to trim the dorsum. Correct method (**A**). Incorrect method (**B**).

resection of tissue is needed, it is recommended that it be deferred until the first few days postoperatively, at which time there will be less question about the viability of the columellar flap. At that time, under local anesthesia, an alar base excision can always be done as an office procedure.

The advent of recent modifications of rhinoplasty technique renders the large alar base excision (with extension into the vestibulum) less often indicated. The large vestibulum can be reduced by resecting a segment of the lateral crus instead. Such a resection reduces the overall perimeter of the ala and minimizes the need to resect skin in the vestibulum.

The patient in Figure 2.49 is a case in point. The patient underwent a primary reduction open rhinoplasty. Preoperatively she had unusually large vestibula and alae, including an abnormal width between the nostrils. At the time of open rhinoplasty, not only was the soft tissue between the medial crura defatted, but a segment of the most convex portion of the lateral crus was resected. This transected lateral crus was then repaired with figure-of-eight 6-0 nylon sutures to

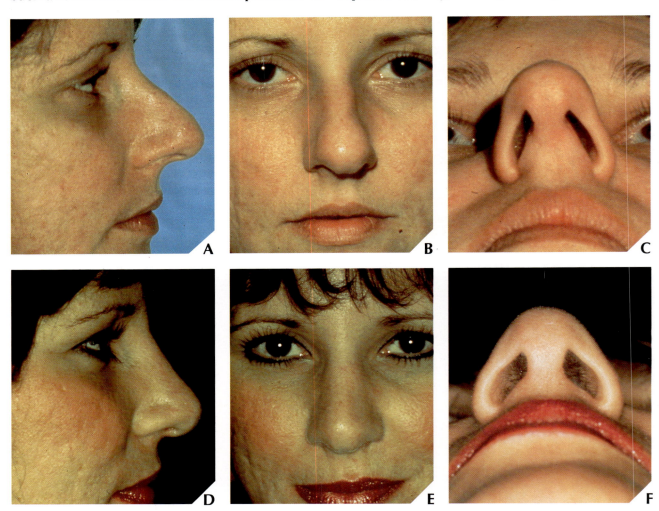

Figure 2.49. Extensive alar base excision (which can affect columellar flap circulation) is avoided by reducing the cartilage of the vestibulum itself. Through the open approach, the tissues between the medial crura are defatted and the most convex portion of the lateral crus is transected. A small segment is removed, which results in a smaller vestibulum. No alar wedge resection is necessary; thus there is no fear of compromising the circulation to the columellar flap. The preoperative (**A–C**) and postoperative (**D–F**) results are shown.

restore the integrity of the arch. With careful undermining of the lateral crus from the vestibular skin, it is often not necessary to even use sutures; the underlying vestibular skin is adherent to the lateral crus and will support the cartilage edges and keep them opposed to one another.

Postoperatively at 16 months one can see that the perimeter of the nostril has been significantly reduced without performing an alar base excision. The lateral crus has not collapsed despite resection of a small segment (2 to 3 mm of cartilage). It must be admitted, however, that some of the reduction of the nostril perimeter is due to the scar tissue high in the dome within the vestibulum. This scar tissue tends to constrict the vestibulum a little bit in some patients. This can be an advantage in patients who have unusually large nostrils but can be a disadvantage in patients with small nostrils.

SUMMARY

The pertinent complications following aesthetic rhinoplasty have been reviewed in detail. Special emphasis was placed on those complications that are specific to open rhinoplasty. These complications include 1) intraoperative problems, such as anesthesia and hypertension; 2) early postoperative problems such as epistaxis, hematoma, edema, infection, and early skin problems; 3) steroid atrophy; 4) late postoperative problems, such as unexpected anatomic complications; 5) implant and allograft rejection; 6) breathing difficulties; 7) the difficult patient; and 8) the columellar scar following open rhinoplasty. Prevention and treatment of these problems were discussed.

BIBLIOGRAPHY

Adamson JE: Constriction of the internal valve in rhinoplasty: treatment and prevention. Ann Plast Surg 18:114-121, 1987.

Broadbent TR, Woolf M: Rhinoplasty. In Courtiss H (ed): Aesthetic Surgery CV Mosby, St. Louis, 1978.

Courtiss EH: Nasal physiology, patient evalauation and effects of surgery. In Rees TD, Baker C, Tabbal (eds): CV Mosby, St. Louis, 1988.

Goldwyn RM: Unexpected bleeding after elective nasal surgery. Ann Plast Surg 2:201-204, 1979.

Gorney M: The septum in rhinoplasty: a few practical hints and technical suggestions. In Rees TD, Baker C, Tabbal N (eds): Rhinoplasty: Problems and Controversy. CV Mosby, St. Louis, 1988.

Guyuron B: Is packing after septal rhinoplasty necessary? A randomized study. Plast Reconstr Surg 184:41-44, 1989.

Hallock GG, Trier WC: Cerebrospinal fluid rhinorrhea following rhinoplasty. Plast Reconstr Surg 71:109-113, 1983.

Jost G, Meyer R, Rees T: The extramucosal technique. In Rees TD, Baker C, Tabbal N (eds): Rhinoplasty: Problems and Controversies. Mosby, St. Louis, 1988.

Kern B: Surgery of the nasal valve. In Rees T, Baker C, Tabbal N (eds): Rhinoplasty: Problems and Controversies. CV Mosby, St. Louis, 1988.

McKinney P, Cook JQ: A critical evaluation of 200 rhinoplasties. Ann Plast Surg 7:357-361, 1981.

Parks ML, Borowiecki B, Binder W: Functional sequelae of rhinoplasty. Ann Plast Surg 4:116-120, 1980.

Peck C: Unfavorable results in rhinoplasty. In Goldwyn RM (ed): The Unfavorable Result in Plastic Surger. Little, Brown, Boston, 1984.

Sheen H: Rhinoplasty complication following the use of banked homologous cartilage. Perspect Plast Surg 4:163-166, 1990.

Slavin SA, Rees TD, Guy CL, Goldwyn RM: An investigation of bacteremia during rhinoplasty. Plast Reconstr Surg 71:196-198, 1983.

Stuzin JM, Kawamoto HK: Saddle nose deformity. Clin Plast Surg 15:83-94, 1988.

Teichgraeber JF, Riley B, Parks DH: Nasal surgery complications. Plast Reconst Surg 85:527-531, 1990.

Tobin G, Shaw RC, Goodpasture HZ: Toxic shock syndrome following breast and nasal surgery. Plast Reconstr Surg 80:111-114, 1987.

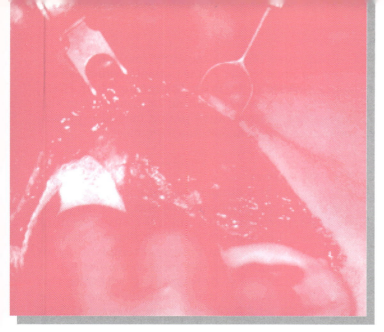

FACELIFT SURGERY

Bernard L. Kaye

CHAPTER 3

The medical and aesthetic challenges of facelift surgery require the plastic surgeon to have the knowledge of a scientist and the sensitivity of an artist. With many patients in their fifties and beyond, the possibility of complications poses an added challenge, even for the most meticulous of surgeons. Fortunately, significant complications following facelift surgery are unusual. When problems do arise, they are generally mild and either disappear over time or can be corrected in a subsequent procedure.

HEMATOMA FORMATION

The most common problem encountered after facelift surgery is hematoma formation, which affects between 1 and 8 of every 100 patients. Hypertension is the major contributing factor, with men more prone to developing hematomas than women. Hematoma formation is often brought on by sudden increases in blood pressure in the hours after surgery, as medications wear off and the patient's adrenergic responses to pain and anxiety become manifest.

Other conditions that predispose patients to hematomas include bleeding diatheses (e.g., von Willebrand's disease) and chronic use of certain medications. For example, aspirin and other nonsteroidal anti-inflammatory agents inhibit platelet aggregation. Other culprits are clofibrate, sulfinpyrazone, dipyridamole, and dextrans. Even topical salicylate compounds that are readily absorbed can produce platelet coagulopathy and result in hematoma.

Premature physical activity may be another cause of hematomas. Some patients resume strenuous physical activity too soon after their surgery. Strenuous vomiting or coughing in the immediate postoperative period may also predispose a patient to hematoma formation.

Prevention

The surgeon should take the patient's blood pressure at the initial consultation and have laboratory tests performed to uncover any bleeding diatheses (i.e., platelet count, prothrombin time, partial thromboplastin time, and template bleeding time). In addition, the surgeon should take a complete history, determining whether the patient is using any drugs that might aggravate bleeding or inhibit platelet aggregation (Fig. 3.1). These medications should be stopped well in advance of the surgery.

Chronic hypertension, a chief cause of hematoma, is usually detected without difficulty. Most hypertensive patients are already under a physician's care and take medication regularly. In patients with undiagnosed or labile hypertension, the condition usually becomes apparent when the plastic surgeon checks the blood pressure at the first consultation. In general, candidates for facelift surgery find this consultation anxiety-provoking and respond with an elevation in blood pressure.

When a patient is found to have hypertension, the surgeon should contact the patient's primary care physician about preoperative management.

Figure 3.1
Examples of Medications that Inhibit Platelet Aggregation

Salicylates*
Other nonsteroidal
  anti-inflammatory agents*
Dextrans
Dipyridamole
Sulfinpyrazone
Clofibrate

*Worst offenders.

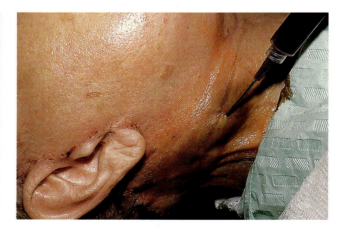

Figure 3.2. Aspiration of liquefied hematoma.

Antihypertensive drugs should be prescribed in doses high enough to keep the systolic blood pressure below 150 mm Hg at all times, even during high-anxiety situations. Patients taking ß-adrenergic blockers should be given a cardiospecific ß$_1$-blocking agent instead (e.g., Tenormin, Lopressor) until after surgery to prevent a paradoxical hypertensive reaction to the ∂-vasoconstrictive properties of epinephrine, used by many surgeons intraoperatively. During surgery, an anesthesiologist can monitor and control blood pressure, leaving the surgeon free to concentrate on procedural details.

Because blood pressure surges are common in hypertensive individuals after their medications wear off, it is wise to hospitalize such patients for at least one night and leave monitoring instructions and medication orders with the nursing staff. In particularly problematic patients, the collaboration of an internist is advisable.

An important intraoperative preventive measure is meticulous hemostasis. The operative field should be closely inspected a number of times and bleeding points electrocoagulated repeatedly. If the patient's head is elevated during surgery, it should be lowered before wound closure to reveal bleeding points. It may even be advantageous to postpone closure until the epinephrine has worn off and vasospasm has ceased.

Treatment

Small hematomas (<30 ml) may take 3 to 5 days to become evident. When the clot liquefies, usually 7 to 14 days postoperatively, the contents may be aspirated through a needle (Fig. 3.2). These hematomas should be drained several times, usually 2 to 3 days apart, either by needle aspiration or a small stab incision. A hematoma close to a suture line may sometimes be rolled out after removal of a few sutures. Left untreated, small hematomas may organize into scar tissue and cause retraction, puckering, and/or discoloration. If any steroids are injected into the lesion, caution must be used to avoid skin atrophy and telangiectasia. Medium-sized hematomas can be removed with equipment designed for suction lipectomy, with the patient under local anesthesia (Fig. 3.3).

Large, expanding hematomas are usually heralded by pain, restlessness, and, possibly, feelings of tightness around the neck and trismus. On palpation, the neck often feels hard on the affected side. Pathognomonic signs are swelling and ecchymosis of the eyelids and buccal mucosa. These hematomas are not in themselves disasters when treated without delay. However, any dyspnea or blistering (indicating circulatory distress) should be regarded as danger signals.

A few sutures at the hematoma site may be removed at the patient's bedside to relieve tension, but generally the patient must be returned to the operating room and given a general anesthetic before the flaps are opened. Clots may be removed with sponge forceps and the site irrigated with normal saline and dilute hydrogen peroxide. When the bleeding is controlled, the flaps may be resutured, often under considerable tension. In cases treated early enough, good healing may be expected although the patient will have considerable temporary edema and ecchymosis.

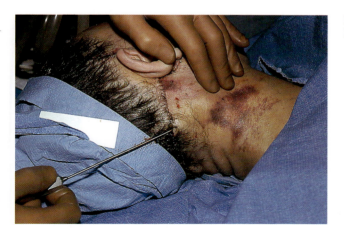

Figure 3.3. Aspiration of clotted hematoma with liposuction equipment.

SENSORY NERVE INJURY

The sensory nerve most often traumatized during facelift surgery is the great auricular nerve that provides sensation to the lower part of the ear and the skin in front of and behind the ear. After nerve damage, the patient has numbness in its area of distribution. A few patients develop painful neuromas or disturbing paresthesias. This nerve is susceptible to injury because, when the patient's head is turned to the side in the usual facelift position, the nerve is almost subcutaneous, covered only by the superficial musculoaponeurotic system in the neck laterally.

The lesser occipital nerve is also susceptible to injury, especially if the dissection is carried into the muscular layer. While the sensory loss after such trauma has little functional significance, some patients report severe pain; in a few, neuroma may develop.

Prevention and Treatment

Intraoperatively, a headlight or fiberoptic retractor should be used when the lateral cervical region is visualized. Only the subcutaneous plane should be dissected. If bare sternocleidomastoid muscle is seen in the area through which the great auricular nerve passes, the nerve (or its severed ends) should be sought. If the nerve has been severed, it should be repaired under magnification. The patient will usually regain sensation within a few months after surgery.

To avoid injury to the lesser occipital nerve, which is most often located 4 to 5 cm below the mastoid process, particular care must be taken during dissection of the posterior neck flap.

If painful neuromas are found after surgery, they should be excised and the nerve ends anastomosed. If significant symptoms persist and no cause can be identified, the surgeon would be wise to search for a neuroma or suture transfixion. Neurolysis may also be performed when the cause of pain cannot be found.

MOTOR NERVE INJURY

Injury to the facial nerve is estimated to occur in fewer than 1 in 150 patients; when it does occur, most patients recover function within 6 months, although recovery periods as long as 2 1/2 years have been reported. The increasing popularity of

---

Figure 3.4
Causes of Facial Nerve Injury During and Immediately Following Facelift Surgery

1. Nerve transection or trauma*
2. Stretching of nerve during tissue traction
3. Pinching with forceps during clamping of bleeding vessels
4. Nerve branches caught during deep suturing or vessel coagulation
5. Nerve branches caught in plication or imbrication sutures
6. Injection of anesthetic agent at the nerve site
7. Pressure on marginal mandibular nerve from tight dressing, producing temporary paresis
8. Development of hematoma or edema within the nerve sheath

If scarring and fibrosis from previous operations are significant, the anatomy may be so distorted that the usual landmarks that the surgeon uses to avoid nerve trauma are no longer clear.

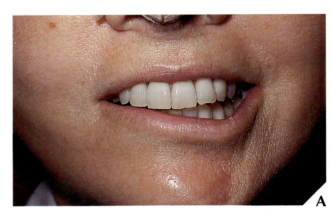
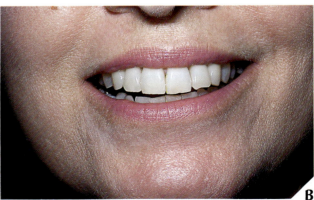

Figure 3.5. (A) Right marginal mandibular injury. **(B)** Spontaneous recovery.

deep dissection techniques may be raising the incidence of this motor nerve injury (Fig. 3.4).

The marginal mandibular nerve is especially vulnerable to damage in facelift surgery because it lies directly below the platysma, which is thin and atrophic in many patients. In patients with several previous facelifts, scarring and fibrosis may obliterate the subplatysmal plane, making the nerve hard to identify. After damage, the patient cannot pull the lower lip down while smiling or talking because innervation of the depressor anguli oris and depressor labii inferioris is interrupted. Figure 3.5 shows such a nerve injury with spontaneous recovery a few weeks later.

The temporal branch is also susceptible to injury. When the nerve is damaged, paresis occurs on the affected side and the patient cannot wrinkle the forehead on that side; also, the eyebrow droops. Figure 3.6 shows such an injury with spontaneous recovery a few months later.

Injury may also involve one of the buccal branches of the facial nerve, although permanent paresis is rare because of numerous intraneural interconnections. Such injury results in decreased motion of the upper lip and, sometimes, paresis in the lower part of the nose, a portion of the cheek, and the angle of the mouth.

Very few rare cases of spinal accessory nerve damage (Fig. 3.7) and damage to the zygomatic branches of the facial nerve have been reported.

Prevention and Treatment

To avoid injuring the temporal branch of the facial nerve, gentle, blunt dissection should be used in the vulnerable tissue between the midzygomatic arch and the lateral canthal area. The surgeon may elevate the medial superficial fascial flap safely using a downward peeling motion, rather than a pushing motion, with a finger wrapped in two layers of gauze sponge (Fig. 3.8). Hydrodissection with a local anesthetic solution may be used to dissect the skin and subcutaneous tissue superior to the zygoma.

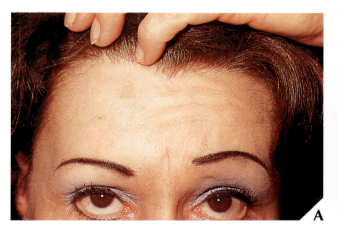
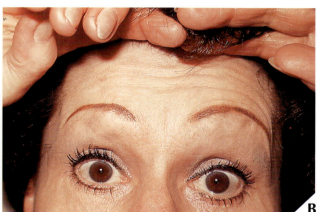

Figure 3.6. **(A)** Right frontal paresis. **(B)** Spontaneous recovery.

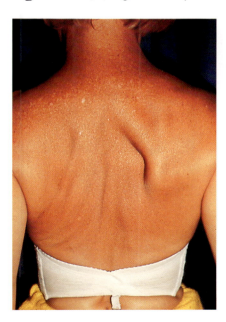

Figure 3.7. Winging scapula from spinal excessory nerve injury.

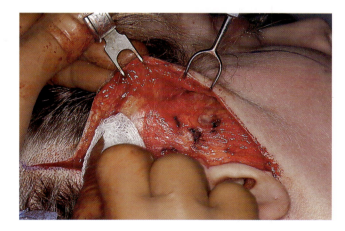

Figure 3.8. Peeling motion for effective gauze-finger dissection.

To prevent injury to the marginal mandibular branch, the surgeon should transect the platysma in a SMAS-platysma facelift surgery at least 5 cm below the inferior border of the mandible. Blunt, gentle dissection should be performed over the course of the nerve using the finger dissection technique described above. Only when the SMAS-platysma flap has been sutured into its new position should the external surface be defatted with a scissors, preventing tenting and inadvertent nerve transection. Another option is to use open liposuction. Particular care must be taken in the patient with previous facelifts, because of probable distortion of tissues along the course of the marginal mandibular nerve.

The buccal nerve or its filaments may be protected by the use of blunt, gentle dissection deep to the SMAS. Fine scissors may be used to spread the tissues (Fig. 3.9A), after which the tissue may be push-dissected with a finger in the yielding plane superficial to the masseteric fasciae and facial nerve branches (Fig. 3.9B). Sharp dissection with scissors or scalpel should be avoided where the buccal branches emerge from the parotid gland. If cheek fat pads are reduced, the fat should be gently teased out, not excised, because the buccal nerve branches cross these pads.

If the temporal branch of the facial nerve is injured, the patient should be followed at regular intervals and offered ongoing support. Any motion on the injured side indicates that recovery has begun. If function does not return within 1 to 2 years, selective neurectomy of the opposite temporal branch may be considered, with electri-cal stimulation used to identify the branches that usually comprise the temporal nerve. Drooping of the brow that follows denervation may be corrected by periodic forehead-brow lifts.

If the buccal nerve is injured, the patient is likely to recover within 3 to 6 months. Occasionally, tics follow buccal branch injury; if they persist, selective neurolysis may be used, or treatment with muscle relaxants or tranquilizers may be tried.

NECROSIS

Necrosis occurs in as many as 1 in 7 patients after facelift surgery. The most susceptible area is the retroauricular mastoid region, where the skin is the most taut and thin and lies farthest from its blood supply. The edge of the temporal flap is also susceptible, as it is often sutured under tension. Necrosis usually becomes apparent within 24 to 48 hours after surgery, when the skin turns bluish (Fig. 3.10). Partial thickness sloughs may show blisters and loss of epidermis. A dark, leathery eschar is typical of full-thickness necrosis (Fig. 3.11).

The incidence of necrosis after facelift is at least 12 to 13 times higher in smokers. Other risk factors include diabetes mellitus, atherosclerosis, Raynaud's disease, and vascular compromise due to prior radiation therapy to the head and/or neck. Intraoperative causes of necrosis include too much traction on skin flaps, tissue trauma due to careless technique, excessive undermining, creasing of flaps, excessively tight dressings,

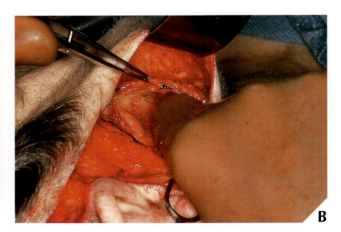

Figure 3.9. (A) Gentle, spreading dissection with small scissors beneath superficial musculoaponeurotic system. A cutting motion is not used. **(B)** Additional dissection of subsuperficial musculoaponeurotic system with gentle, finger-pushing motion.

and overenthusiastic trimming of skin flaps producing excessive skin tension.

A large, expanding hematoma is the most common postoperative cause of skin necrosis, because the clot occludes circulation and blocks neovascularization. There are humeral factors in the clot that also affect circulation adversely. Other postoperative causes of necrosis may be tight dressings, excessive neck flexion, smoking, and severe edema that puts tension on skin flaps and hampers circulation.

Prevention

Smokers should give up their habit for about 2 weeks before and after surgery. Some surgeons suggest abstinence for only a few days before surgery, arguing that carboxyhemoglobin is the agent lowering oxygen availability and its half-life is only 4 hours; also patients are more likely to comply with a short period of abstinence.

Patients with Raynaud's disease must be managed with extreme caution, not only in the surgical approach used but in the administration of vasoconstrictive agents such as epinephrine.

Intraoperative preventive measures include gentle handling of tissues, moderate traction, sufficient flap thickness, and conservative undermining and devascularization of flaps. Tight dressings should be avoided. Postoperatively, inhaled oxygen may be administered to the hospitalized patient who has continued smoking up to the time of surgery; it also prevents the patient from smoking for a day or so postoperatively. Because

the effects of "passive smoking" are now recognized, members of the patient's household should not smoke in the patient's presence until healing is complete.

Finally, the patient should be told to avoid turning the head or bending the neck very much during healing. The patient should not use pillows, or only a relatively flat one, while sleeping. Some surgeons suggest a vertically oriented pillow.

Treatment

Suspected circulatory compromise should be treated by removal of tight dressings and any sutures that are under excessive tension. Oxygen inhalation or treatment with hyperbaric oxygen should be considered. Isoxsuprine (Vasodilan) may improve skin flap circulation somewhat, but its effects are more likely to benefit muscle than skin. Nitroglycerin ointment may be applied to the compromised flap.

If an eschar has formed, the process is irreversible; management should be conservative and expectant. Debridement should be done only when liquefaction is evident beneath the eschar. Povidone-iodine ointment (Betadine) may be helpful until eschar separation and epithelialization take place. In the absence of simultaneous epithelialization, the remaining granulation tissues can be managed with simple daily dressings until healing occurs. Some authors suggest closure with simple split-thickness grafts from adjacent scalp tissue if granulation persists. Psychological support is extremely important to

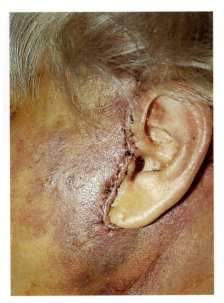

Figure 3.10. Bluish discoloration in a smoker. Such areas may become necrotic.

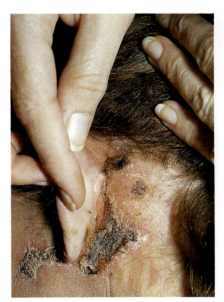

Figure 3.11. Dark, leathery eschar of full-thickness necrosis.

patients during the healing period; frequent office visits should be scheduled.

After the wound has healed and matured, surprisingly little scarring may be evident. Most areas of necrosis and slough eventually heal on their own. If significant scarring remains, it may be treated by revision or a secondary facelift procedure.

EDEMA

Mild or moderate edema is inevitable after facelift surgery and appears to do no harm to the patient or the results. However, severe edema (Fig. 3.12) may compromise the aesthetic outcome and contribute to early recurrence of facial laxity. Possible intraoperative causes of postoperative edema include extensive undermining, rough handling of tissues, pinching or squeezing of the flap, and the use of suction. Excessive neck flexion and failure to keep the head elevated postoperatively may also be factors.

Prevention and Treatment

The patient's head and shoulders should be elevated above the rest of the body during sleep; there should be no bending of the neck. Cold compresses for 24 to 48 hours after the procedure help and also relieve discomfort. If edema advances beyond the mild stage, steroids may help reduce the swelling.

INFECTION

Infection is rare after facelift surgery (fewer than 1 in 100 patients) probably because of the rich blood supply to the area. Infections that do arise are generally minor, involving abscessed stitches. When the stitches are removed, the infection disappears. Significant infections are generally associated with unevacuated hematomas. Postoperative staphylococcal infections, while rare, may cause ischemic necrosis of overlying skin. Figure 3.13 illustrates such an infection with complete recovery after treatment. Common signs and symptoms are pain, swelling, tenderness, erythema, and fever. Streptococcal infections are more often systemic, causing fever and generalized illness.

Prevention and Treatment

When prophylactic antibiotics are used, they should be administered 20 minutes to 2 hours before surgery and be stopped within 24 to 48 hours afterward. If staphylococcal infection is suspected, the site should be cultured if possible

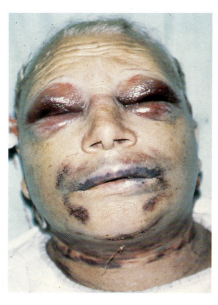

Figure 3.12. Massive postoperative edema masquerading as hematoma.

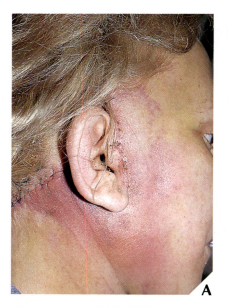
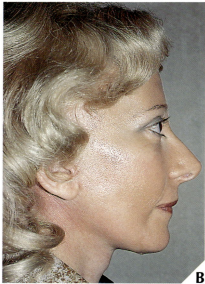

Figure 3.13. (A) Full-blown purulent staphylococcal infection. (B) Complete recovery after daily treatment by local irrigation with nafcillin sodium and dilute hydrogen peroxide, as well as systemically administered nafcillin sodium and probenicid to maintain antibiotic blood levels. Currently most infectious disease specialists no longer recommend topical irrigation with antibiotic solution, preferring the antibiotic therapy be given systemically. Hydrogen peroxide–saline irrigation is still considered efficacious, provided the skin around the irrigation is protected with petroleum jelly.

SKIN PERFORATION

Inadvertent perforation of the patient's skin during facelift usually results from the use of scalpel blades or sharp scissors during dissections.

Prevention and Treatment

When cutting with a scalpel, the surgeon can use a Millard thimble thumb hook, which allows the middle and ring fingers to feel the position and direction of the knife blade (Fig. 3.24). Scissors with rounded points are also helpful. When curved scissors are used, the tips should point away from the skin. An open scissors/push technique allows the surgeon to tent the flap with the convex rounded scissor blades while ensuring that the tips do not perforate the skin. Whenever possible, blunt dissection should be done with a gauze-wrapped finger.

If perforation does occur, the skin must be closed meticulously in two layers. The surgeon should trim the flap behind the perforation more conservatively than usual to minimize tension on the repair.

PAIN AND DISCOMFORT

Pain is uncommon after facelift surgery because many sensory nerves are divided during surgery and the procedure is relatively superficial, unlike operations performed on deep structures. Any pain that does occur along sensory nerve pathways usually disappears within 3 months. If a patient has persistent localized pain at a trigger point or in a palpable nodule, a neuroma may be responsible.

Minor discomforts may accompany postoperative healing of sensory nerves: sharp shooting sensations, itching, and so on. Patients whose platysma has been shifted laterally, with suturing to the sternocleidomastoid, may feel suture knots under the skin. Feelings of tightness are not uncommon after significant repositioning of tissue.

Prevention and Treatment

Preoperative counseling and explanations of why pain is uncommon after facelift surgery can reduce patients' anxiety and serve as a form of preoperative suggestion. If patients have persistent pain along sensory nerves, repeated nerve blocks may be performed. Patients with tightness may be helped by muscle relaxants. Suture knots made with resorbable sutures will disappear on their own. It is important that the surgeon have an appreciation of the psychological components of pain and be willing to counsel and reassure patients in order to help them through a trying period.

EARLY RECURRENCE OF DEFORMITY

Contributing factors to early recurrence include age, genetic makeup, race (with fair-skinned patients being more susceptible), previous acne, and, in women, decreased ovarian function.

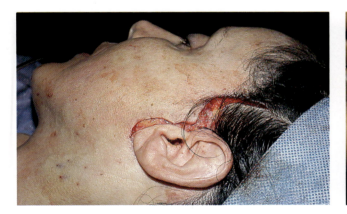

Figure 3.23. Pre-sideburn incision to prevent sideburn from disappearing upward.

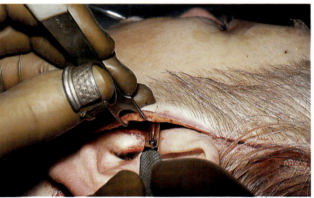

Figure 3.24. Retraction with Millard thimble hook, which permits tactile appreciation of scalpel depth.

Patients with deformities such as fat neck, severe turkey-gobbler deformity, or sun-damaged skin are more prone to early recurrence, as are those with severe postoperative edema whose skin is overstretched. Other contributing factors include significant weight loss after surgery, continued overexposure to the sun, smoking, and excessive alcohol consumption.

Prevention and Treatment

Preoperative counseling is the key to effective management in the recurrence-prone patient. Patients should be told that a facelift will turn back the clock, but that the clock resumes ticking as soon as the procedure ends. To maintain the results of facelift surgery requires renewal operations—although the interval between procedures gets increasingly longer. Figure 3.25A illustrates a patient preoperatively at age 71. In Figure 3.25B, she is three years older, but has had two facelifts during that interval. The claim made in popular magazines that a first facelift lasts 7 years is simply not true.

Intraoperative measures that have been suggested to delay recurrence include: 1) dividing both the platysmal muscle and posterior sheath in the neck, as well as excising parts of the platysma not connected to the sheath; 2) interrupting band continuity satisfactorily; 3) avoiding excess tension on the suture line; 4) avoiding tight sutures that might cut through the medial borders of sutured muscle; and 5) avoiding excess tension on the lateral platysmal border, which might also make the medial sutures cut

through the muscle edges. It has also been suggested that interrupting the medial platysma border by wedge resection and not partial transection by incision, will widen the muscle gap and make it less possible for vertical fibers to reconnect.

PATIENT DISSATISFACTION

Patients who express dissatisfaction in the early postoperative period are often anxious about the ultimate result. Some are disappointed 2 to 3 weeks postoperatively when they see the limitations of aesthetic surgery. Others express disappointment 2 to 3 months after the procedure, when their lives have failed to change in the major ways they expected as a result of surgery. Some patients are the victims of psychological sabotage at home or by friends or relatives who are jealous or threatened.

Prevention and Treatment

Immediately after surgery, the plastic surgeon should reassure the patient about the temporary nature of any regression. Later disappointment may be dealt with by sympathetic inquiry and discussion of any unrealistic goals the patient may have had. The degree of improvement can be documented by showing the patient both pre- and postoperative photographs. If the patient has a justifiable complaint, the surgeon should recognize it openly and honestly, offering a logical plan for correcting the problem

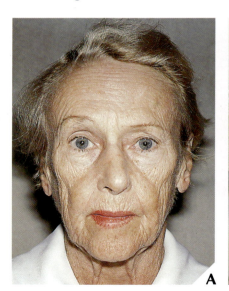 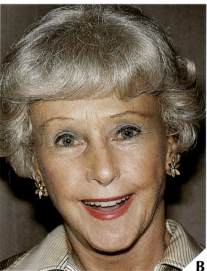

Figure 3.25. Good results in older patient achieved through two operations in 3 years. **(A)** Preoperative view. **(B)** Postoperative view.

BIBLIOGRAPHY

Angel MF, Ramastry SS, Swartz WM, et al: Free radicals: basic concepts concerning their chemistry, pathophysiology and relevance to plastic surgery. Plast Reconstr Surg 79:990, 1987.

Aston SJ: Problems and complications in platysma-SMAS cervicofacial rhytidectomy. In Kaye BL and Gradinger GP (eds): Symposium on Problems and Complications in Aesthetic Plastic Surgery of the Face, pp. 132–145. CV Mosby, St. Louis, 1984.

Baker TJ and Gordon HL: Surgical Rejuvenation of the Face. CV Mosby, St. Louis, 1986.

Converse JM and Coburn RJ: The twitching scar. Br J Plast Surg 24:272, 1971.

Ellenbogen RL and Karlin JV: Regrowth of platysma following cervical lift: etiology and methodology of prevention. Plast Reconstr Surg 67:616, 1981.

Fodor PB and Liverette DM: Sideburn reconstruction for post rhytidectomy deformity. Plast Reconstr Surg 74:430, 1984.

Hugo NE and Starke RB: Complications after rhytidectomy. In Starke RB (ed): Plastic Surgery of the Head and Neck, p. 897. Churchill Livingstone, New York, 1987.

Kaye BL: Complications of face lift. Adv Plast Reconstr Surg 6:125, 1990.

Kaye BL: Facial Rejuvenative Surgery: A Color Photographic Atlas. JB Lippincott, Philadelphia, 1987.

Kaye BL and Gradinger GP (eds): Symposium on Problems and Complications in Aesthetic Surgery of the Face. C. V. Mosby, St. Louis, 1984.

Mulliken JB and Healey NA: Pathogenesis of skin flap necrosis from an underlying hematoma. Plast Reconstr Surg 1979; 63:540, 1979.

Rees TD, Liverett DM, and Guy CL: The effect of cigarette smoking on skin flap survival in the face lift patient. Plast Reconstr Surg 73:911, 1984.

Zaworski RE and Noriega CJ: Massive postoperative facial edema in a rhytidectomy. Plast Reconstr Surg 62:622, 1978.

FIGURE CREDITS

Figures 3.2, 3.3, 3.5, 3.6, 3.13, 3.14 are reprinted with permission from Salisbury CC, Kaye BL: Complications following rhytidectomy. Plast Surg Nurs 76-83, 1987; Figure 3.7 is reprinted with permission from McGregor MW, Greenburg RL: Rhytidectomy. In Goldwyn RM (ed): The Unfavorable Results in Plastic Surgery. Little Brown, Boston, 1972; Figures 3.8, 3.9, 3.25 are reprinted with permission from Kaye BL: Facial Rejuvenative Surgery: A Color Photographic Atlas. JB Lippincott, Philadelphia, 1987; Figures 3.10, 3.11, 3.15, 3.16, 3.17, 3.18, 3.19, 3.21, 3.22, 3.23, 3.24 are reprinted with permission from Kaye BL: Complications of face lift. Adv Plast Reconstr Surg 6:125–176, 1990; Figure 3.12 is reprinted with permission from Zaworsky RE, Noriega CJ: Massive postoperative facial edema in a rhytidectomy. Plast Reconstr Surg 62:622–625, 1978.

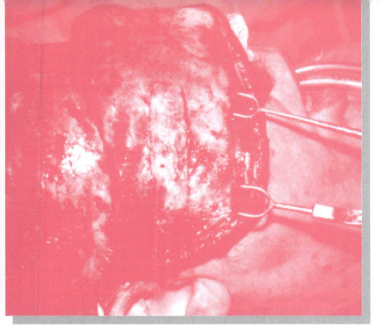

FOREHEAD LIFT
SURGERY

Bernard L. Kaye

C H A P T E R

4

Forehead, or brow, lift surgery is relatively free of complications. Those that do occur usually tend to be mild and transient, requiring only routine management.

POSTOPERATIVE PAIN

Frontal pain is a problem in some patients, usually occurring within the first few hours after surgery. Patients often describe a severe headache over the forehead. The cause is probably intraoperative stretching of the supraorbital and supratrochlear nerves.

Treatment

The onset of frontal headache can be delayed and its intensity lessened by the injection of a long-acting local anesthetic agent such as bupivacaine (Marcaine) or etidocaine (Duranest) at the end of the procedure. The anesthetic solution is injected around the supraorbital and supratrochlear nerves where they emerge from their foramina. Usually, a single injection suffices. Systemic analgesics are less helpful.

SCALP NUMBNESS

Loss of sensation in the anterior scalp is common after brow lift because the coronal incision divides the supraorbital and supratrochlear nerves as they run from the forehead into the scalp. This probability should be discussed with the patient during preoperative counseling. While sensation returns in most cases, occasionally a partial deficit becomes permanent.

Numbness in the middle of the forehead, if it occurs at all, is usually mild, even when the surgeon has excised the origins of the corrugator muscles to reduce frowning—a procedure that is certain to divide some fine branches of the supratrochlear nerves because they are intertwined with muscle fibers. Absence of numbness is probably due to the abundance of crossover nerves linking the supratrochlear and supraorbital areas of sensation in the mid-forehead.

Prevention and Treatment

To help maintain sensation in the scalp, the levels of division of the supraorbital nerves can be limited. The surgeon should interrupt frontalis muscle strip excisions directly over the courses of these nerves when excising strips of frontalis to reduce muscle pull on the raised forehead flap. This leaves vertical bridges of muscle intact over the area (Fig. 4.1).

PARESTHESIAS AND ITCHING

A few weeks to several months after surgery, itching and paresthesias are common. Patients who are warned about this minor sequela of surgery rarely need treatment; they realize that it is a normal part of recovery. Persistent itching may cause problems in patients who do not restrain themselves from scratching the scalp. While scratching can produce ulcerations (Fig. 4.2), healing usually commences after the patient stops scratching.

Treatment

If itching is severe, trimeprazine tartrate (Temaril) may be prescribed, 2.5 mg four times daily. Cyproheptadine hydrochloride (Periactin) may also be helpful, 4 mg four times daily.

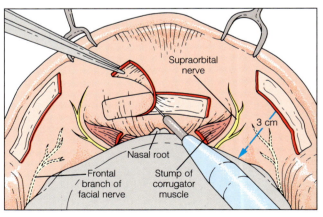

Figure 4.1. Interrupted strips of frontalis excised with intact bridges over courses of supraorbital nerves.

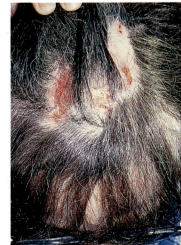

Figure 4.2. Ulceration produced by scratching because of itching.

HIGH FRONTAL HAIRLINE

A conventional brow lift, in which the incision is made in the hair-bearing portion of the scalp, inevitably raises the frontal hairline, although less skin is generally removed in the center of the forehead flap than at the sides.

Prevention

If the patient already has a high frontal hairline, the surgeon may elect not to make an incision that travels behind the hairline (Fig. 4.3A,B), but rather to make the central part of the incision between the temporal areas just in front of the hairline (Fig. 4.3C). In this way, the middle of the frontal hairline is not raised. Also, if a secondary forehead lift is performed, the center front of the hairline will stay at the same level.

The disadvantage of this approach is that an incision line is located at the edge of the hairline. It is important not to make the incision too far in front of the hairline, lest it be visible after healing. The anterior incision should be made directly against the frontal hairline; with a carefully, layered closure; it normally heals very well (Fig. 4.4). If necessary, it can be covered by a slight overlap of hair; many patients with high frontal hairlines already wear their hair in styles that cover some of the forehead. The incision should always be made just at the hairline; it is even acceptable to sacrifice a small segment of hairbearing skin. If an intervening strip of hairline skin is left, the incision line will be harder to cover.

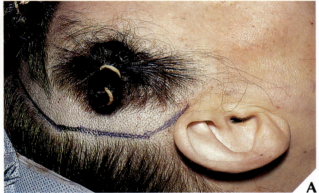

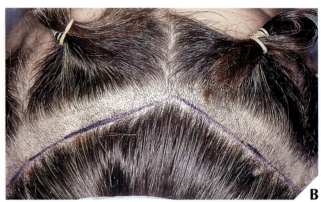

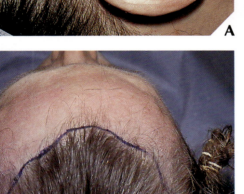

Figure 4.3. (A , B) Forehead incision made posterior to hairline.(C) Central portion of forehead incision made anterior to hairline in patient with high frontal hairline.

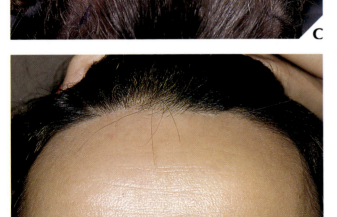

Figure 4.4. Healed anterior forehead incision.

TEMPORARY HAIR LOSS

A few weeks after a brow lift, some of the hair follicles in the flap may enter a resting phase, possibly due to tension after suturing. This can produce temporary thinning of the hair in front of the incision; normal regrowth usually occurs within 2 to 3 months.

Prevention

To avoid this problem, the edges of the forehead flap should be trimmed conservatively so that there is little or no tension on the suture line. The galea should be closed as one layer, and the skin and subcutaneous tissue as another. When strips of lateral frontalis muscle under the temporal, hair-bearing portions of the forehead flap are excised, one should avoid cutting hair follicles.

TEMPORARY FOREHEAD LAG

If frontalis strip excisions are placed too low in the lateral portions of the flap, temporary forehead lag may result. The surgeon can usually avoid this type of frontal motor nerve injury by keeping in mind the anatomy of the frontal branches of the facial nerve when excising or incising strips of frontalis muscle in the lateral portions of the forehead flap. Frontal nerve branches course along a path beginning about 0.5 cm below the tragus of the ear and pass 1.5 cm above the lateral edge of the eyebrow (Fig. 4.5).

Prevention and Treatment

By keeping lateral frontalis strip excisions at least 3 cm above the eyebrow and orbital rim, the surgeon can usually avoid injury to these nerves (Fig. 4.6).

If the forehead lift surgery is being combined with a facelift, the surgeon can reconcile the deep plane of the forehead lift with the superficial plane of the facelift. This is done by surgically defining a fascial web that contains the frontal branches of the facial nerve (Fig. 4.7A). The web is defined by gentle, blunt dissection using a peeling motion with a finger wrapped in a gauze sponge (Fig. 4.7B). This method is effective because nerve branches are tougher than connec-

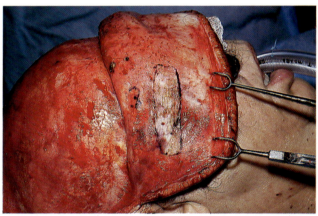

Figure 4.6. Lateral frontalis strip excision made at least 3 cm above superorbital ridge to avoid injury to frontal nerve branch.

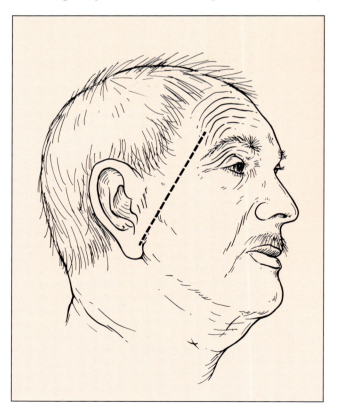

Figure 4.5. Course of frontal branch of facial nerve, starting 0.5 cm inferior to tragus and passing 1.5 cm superior to lateral end of eyebrow.

The occurrence of some complications is inevitable if one performs enough blepharoplastic procedures. The incidence and severity of permanent complications are reduced by careful preoperative evaluations, including a medical and ophthalmologic history and physical examination of the patient. Preoperative clinical photography is essential in documenting existing eyelid and periocular anatomy.[24,40] The photographs are used for preoperative surgical planning and intraoperative decision making (Fig. 5.4).

THE CONSULTATION

Medical History

It is important to determine the general health of the patient and the specific purpose for the consultation. The patient should describe what he would like corrected and what degree of expectation he has that this aesthetic goal will be achieved. It is important to record previous evaluations or treatments by other plastic surgeons.

The patient should list previous surgical procedures (especially those that were cosmetic) and whether he is satisfied with the results. The surgeon directs questions to the patient to detect whether there is any possibility of chronic illness, psychiatric disturbance, hypertension, diabetes, or cardiovascular or cerebrovascular disease. Thyroid function and general endocrine status are also determined. Further questioning elicits whether the patient has had hepatitis, liver disease, blood clots, bleeding disorders, arrhythmias, heart disease, or cancer. The patient should list any medication he has taken in the past, especially any steroids, hormones, beta blockers, or aspirin-containing medication. He should also list currently administered medications, including dosage, frequency, and purpose. Any allergic reactions are carefully documented. The amount and type of alcohol ingested on a daily or weekly basis is noted. If the patient smokes, the number of cigarettes smoked daily and the duration in years of his habit are recorded. Drugs used for recreational purposes, such as marijuana, LSD, cocaine, or heroin, must be listed.

Figure 5.3 Major Complications of Blepharoplasty

I. Visual Loss
A. Globe Penetration
B. Retrobulbar Hemorrhage
C. Glaucoma
D. Extraocular Muscle Disorder
E. Corneal
  1. Exposure
    a. Ulcer
    b. Filaments
    c. Scar
    d. Neovascularization
  2. Refractive
    a. Astigmatism
    b. Tear film abnormality
    c. Contact lens intolerance
  3. Basement membrane disorder

II. Permanent Eyelid Deformities and Functional Disorders
A. Lacrimal Disorders
  1. Dry eye
  2. Epiphora

a. Tear film abnormality (reflexly stimulated)
b. Tear distributional abnormalities
  i. Lid eversion
  ii. Lid retraction
  iii. Ectropion
  iv. Entropion
c. Tear drainage abnormalities
  i. Lid paralysis
  ii. Medial punctal eversion
  iii. Obstruction of nasolacrimal system
B. Eyelid Malpositions
  1. Upper eyelid
    a. Ptosis
    b. Retraction
    c. Contour changes
    d. Marginal abnormalities
  2. Lower eyelid
    a. Scleral show
    b. Retraction
    c. Laxity
    d. Paralysis

e. Marginal abnormalities
f. Ectropion
g. Entropion
C. Eyelid Deformities
  1. Palpebral aperture assymetry
    a. Unveiled, pre-existing condition
    b. Iatrogenic
  2. Upper eyelid fold
    a. Assymetric
    b. Absent
    c. High
    d. Low
    e. Multiple
  3. Epicanthal folds
  4. Cicatrix
  5. Inadequate fat removal
  6. Excessive fat removal
  7. Suture tunnels
  8. Dermal pigmentary changes
  9. Festoons
  10. Malar pads

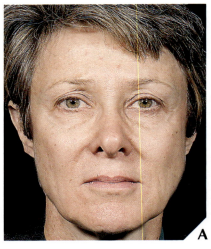

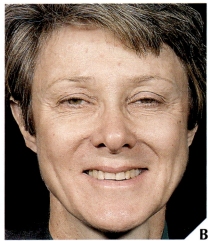

Figure 5.4. Standard preoperative photography for blepharoplasty. **(A,B)** Full face in repose and smiling. **(C,D)** Close-up view of eyelids and periorbital structures in repose and smiling. **(E,F)** Close-up view of eyelids in up gaze and down gaze. **(G,H)** Close-up lateral views of eyelids and periorbital structures.

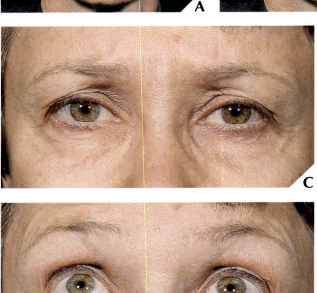

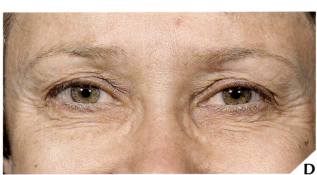

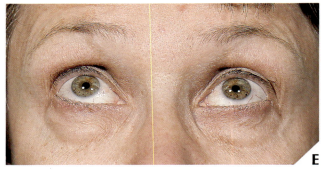

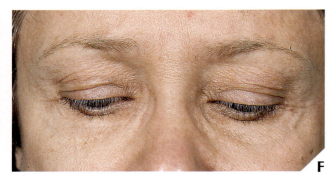

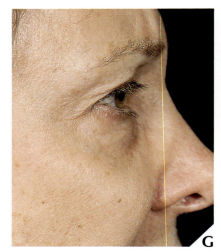

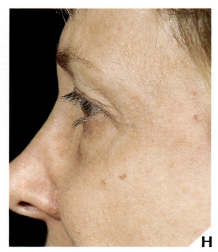

Ophthalmologic History

The use of eye glasses or contact lenses is determined and then vision of each eye is checked. Previous surgery for the eyes, especially glaucoma, strabismus, or cataract procedures, is recorded. The patient should be asked if his vision is decreased by overhanging skin from the upper eyelids because this can be documented by visual field examinations (Fig. 5.5). A history of any facial muscle weakness (previous Bell's palsy, trauma, facial nerve surgery) is specifically elicited, because incomplete return can adversely affect the expected results from a cosmetic blepharoplasty[43] (Fig. 5.6). A past history of recurrent, periodic, severe eyelid and periorbital edema may

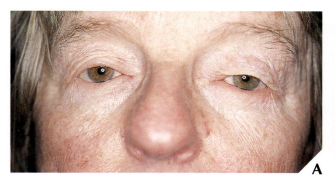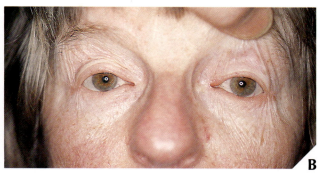

Figure 5.5. (A) Patient with apparent bilateral ptosis. **(B)** Elevation of the upper lid skin reveals normal upper eyelid levels. The pseudoptosis is caused by the excess, lax upper lid skin hanging over the lid margin obstructing the visual fields.

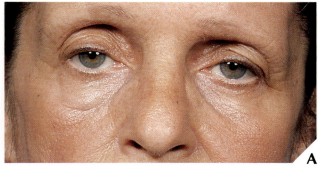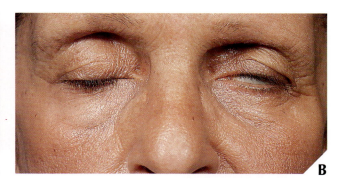

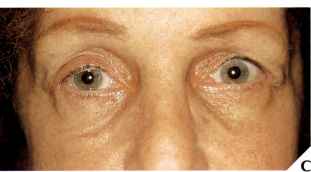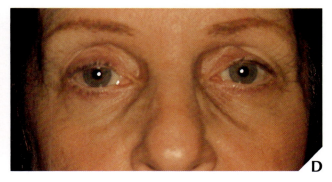

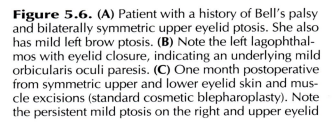

Figure 5.6. (A) Patient with a history of Bell's palsy and bilaterally symmetric upper eyelid ptosis. She also has mild left brow ptosis. **(B)** Note the left lagophthalmos with eyelid closure, indicating an underlying mild orbicularis oculi paresis. **(C)** One month postoperative from symmetric upper and lower eyelid skin and muscle excisions (standard cosmetic blepharoplasty). Note the persistent mild ptosis on the right and upper eyelid retraction on the left. The retraction is caused by the normal levator muscle working to open the eyelid against a slightly paretic orbicularis oculi muscle working to keep the eyelids tense. **(D)** After an appropriate waiting period (6 months), the upper eyelids usually adjust to acceptable levels. If the retraction persists, it can be corrected with a levator recession.

represent blepharochalasis, a chronic familial allergic situation that responds poorly to surgery[15] (Fig. 5.7). The presence of skin conditions that may compromise eyelid surgery, such as atopy, acne rosacea, pemphigoid, and psoriasis, is determined. Questions are asked to determine any signs and symptoms of dry eye, allergic conjunctivitis, or chronic blepharitis (tearing, mucous discharge, crusting of the lid margins, red eye, eyelid edema, itching, or burning). If the patient is able to tolerate the use of contact lenses, there is little chance of a significant dry eye condition.[40] A patient with a chronic red eye who complains of frequent irritation or contact lens intolerance warrants an ophthalmologic evaluation prior to blepharoplasty.[41,71,74,75,77]

THE PHYSICAL EXAMINATION

A record of a recent general and ophthalmologic examination is helpful prior to eyelid surgery. The age and physical condition of the patient will determine the necessity of obtaining a general medical examination prior to surgery. If necessary, permission to consult with the patient's physician is obtained.

The patient's best corrected visual acuity in each eye (with glasses or contact lenses) is determined and recorded using either a wall-mounted or hand-held chart. Occasionally a person has an unrecognized loss of vision in one eye for a variety of reasons. The most common cause, ambly-

Figure 5.7. Blepharochalasis. The patient presents with a history of recurrent eyelid and periorbital edema since teenage years. Surgery is not a definitive treatment for this familial condition.

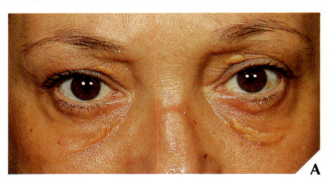

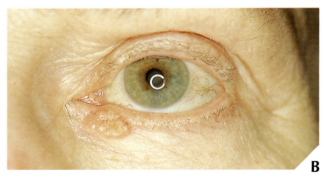

Figure 5.8. (A) Patient with benign xanthelasma lesions of all four eyelids. Excision is performed with modifications of the cosmetic blepharoplastic operation. (B) Patient with a basal cell lesion of the medial left lower lid. It must be removed prior to cosmetic surgery.

blocks of the supraorbital and supratrochlear nerves do not offer relief. Swelling in the forehead, while obvious, does not correspond with the severity of pain. The swelling is limited by the inelasticity of the forehead flap, causing intense pressure underneath. The resulting blockage in circulation can threaten the viability of the flap.

Minor hematomas take longer to appear, usually several days, and may not be painful.

Treatment

The only way to relieve the pain caused by a major hematoma is by decompressing and evacuating the hematoma (Fig. 4.10B). The suture line should be opened enough to allow the surgeon to remove clots and tie off any bleeding vessels. Fortunately this can be done easily and rapidly, and the patient responds favorably almost immediately (Fig. 4.10C). If treatment is prompt, healing should be uneventful and without sequelae.

In patients with small hematomas (Fig. 4.11), the blood in the hematoma should be allowed to liquefy and then should be aspirated every few days. The patient should wear a gentle compression bandage after each aspiration. Aspiration should be repeated until no more fluid is found.

NECROSIS

While unusual, necrosis may occur as a consequence of hematoma formation, an overly tight bandage, or infection. Necrosis in forehead flaps has been reported, but the situation is undoubt-

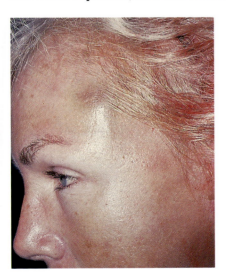

Figure 4.11. Small hematoma that will resolve with multiple aspirations.

edly rare. Patients of mine who have had previous direct brow lifts have suffered no ill effects in flap circulation after coronal forehead lifts.

LAGOPHTHALMOS

When a brow lift is performed too aggressively in a patient who has had an upper lid blepharoplasty, the possibility exists that the palpebral fissures may not close completely postoperatively, exposing the patient to the potential risk of damage to the cornea and bulbar conjunctiva.

Prevention

Preoperative evaluation must be particularly thorough in patients who have had a prior upper lid blepharoplasty. During the office consultation, the surgeon should elevate the patient's forehead manually into the anticipated new position and make sure that the patient's eyes will still close. The patient in Figure 4.12 could not close her eyes. No forehead lift was done.

The evaluation should be repeated just before surgery, when the patient's upper lids have relaxed under sedation or general anesthesia. If, when relaxed, the eyes remain open enough to expose the corneas, the surgeon should limit the scalp excision to the most lateral parts of the flap, or the procedure should be abandoned.

If an upper lid blepharoplasty is being performed at the same time as the brow lift, the brow lift should be done first. The amount of excess skin in the upper lids can be assessed accurately

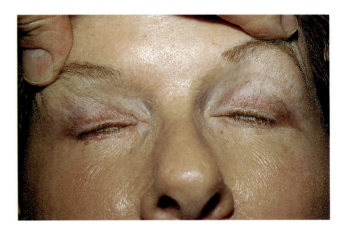

Figure 4.12. Simulated forehead lift in patient who had previous upper lid blepharoplasty and cannot close eyes. Forehead lift was not performed.

after the brow lift. In many patients, the brow lift will provide all the correction needed and an upper lid blepharoplasty may not be necessary. When anticipating both a forehead lift and an upper lid blepharoplasty, many surgeons elect to defer the blepharoplasty for a few months.

INFECTION

Infection is unusual after forehead lifts because of the excellent vascularity of the forehead flap.

Prevention and Treatment

Precautions include having the patient shampoo the hair before surgery with an antibacterial soap such as chlorhexidine gluconate (Hibiclens), povidone iodine (Betadine Surgical Scrub), or hexachlorophene detergent cleanser (pHisoHex). The surgeon may also wish to prescribe preventive antibiotics just before surgery and for a day or two afterward.

CHANGES IN FACIAL EXPRESSION

If too much skin is trimmed from the forehead flap or tension on the flap is excessive in some part of the flap, the patient's facial expression may be altered in a way that was not intended. If the medial portions of the eyebrow are too high, the eyebrows may slant downward from the center, giving the patient a sad appearance. Eyebrows that are raised too high centrally or totally give the patient a startled or surprised expression. The maximum elevation should be above the most lateral parts of the eyebrows (Fig. 4.13).

Because a forehead lift raises the forehead and brows as a unit, it is less likely to cause unfavorable alterations in facial expression than a direct eyebrow lift. Because the brows are raised naturally, the normal facial expression is retained. However, the surgeon may also correct pre-existing problems of facial expression. For example, the surgeon can alter a constantly angry expres-

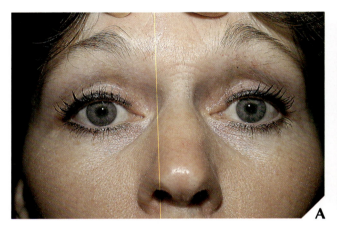

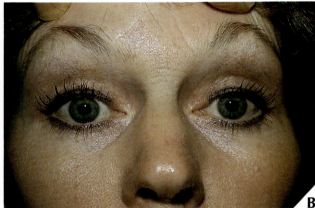

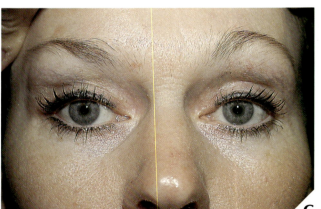

Figure 4.13. Changes in facial expressions that may be produced when brows are raised inappropriately. **(A)** Excess elevation medially produces a sad look. **(B)** Over-elevation centrally gives a startled or suprised look. **(C)** Maximum elevation should be over lateral parts of eyebrow.

sion by raising the central portion of the flap slightly higher than usual. If the patient had a pre-existing sad expression, the surgeon can raise the lateral part of the flap.

Prevention

While some surgeons have suggested mathematical formulas for determining the amount of skin that should be trimmed from the flap during a brow lift, I believe that patients are better served when plastic surgeons rely on their intuitive aesthetic sense, as well as their surgical knowledge—erring on the conservative side, if necessary. In general, excision of scalp at the center of the flap should not exceed 1 cm; laterally, it should not exceed 2 cm.

REFERENCES

Connell BF: Eyebrow, face and neck lifts for males. Clin Plast Surg 5:15, 1978.

Connell BF: Finesse in rhytidectomy. Rec Adv Plast Surg 3:137, 1985.

Connell BF, Lambros VS, Neurohr GH: The forehead lift: techniques to avoid complications and produce optimal results. Aesth Plast Surg 1313:217, 1989.

Kaye BL: The forehead lift: a useful adjunct to face lift and blepharoplasty. Plast Reconstr Surg 60:161, 1977.

Kaye BL: The forehead lift. In Goldwyn RM (ed): Long-Term Results: Plastic & Reconstructive Surgery. Little, Brown, Boston, 1980.

Kaye BL: Facial Rejuvenative Surgery: A Color Photographic Atlas. JB Lippincott, Philadelphia, 1987.

Pitanguy I, Silveria Ramos, A: The frontal branch of the facial nerve. The importance of its variations in face lifting. Plast Reconstr Surg 38:352, 1966.

Reifkohl R: The forehead-brow lift. Ann Plast Surg 8:55, 1982.

Vinas JC, Caviglia C, Cortinas JL: Forehead rhytidoplasty and brow lifting. Plast Reconstr Surg 57:445, 1976.

FIGURE CREDITS

Figures 4.1, 4.7B are reprinted with permission from Kaye BL: Facial Rejuvenative Surgery: A Color Photographic Atlas. JB Lippincott, Philadelphia, 1987; Figures 4.2, 4.9, 4.10, 4.11 are reprinted with permission from Kaye BL: Problems and complications in the forehead lift. In Kaye BL, Bradinger GP (eds): Symposium on Problems and Complications in Aesthetic Plastic Surgery of the Face, CV Mosby, St. Louis, 1984.

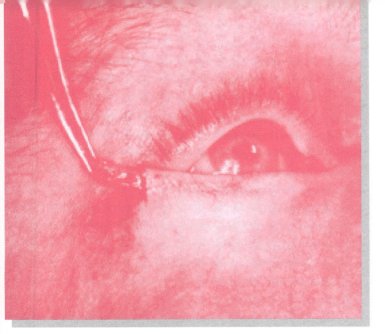

BLEPHAROPLASTY

Glenn W. Jelks
Elizabeth B. Jelks

C H A P T E R 5

Several thousand cosmetic blepharoplasties are performed throughout the world each year. This discussion describes the complications and unfavorable results that may occur with cosmetic blepharoplasty with an emphasis on their prevention.[2,11-14,17,49,57,58,68,80-82] Methods useful in managing evolving and established problems are demonstrated. The eyelids and periorbital tissues are divided into anatomic zones to help in the categorization and identification of complications (Fig. 5.1). Minor complications are temporary and self-limiting with minimal visual disturbance or aesthetic consequence (Fig. 5.2). Major complications, however, include visual loss, fixed eyelid deformities, and significant aesthetic compromise (Fig. 5.3).

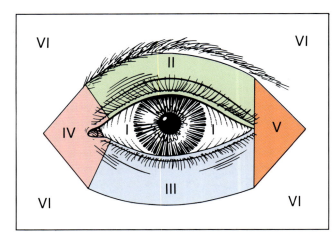

Figure 5.1. Orbital and eyelid anatomy.

ZONE I: Ocular/Orbital
ZONE II: Upper Eyelid
  A. Preseptal
  B. Postseptal
ZONE III: Lower Eyelid
  A. Preseptal
  B. Postseptal
ZONE IV: Medial Canthus including Lacrimal Drainage System
  A. Preseptal
  B. Postseptal
ZONE V: Lateral Canthus (Retinaculum)
  A. Preseptal
  B. Postseptal
ZONE VI: Contiguous Structures
  Nasal
  Glabellar
  Brow
  Forehead
  Temple
  Malar
  Nasojugal

Figure 5.2 Minor Complications of Blepharoplasty*

A. Retrobulbar Hemorrhage
B. Pupil Changes
C. Glaucoma
D. Extraocular Muscle Disorder
E. Corneal Changes
  1. Exposure
    a. Keratitis
    b. Erosion
    c. Ulcer
  2. Refractive
    a. Astigmatism
    b. Edema
    c. Tear film abnormality
  3. Basement membrane disorder
F. Lacrimal Disorder
  1. Dry eye
  2. Epiphora
    a. Tear film abnormality
    b. Reflexly stimulated tears
    c. Tear distributional abnormalities
      i. Lid margin eversion
      ii. Lid retraction

      iii. Lid ectropion
      iv. Lid entropion
      v. Lid paresis
    d. Tear drainage abnormalities
      i. Punctal eversion
      ii. Obstruction of nasolacrimal system
      iii. Lid paresis
  3. Dacryocystitis
G. Conjunctival Changes
  1. Chemosis
  2. Prolapse
  3. Incarceration
  4. Hemorrhage
H. Eyelid Malposition
  1. Upper eyelid
    a. Ptosis
    b. Retraction
    c. Contour change
    d. Marginal rotation
  2. Lower eyelid
    a. Scleral show
    b. Lid retraction
    c. Lid paresis

    d. Marginal rotation
    e. Ectropion/entropion
I. Eyelid Deformities
  1. Hematoma
  2. Epicanthal folds
  3. Cysts
  4. Wound separation
  5. Eyelid numbness
  6. Eyelid discoloration
  7. Scars
  8. Loss of eyelashes
J. Inflammatory Conditions
  1. Infectious
    a. Cellulitis
    b. Abscess
    c. Hordeolum
    d. Chalazion
    e. Blepharitis
  2. Non-infectious
    a. Allergic
    b. Chemical
    c. Blepharitis

*These are temporary or self-limiting conditions.

opia (lazy eye), has an incidence of 2% in the general population.[27] Occluding the fellow eye, while testing vision, is the only way that unrecognized visual loss is determined.

Careful observation of the skin and subcutaneous tissue of the eyelids and periorbital area is essential to rule out the presence of any tumors or lesions that must be removed (Fig. 5.8). Surgical removal of eyelid and periorbital lesions requires preservation of local tissue to perform the necessary reconstructions (Fig. 5.9). This may postpone or eliminate the possibility of performing a cosmetic blepharoplasty.

Evaluation of the surface anatomy of the orbital region includes observation and documentation of the size, shape, and configuration of the bony orbit, eyebrows, malar eminences, and eyelids. To facilitate this analysis, the eyelids and periorbital structures are divided into zones (see Fig. 5.1). Zone I includes the ocular globe and orbital struc-

tures behind the orbital septum. Zones II and III include the upper eyelid and lower eyelid, respectively, from the lateral commissure to just temporal to the canalicular puncti. Zone IV is the medial canthus with the lacrimal drainage system, and Zone V is the lateral retinaculum. Zones II through V are further subdivided into structures that are anterior (preseptal) or posterior (postseptal) to the septum orbitale. Zone VI includes contiguous structures such as the nasal, glabellar, brow, forehead, temple, and malar and nasojugal regions, which merge with Zones II to V.

The palpebral aperture varies considerably in shape, size, and obliquity due to hereditary, racial, traumatic, or other acquired situations. The surrounding bony orbital anatomy, the internal orbital volume, and the integrity of the eyelids, with their muscular and tarsoligamentous supports, are some of the factors that influence the palpebral aperture. It is also influenced by the

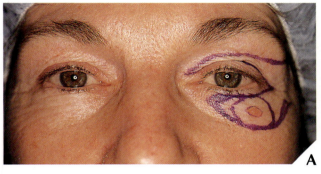

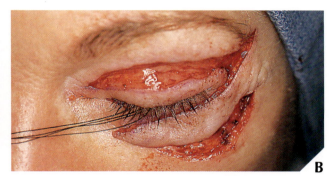

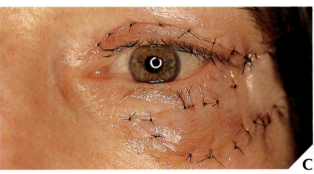

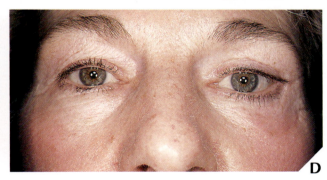

Figure 5.9. (A) Patient with melanoma in situ of the left lower eyelid and cheek prior to excision. Identifying potentially malignant lesions prior to cosmetic surgery is important so that valuable local tissue is not sacrificed. **(B)** A vascularized, laterally based skin-muscle pedicle flap from the upper eyelid is used to reconstruct the skin and muscle defect following excision of the lesion. A lateral canthalplasty was also performed to support the lower eyelid reconstruction. **(C)** One week postoperatively. **(D)** One year postoperatively.

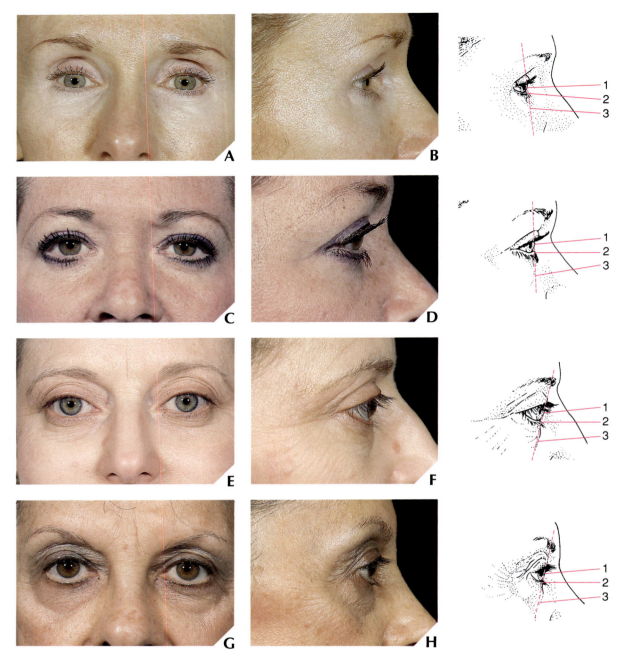

Figure 5.10. Comparison of the variable anatomic relationships of the orbital region that influence the palpebral aperture. Cosmetic blepharoplasty may have to be combined with other surgical procedures to prevent complications. **(A,B)** Young woman with high lid folds, deep set eyes (large, bony orbital volume with small ocular globes), and well-developed malar eminences. The most anterior projection of the ocular globe lies behind the lower eyelid margin and the malar eminence. This is a favorable anatomic situation since there is good eyelid and tarsoligamentous integrity with normal eyelid contours and levels. **(C,D)** Woman presenting for cosmetic blepharoplasty with prominent ocular globes and increased periorbital skin and fat. Since the most anterior projection of her ocular globes are posterior to the lower eyelid margin and inferior orbital margin (malar eminence), she is at minimal risk for lower eyelid malposition. **(E,F)** Woman with prominent ocular globes, slight scleral show, and malar hypoplasia. The lateral view demonstrates the influence of the globe on the lower eyelid position and the lack of eyelid support from the inferior orbital rim. This negative support relationship requires alterations in the cosmetic blepharoplastic procedure to prevent lower eyelid malposition. **(G,H)** Middle-aged woman with excess eyelid skin and fat, normal ocular globe position, marked inferior scleral show, lower eyelid laxity, and malar hypoplasia. She is at risk for an unfavorable result from lower eyelid surgery. A lower eyelid and lateral canthal tightening with repositioning (lateral canthalplasty) should be combined with the cosmetic blepharoplasty.

relative amount of associated periorbital skin, fat, and soft tissues. Unique individual combinations of the above eyelid and orbital anatomy can cause variations in the palpebral aperture[24,40] (Fig. 5.10).

The Upper Eyelid

The normal periorbital and eyelid anatomy of a Caucasian will be described here to simplify understanding variations in the palpebral aperture that may be present in the candidate for blepharoplasty. When the eyelids close, the aperture forms a palpebral fissure with the outer canthus lying 2 to 3 mm below the inner canthus. When the eyelids open, the palpebral aperture assumes the shape of an asymmetric ellipse that is 30 mm wide and 10 mm high. With the eyelids open, the outer canthus is 1 to 2 mm higher than the inner canthus due to the greater mobility of the lateral canthal structures. The lower eyelid normally does not allow for a visible scleral rim between the lid margin and the inferocorneal limbus. However, considerable physiologic and anatomic variations appear in patients. The normal upper eyelid level covers 2 to 3 mm of the superior limbus or lies at a level midway between the superior edge of a 4-mm pupil and the superior corneal limbus. If the upper eyelid is higher than this arbitrary position, lid retraction is present. Similarly, ptosis is present if the lid is lower than this position[19,40,92,96] (Fig. 5.11). There are some individuals who normally have upper eyelid

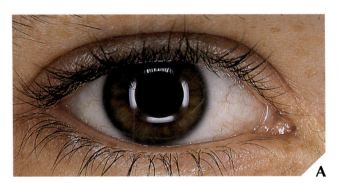

A

Figure 5.11. **(A)** Normal palpebral aperture. **(B)** I. The upper eyelid is normally 1 to 2 mm below the superior corneal limbus. II. Ptosis is seen when the upper eyelid level is below that in I., interfering with the superior visual field. III. Lid retraction is seen when the elevation of the upper lid is at or above the superior corneal limbus.

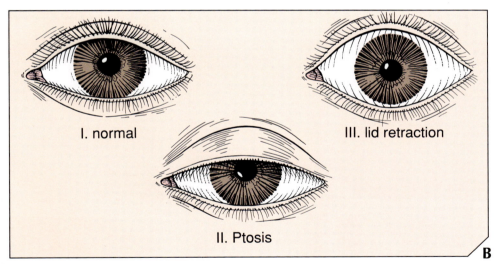

I. normal   III. lid retraction

II. Ptosis

B

levels at or above the superior corneal limbus (Fig. 5.12A). Variations in upper eyelid levels may be due to alertness, pharmacologic agents, direction of gaze, size of the ocular globe, orbital volume, visual acuity, and extraocular muscle balance.

The most common cause of pathologic upper eyelid retraction is thyroid infiltrative ophthalmopathy, a condition in which foreshortening of the levator palpebrae superioris, thickening and contracture of Müller's muscle, and enlargement of the extraocular muscle and other intraorbital structures occur. Whenever the upper eyelid level is above the superior corneal limbus, a thorough evaluation of thyroid function should be considered.[8,18,40,42,90] The most reliable findings in the patient with thyroid ophthalmopathy are the presence of upper lid retraction with a staring appearance. The upper eyelid retraction may be unilateral (Fig. 5.12B) or it may be bilateral and symmetric or asymmetric (Fig. 5.12C). Other findings in the patient with thyroid ophthalmopathy include lymphoid infiltration of the orbital fat and extraocular muscles (producing ocular motility problems), eyelid fullness, proptosis, prominent scleral blood vessels, and lid lag or the inability of the upper eyelids to relax adequately to cover the corneas on down gazing[90] (Fig. 5.12D).

The upper eyelids (Zone II) merge with the eyebrow and forehead (Zone VI). In the Caucasian patient, the upper eyelid fold is normally 8 to 10 mm above the lid margin. This corresponds to the superior attachments of the levator aponeurosis into the subcutaneous tissue of the eyelid. Above the lid fold, the aponeurosis does not attach to the preseptal or orbital subcutaneous tissue, and the overhanging skin forms a fold. Inferior to the lid fold, there are levator attachments to the subcutaneous tissue overlying the tarsus (Fig. 5.13A,B). In the Asian, the orbital septum inserts more inferiorly onto the distal expansion of the levator aponeurosis. This inferior extension of the orbital septum allows more preaponeurotic fat to descend into the upper eyelid. The combination of more pretarsal and preseptal suborbicularis oculi fat inhibits the anterior extension of the levator into the pretarsal subcutaneous tissue. The result is an absent, inferiorly placed or variably positioned upper eyelid fold[20,40] (Fig. 5.13C,D).

Ptosis and lid retraction are conditions that alter the palpebral aperture by affecting the anatomic position of the upper eyelid. Ptosis of the upper eyelid is detected by eliciting an abnormally low eyelid level in straight-ahead gaze. The position of the upper eyelid interferes with the field of vision (see Fig. 5.11B). Ptosis is classified as congenital or acquired and is caused by neurogenic, myogenic, aponeurotic, and mechanical mechanisms.[6,9,10,25,54] Ptosis is considered mild at 1 to 2 mm, moderate at 2 to 3 mm, and severe at 4+ mm. Whenever ptosis is diagnosed the

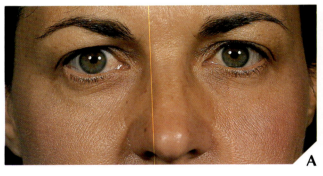
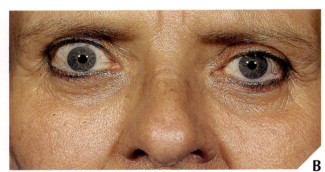
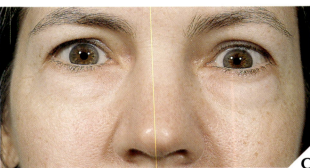
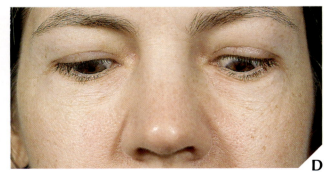

Figure 5.12. (A) Patient with physiologic upper eyelid retraction and no systemic disorders. **(B)** Patient with known thyroid ophthalmopathy and asymmetric upper eyelid retraction in conjunction with a more prominent right globe. **(C)** Patient with thyroid ophthalmopathy and asymmetric upper eyelid retraction. **(D)** The infiltrated, tight upper eyelids have abnormal excursions in down gaze (lid lag).

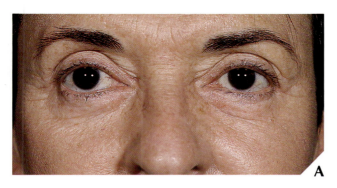

A

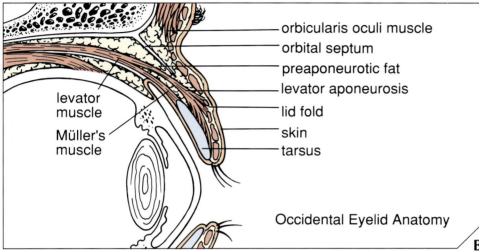

- orbicularis oculi muscle
- orbital septum
- preaponeurotic fat
- levator aponeurosis
- lid fold
- skin
- tarsus

levator muscle

Müller's muscle

Occidental Eyelid Anatomy

B

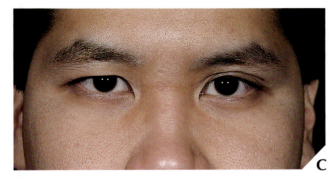

C

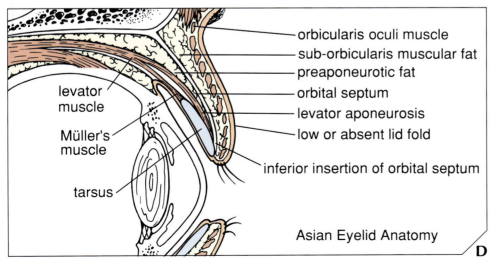

- orbicularis oculi muscle
- sub-orbicularis muscular fat
- preaponeurotic fat
- orbital septum
- levator aponeurosis
- low or absent lid fold

inferior insertion of orbital septum

levator muscle

Müller's muscle

tarsus

Asian Eyelid Anatomy

D

Figure 5.13. (A,B) Caucasian eyelid anatomy. The upper eyelid fold is normally 8 to 10 mm above the lid margin. This corresponds to the superior attachments of the levator aponeurosis into the subcutaneous tissue of the eyelid. Above the lid fold, the aponeurosis does not attach to the preseptal or orbital subcutaneous tissue, and the overhanging skin forms a fold. Below the lid fold, there is firm attachment of the subcutaneous tissue to the tarsus. **(C,D)** In the Asian patient, the upper eyelid has more sub-orbicularis oculi fat and the orbital septum inserts more inferiorly onto the distal expansion of the levator aponeurosis, allowing preaponeurotic fat to descend more inferiorly in the upper eyelid. The result is an absent, inferiorly placed, or variably positioned upper eyelid fold.

amount of levator function is measured in millimeters in order to plan surgical correction. The test is performed by examining the upper eyelid excursion from complete down gaze to up gaze while blocking any contribution to upper eyelid elevation by the eyebrow (Fig. 5.14). The vertical dimensions of the palpebral apertures at the mid-pupillary line are also measured.[9]

Minimal acquired ptosis with good levator function (greater than 10 mm) may be corrected at the same time as cosmetic blepharoplasty with a high degree of success. Aponeurosis disinsertion, or dehiscence, is the most common form of acquired ptosis that is repaired with cosmetic blepharo-

plasty.[3,4,65] The typical clinical presentation is a mild (1 to 2 mm) to moderate (2 to 4 mm) case of ptosis associated with thin upper eyelids, high lid folds, and good levator excursion. These conditions occur because the normal levator attachment to the anterior two thirds of the tarsus is disrupted by posterosuperior displacement of the levator complex inclusive of its lid fold fibers (Fig. 5.15). The condition is repaired by levator exploration and advancement of the aponeurotic structures to the anterior tarsus[4,42] (Fig. 5.16). The Fasanella-Servat technique or variations of a tarsomüllerectomy procedure are also excellent approaches to correct minimal ptosis with good

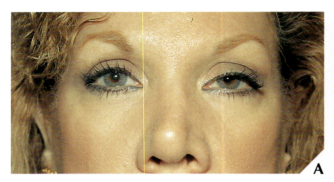

A

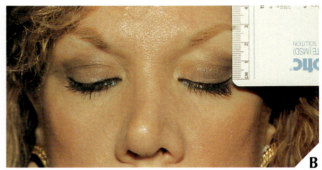

B

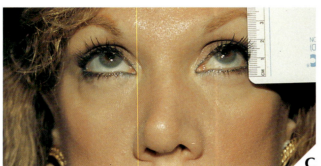

C

Figure 5.14. **(A)** Woman with acquired ptosis of the left upper lid. **(B,C)** Levator function of 15 mm was measured with a ruler from down gaze to up gaze while manually blocking brow elevation of the upper eyelid. Levator function greater than 10 mm is considered good.

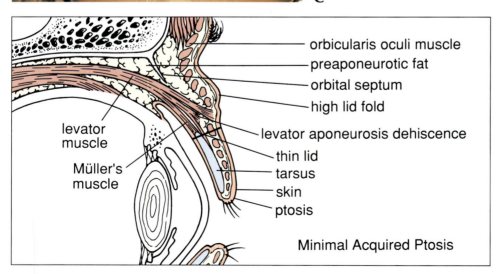

Figure 5.15. Levator aponeurosis dehiscence produces a high upper lid fold, thin upper eyelid, and ptosis.

levator function. These procedures are performed at the same time as cosmetic blepharoplasty.

The patient with congenital or severe acquired ptosis is best managed prior to cosmetic blepharoplasty.[9] Testing of visual field acuity is necessary to document visual loss from obstruction by excess upper eyelid skin or from true lid ptosis. The examination should be performed with the lid in a relaxed, straight-ahead position and again with the hooded skin elevated or the ptotic eyelid held at a level just below the superior limbus. The visual field test is performed by the direct confrontation, tangent screen, or perimeter method.

The Lower Eyelid

The lower eyelids (Zone III) extend from the lid margin to the cheek area. The nasojugal fold runs inferiorly and laterally from the inner canthus along the side of the nose. An inferior eyelid fold can extend 3 to 4 mm inferior to the eyelid margin medially and 5 to 6 mm inferior to the lid margin laterally. This inferior eyelid crease is seen more frequently in children and is created by greater adherence of the pretarsal orbicularis oculi muscle to the overlying skin. A malar fold may run inferiorly and medially from the outer canthus toward the inferior aspect of the nasojugal fold.

Figure 5.16. (A) Woman with bilateral upper eyelid levator disinsertions. (B) Intraoperative photograph demonstrating the inferior edge of the disinserted levator aponeurosis [a] and the structures adjacent to the superior border of the tarsus [b]. (C) Intraoperative photograph demonstrating advancement of levator aponeurosis to the point of detachment at the superior border of the tarsus where suture fixation was performed. (D) Patient 9 months postoperatively with a satisfactory result.

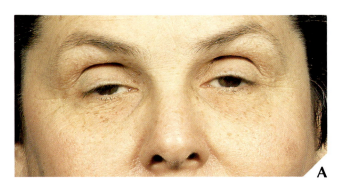

A

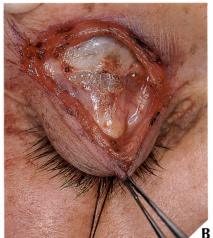

B

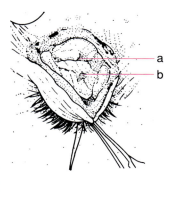

a
b

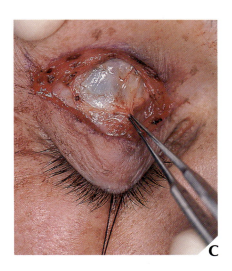

C

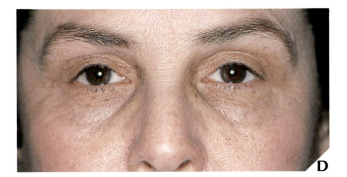

D

Loose folds of skin can form at the junction of loose connective tissue of the eyelids and the more dense connective tissue of the cheek[19,96,97] (Fig. 5.17).

Medial and Lateral Canthi and Contiguous Structures

The medial canthal area (Zone IV) includes the medial canthal structures, the lacrimal drainage system, and the overlying tissue.[42,48] The lateral aspect of the eyelids (Zone V) is an integral anatomic unit. The lateral canthus, which is more correctly termed *lateral retinaculum*, consists of: (1) the lateral horn of the levator palpebrae superioris muscle, (2) the continuation of the preseptal and pretarsal orbicularis oculi muscle (the lateral canthal tendon), (3) the inferior suspensory

ligament of the globe (Lockwood's ligament), and (4) the check ligaments of the lateral rectus muscle[97,98] (Fig. 5.18). Zone VI includes the areas adjacent to Zones II to V, i.e., the nasal, glabellar, forehead, brow, temple, and malar and nasojugal regional structures (see Figs. 5.1 and 5.17).

The Ocular Globe and Orbit

The ocular globe and retroseptal structures (Zone I) require careful examination to identify potential problems that could produce a complication to cosmetic blepharoplasty. The size, shape, and clarity of the sclera, cornea, and iris are noted. The pupils are evaluated for a normal, direct, and consensual response to light. The extraocular muscles are tested to determine the presence of any eye deviations or diplopia. It is also important

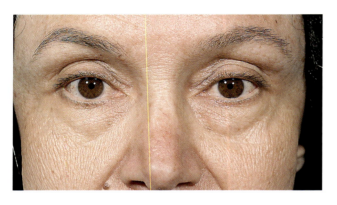

Figure 5.17. Topographic anatomy of the eyelids and cheeks. (1) Superior eyelid fold, (2) inferior eyelid

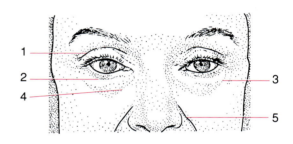

fold, (3) malar fold, (4) nasojugal fold, and (5) nasolabial fold.

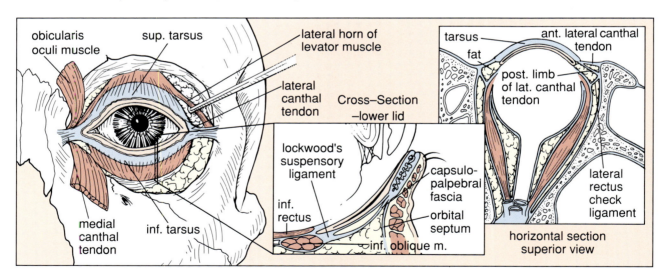

Figure 5.18. The lateral canthal structures or the lateral retinaculum (LR) consists of: (1) the lateral horn of the levator palpebrae superioris muscle, (2) the continuation of the preseptal and pretarsal orbicularis oculi

muscle (the lateral canthal tendon), (3) the inferior suspensory ligament of the globe (Lockwood's ligament), and (4) the check ligaments of the lateral rectus muscle.

to determine if the patient has an intact Bell's reflex, i.e., rotation of the globe upward and outward with eyelid closure. Gentle forced opening of the eyelids is performed to observe the position of the cornea. Because temporary inability to close the eyelids occurs following blepharoplasty, this reflex helps protect against corneal injury and exposure keratitis.[27,28,71,74]

A light held parallel to the plane of the iris allows a view of the anterior chamber of the eye. This technique is used to look for a shallow anterior chamber and to determine if the iris is very close to the posterior surface of the cornea. These findings, combined with a small pupil, suggest the patient is prone to developing angle-closure glaucoma if the pupil dilates (Fig. 5.19). Pupillary dilation may occur during blepharoplasty from emotional, physiologic, or pharmacologic causes. Hyperopic, or farsighted, patients have a higher incidence of angle-closure glaucoma because the depth of their anterior chambers are often decreased.

An ophthalmoscopic examination is performed to assess the clarity of the ocular media and the status of the macula, retinal vascular structures, and optic nerve head. An ophthalmologist is consulted if any abnormalities are found. Patients who desire cosmetic blepharoplasty occasionally have undiagnosed problems in tear production or tear film maintenance. A common manifestation of abnormal tear production is keratoconjunctivitis sicca, or the "dry eye syndrome."[29,41,43,50] Sjögren's syndrome, ocular cicatricial pemphigoid, Stevens-Johnson syndrome, acne rosacea, radiation-induced xerosis, vitamin A deficiency, and chemical or thermal burns are other conditions that alter the production of tears and can lead to significant ocular symptoms. These symptoms are worsened by cosmetic blepharoplasty.[75]

The basic precorneal tear film, produced by the lacrimal secretory system, is composed of three distinct layers (Fig. 5.20). The inner layer is made of mucoprotein secretion, which helps to stabilize the tear film and is formed from the mucin-secreting goblet cells of the conjunctiva, tarsus, and limbal areas. The intermediate aqueous layer is produced by the subconjunctival accessory lacrimal exocrine glands of Krause and Wolfring. This secretion changes the corneal surface from a

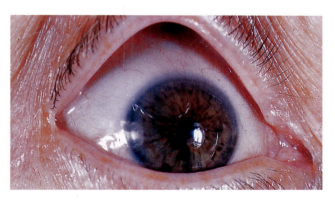

Figure 5.19. Patient with small pupil, shallow anterior chamber, and farsighted (hyperopic) vision. A light is directed parallel to the plane of the iris, revealing the shallow anterior chamber with the iris in close proximity to the corneal endothelium. This patient is at potential risk for angle-closure glaucoma.

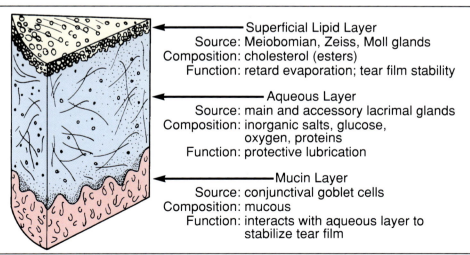

Superficial Lipid Layer
Source: Meiobomian, Zeiss, Moll glands
Composition: cholesterol (esters)
Function: retard evaporation; tear film stability

Aqueous Layer
Source: main and accessory lacrimal glands
Composition: inorganic salts, glucose, oxygen, proteins
Function: protective lubrication

Mucin Layer
Source: conjunctival goblet cells
Composition: mucous
Function: interacts with aqueous layer to stabilize tear film

Figure 5.20. Composition of the precorneal tear film. (Adapted from Holly FJ, Lemp MA: Tear physiology and dry eyes. Surv Ophthalmol 22 (2):70,1977)

hydrophobic to a hydrophilic state. The overlying aqueous layer is thus able to spread more uniformly. The aqueous layer is 98% water and accounts for 90% of the thickness of the precorneal tear film. The outermost layer of the tear film retards evaporation and is composed of lipids secreted from the Meibomian, Zeis, and Moll glands of the lids. The precorneal tear film is the product of the basic tear secretory system.

The basic secretor glands can produce all three layers of the tear film without the assistance of the reflex lacrimal gland system. However, the volume of the basic tear secretion decreases with age. This predisposes the older patient who undergoes blepharoplasty to a symptomatic dry eye condition. Symptoms of itching, foreign body sensation, burning, mucoid secretions, frequent blinking, and conjunctival infection suggest dry eye problems. The clinical diagnosis is confirmed by mucous filaments on a dull gray-appearing cornea, a precorneal tear film that evaporates more rapidly, characteristic corneal staining to fluorescein or rose bengal dye, and a positive Schirmer's test[74] (Fig. 5.21A). Other tests that may be utilized to confirm deficiencies in tear quality and/or quantity include the fluorescein dilution, lysozyme assay, tear osmolality, and conjunctival scraping for histologic analysis.[41,42] Symblepharon, contraction, and scarring of the conjunctival surfaces of the upper (Fig. 5.21B) and lower (Fig. 5.21C) eyelids are associated with significant tear film abnormalities.

Deficiencies of the tear film are difficult to diagnose with a high degree of accuracy. It is necessary to perform repeated examinations to document clinical symptoms and physical findings that are consistent with tear film deficiencies. The Schirmer's test is the most useful procedure to verify suspected tear deficiencies. Schirmer's tear test is performed in a dimly lit room since retinal stimulation can increase reflex tearing. The filter paper test strips are evaluated after 5 minutes of contact with the lateral lower eyelid and conjunctiva (Fig. 5.22). Normal wetting of the strips is between 15 to 30 mm. Less than 10 mm is considered hyposecretion of both basic and reflex secretion. To document the consistency of the findings, it is recommended that several Schirmer's tests be performed. If the wetting is consistently 5 mm or less, a tear deficiency state, such as keratoconjunctivitis sicca, should be considered.

Blepharoplasty in patients with signs and symptoms of poor tear film maintenance may alter the eyelid anatomy enough to cause a subclinical condition to become a full-blown case of keratoconjunctivitis sicca.[74] Rees and La Trenta emphasize that assessment of the Schirmer's tear test in relationship to the eyelid and periorbital anatomy is a highly reliable method to identify those patients at risk of developing dry eye postoperatively (see Fig. 5.10). The patient prone to a dry eye condition may still have blepharoplastic surgery performed if adequate ocular protection is provided and the procedure is altered to include a variety

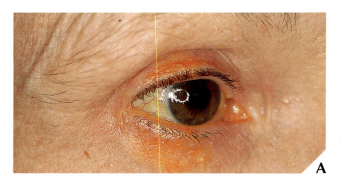

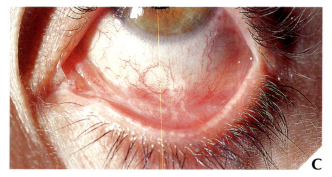

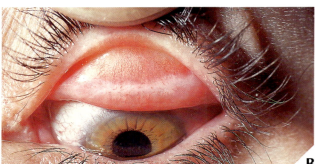

Figure 5.21. (A) Patient with keratoconjunctivitis sicca with mucous filaments on a dull-appearing cornea that is stained with fluorescein dye. (B) Cicatricial changes of the upper eyelid conjunctival and tarsal glands in a patient with dry eye and previous history of Stevens-Johnson's keratoconjunctivitis. (C) Symblepharon, contraction, and scarring of lower lid conjunctival surfaces in a patient with ocular pemphigoid.

of reconstructive procedures, such as levator recession, medial canthoplasty, lateral canthoplasty, and horizontal lower lid shortening.

COMPLICATIONS

Figures 5.2 and 5.3 list minor and major complications that may occur as a result of blepharoplasty. Complications of cosmetic blepharoplasty are rare but when they do occur the patients are usually distraught. When the cosmetic surgical procedure a patient electively underwent to improve his appearance produces the opposite result, he becomes a more difficult patient to manage. The surgeon must devote more time to helping the patient through this disappointing situation. Management of patient dissatisfaction is much easier when the patient is informed of the possibilities of complications during the preoperative consultation.

Pre-existing Conditions

The easiest complication to avoid is a pre-existing condition that will increase the likelihood of unfavorable results following blepharoplasty. These conditions include underlying medical problems that may increase the risk of visual loss, anatomic variations that may be accentuated after eyelid skin and fat excision, and most important, the psychological ability of the patient to deal with the postoperative discomfort and possibly a less-than-perfect cosmetic outcome. The presence of pre-existing conditions does not preclude the performance of cosmetic blepharoplasty; however, the surgical technique must be altered. More conservative skin and fat resec-

tions, facial suspension, and inclusion of reconstructive eyelid procedures may be necessary (see Fig. 5.10).

Intraoperative Complications

Complications that occur intraoperatively result from untoward effects of the administration of sedatives, general anesthesias, and local anesthesia. The patient with narrow angles and flat anterior chambers may have an episode of angle-closure glaucoma if the pupil dilates[11,55] (see Fig. 5.19). The pupil dilates when systemic atropine is used during general anesthesia and when the vasopressor epinephrine (used in local anesthetic) is absorbed by the dilator pupillae muscle. The acute rise of intraocular pressure is caused by crowding of the peripheral iris into the region inside the eye that drains the aqueous humor. Intraocular pressure can rise to greater than 60 mm Hg. Severe pain, corneal edema, and visual loss associated with nausea and vomiting follow. Treatment entails the administration of oral or intravenous acetazolamide (500 mg), oral isosorbide (1 to 2 mg/kg), or intravenous mannitol (1 to 2 g/kg) and one drop of topical timolol (0.5%), followed by serial intraocular pressure measurements. The surgery should be discontinued. Immediate consultation with an ophthalmologist is recommended.

One of the most feared intraoperative complications is inadvertent penetration of the ocular globe with the needle used to inject the local anesthesia (Fig. 5.23). The visual consequences of this event are usually catastrophic with chemosis, subconjunctival hemorrhage, retinal detachment, traumatic cataracts, choroidal ruptures, intraocu-

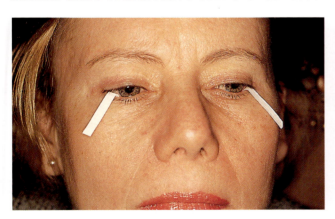

Figure 5.22. Patient undergoing the 5-minute Schirmer's tear test to evaluate tear production.

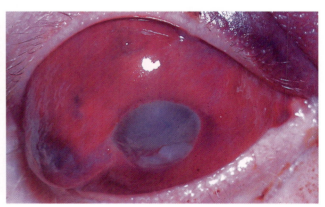

Figure 5.23. Corneal opacity, chemosis, subconjunctival hemorrhage, and blindness caused by inadvertent penetration of the ocular globe with local anesthetic solution.

lar fibrosis, and glaucoma reported.[26,33,34,36,46] Necrosis of the eyelid skin has been reported following the inadvertent injection of formaldehyde instead of a local anesthetic agent.[50,83]

Corneal injury during surgery can be prevented by careful attention to surgical technique, frequent application of a balanced saline solution to the cornea, and protection of the eye from sharp instruments, cautery devices, and gauze sponges. The routine use of a protective acrylic corneal shield is strongly advised. Corneal shields can be manufactured with a flat peripheral curve and a steeper central curve so that the cornea does not contact the shield (Fig. 5.24). Instillation of a topical ophthalmic anesthetic agent is required prior to placing the shield on the eye. If a corneal injury occurs, fluorescein staining and high magnification examination are necessary to determine the depth of the wound. Large and deep corneal wounds require treatment by an ophthalmologist. Superficial corneal defects, erosions or de-epithelializations are treated with topical antibiotic solutions and ointments and patching of the eye. Examination in 12 to 24 hours or whenever the patient complains of pain is mandatory.

Bleeding is usually minimal during cosmetic blepharoplasty. When it is excessive or difficult to control, the patient may bleed postoperatively with resultant ecchymoses and potential retrobulbar hemorrhage. Visual loss is thought to be caused by hemorrhage into the orbit with resultant increased intraorbital and intraocular pressure, which causes central retinal artery occlusion and ischemia of the retina and/or nutrient vessels of the optic nerve.[11,13,32,34,45,47,52,64] Patients with a history of bleeding disorders, previous ocular or orbital surgery,[11] hypertension, arteriosclerosis, and thyroid ophthalmopathy are likely candidates for retrobulbar hemorrhage during retroseptal periocular surgery.[32,34,91]

There has been a total of 60 reported cases of permanent partial or total visual loss in cosmetic blepharoplastic patients.[55] De Mere et al. surveyed 3,000 surgeons reporting 98,000 blepharoplastic procedures in which 40 cases of visual loss occurred.[17] Although this incidence of 0.04% may seem statistically insignificant, the devastating consequences of the complication makes each occurrence a major event for patient and physician. In all cases, the orbital septum was opened and fat dissected for excision. It is known that traction on the anterior orbital structures by dissection is transmitted to the posterior orbit with potential vascular disruption.[20,92,97] Furthermore,

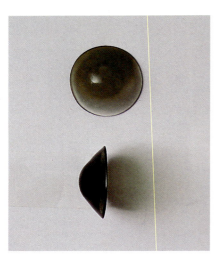

Figure 5.24. Corneal protective shields manufactured with a steep central radius of curvature and a flat peripheral radius of curvature. This configuration prevents direct corneal contact.

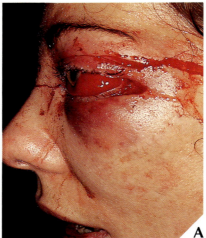

Figure 5.25. (A) Patient 2 hours postoperatively who developed a retrobulbar hemorrhage without visual loss, requiring removal of sutures, opening of orbital septum, lateral canthotomies, and drainage of blood. (B) Note the marked chemosis, subconjunctival hemorrhage, proptosis, and pupillary dilation.

visual loss due to tractional avulsion of the fine nutrient blood vessels to the optic nerve as it enters the orbit can occur.[49] Orbital fat has a sparse blood supply, except in the medial and lateral regions of upper and lower eyelids.[85] Vascular pedicles from the infratrochlear and lacrimal vessels pass within the medial and lateral fat, respectively, to supply the overlying muscle and skin. Careful control of bleeding from these vessels is necessary to prevent retrobulbar hemorrhage. Symptoms and signs of retrobulbar hemorrhage include visual loss, pain, proptosis, periorbital ecchymosis and edema, chemosis, and subconjunctival hemorrhage (Fig. 5.25).

If there is significant bleeding in the orbit during surgery or if visual loss occurs in either eye, emergent ophthalmologic consultation is obtained. When there is a retrobulbar hemorrhage without visual loss, the wounds are opened and identifiable sources of bleeding controlled. Usually the source of bleeding is not found. The priority is to decrease the intraorbital pressure, which is assisted by inserting neurosurgical cottonoids into the wounds to serve as drains. Frequent blood pressure measurements, vision assessment, and ophthalmoscopic evaluation of the retinal vasculature are necessary. If visual loss occurs, immediate lowering of the intraocular pressure and surgical decompression of the orbit are instituted. Mannitol (20%) is given intravenously at a dosage of 1 to 2 g/kg of body weight. In healthy patients, 12.5 g is administered over 3 minutes and the remainder over 30 minutes. Acetazolamine, 500 mg intravenously, may also be given to reduce intraocular pressure by decreasing the secretion of fluid into the anterior chamber of the eye.[39] Pressure on the globe can be further relieved by a lateral canthotomy and cantholysis of the superior and inferior components of the lateral canthal tendon[32,36] (Fig. 5.26). If visual deterioration persists, lateral and inferior bony decompression of the orbit is performed. Paracentesis of the anterior chamber of the eye has been suggested to decrease the intraocular pressure; however, this is not recommended.[36,55] Assessment of visual acuity, pupillary reactions, and retinal structures are repeated for several days following the retrobulbar hemorrhage.

Temporary extraocular muscle imbalance with subjective diplopia occurs when the local anesthetic causes paresis of the muscles following retroseptal injection. This often happens when the fat is injected prior to resection. Direct surgical trauma to the extraocular muscles may result in permanent diplopia.[1,7,95] The inferior oblique muscle originates from the anterior medial orbit and passes under the ocular globe within the orbital fat; it is at risk for injury.[31,35] Permanent diplopia has resulted from damage to the superior oblique muscle directly or indirectly by disturbing the trochlea, which is just beneath the deep nasal fat in the superior medial orbit.[49,95]

Postsurgical Complications

Varying degrees of corneal exposure, with symptoms of pain, dryness, grittiness, and blurred vision, occur after blepharoplasty. Frequent instillation of ocular solutions and ointments to protect the corneas is usually adequate treatment. The combination of corneal exposure, lagophthalmos, poor Bell's phenomenon, and pre-existing poor tear film can produce severe visual disturbances. Mild corneal epithelial disruption can rapidly progress to confluent erosions and purulent ulcers.[60,73] Immediate ophthalmologic treat-

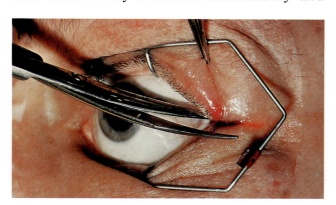
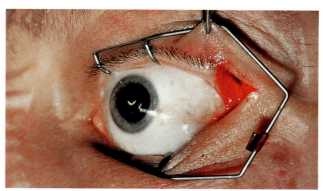

Figure 5.26. Lateral canthotomy is performed by cutting the lateral canthal tendon horizontally to the bony orbital rim. This divides the lateral canthal tendon into superior and inferior components, which can then be selectively lysed to allow decompression of the orbit.

ment usually results in corneal salvage. Severe exposure keratopathy (Fig. 5.27A), corneal ulcers (Fig. 5.27B), and filamentary keratitis (see Fig. 5.21A) may heal, but with permanent scarring and decreased vision. The underlying cause of the corneal damage must be corrected.

The patient with dry eye is managed with ocular tear film stabilizers, ophthalmic solutions and ointments, lid taping, puntal occlusion, soft contact lenses, humidified eyelid chambers, tempo-

rary eyelid suture closure, or permanent surgical tarsorrhaphy, depending upon the severity of the condition. Obviously, it is best to identify the dry eye patient preoperatively to avoid this situation.

Lid malpositions, such as marginal eversion, retraction, entropion, ectropion, paresis, or punctal eversions, contribute to corneal exposure. Most lid malpositions are temporary and resolve within 4 to 6 weeks postoperatively. It is impor-

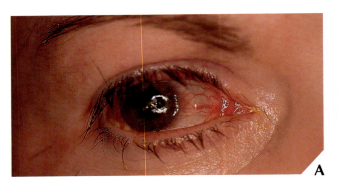
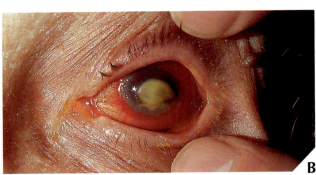

Figure 5.27. (A) Patient with epithelial break-down of the cornea and conjunctival inflammatory changes caused by exposure aggravated by lagophthalmos.

(B) Patient with complete disruption of the corneal epithelium and a purulent bacterial corneal ulcer.

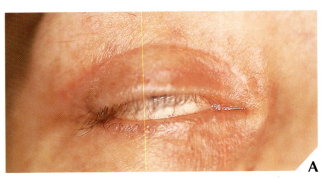
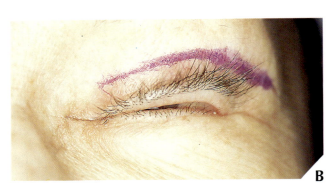
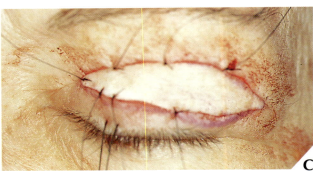
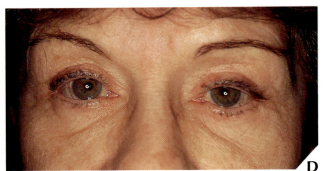

Figure 5.28. (A) Patient with excessive skin removal from the upper eyelid and lagophthalmos. Bell's reflex is fair. **(B)** Patient with upper eyelid retraction, lid margin eversion, and exposure keratopathy due to excessive upper eyelid skin excision. Note the surgical

marking for the proposed incision to release the scar and create a wide defect. **(C)** Retroauricular full-thickness skin graft sutured to the defect. **(D)** Patient 9 months postoperatively.

tant to protect the cornea during this time. If the lid malpositions aggravate and contribute to corneal decompensation, they should be corrected as soon as possible.[67,93,94] Lid malpositions that do not compromise visual function may be corrected after scar maturation.[79–81]

Excessive skin removal from the upper eyelid results in lagophthalmos and lid retraction which prevents the eyelids from complete closure (Fig. 5.28A). Varying amounts of lid margin eversion may also be present (Fig. 5.28B). Surgical correction requires release of the retraction by recreating the defect in the upper eyelid and application of a retro- or preauricular full-thickness skin graft[7,8,10,27] (Fig. 5.28C,D). Adhesion, fibrosis, and foreshortening of the mid-lamellar structures of the upper lid (levator aponeurosis, orbital septum, and tarsus) can cause upper eyelid retraction (Fig. 5.29A). Treatment requires surgical release of the adhesion, levator aponeurosis recession, interpositional fascial grafts, and lid traction sutures, which should create a minimal amount of ptosis of the involved lid[8] (Fig. 5.29B). Subsequent ptosis correction by a levator aponeurosis advancement or (as in this case) par-

tial tarsomüllerectomy usually produces an acceptable result (Fig. 5.29C).

Ptosis of the upper eyelid can result from damage to the levator complex during retroseptal dissection by direct trauma, hematoma, edema, or septal adhesion. The levator muscle originates from the apex of the orbit and passes anteriorly, becoming aponeurotic at the superior orbital margin to insert onto the anterior two thirds of the anterior tarsal surface. Some fibers of the aponeurosis extend to the orbicularis fascia to attach to the dermis of the upper eyelid, forming the upper lid crease. In the Caucasian patient, the orbital septum blends with the aponeurosis at the level of the superior border of the tarsus, or 5 to 10 mm superiorly (see Fig. 5.13B). The anterior orbital fat removed during upper blepharoplasty lies posterior to the septum and anterior to the levator aponeurosis. Inadvertent penetration or detachment injury to the levator aponeurosis can occur during removal of the preseptal orbicularis oculi muscle or retroseptal fat. If this is noted at the time of blepharoplasty, reattachment of the injured levator aponeurosis is indicated. If the injury is not repaired, the ptosis that results is

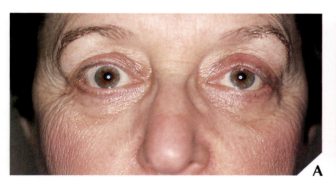

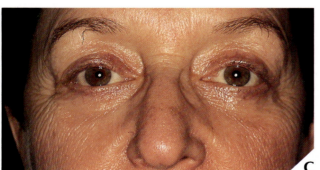

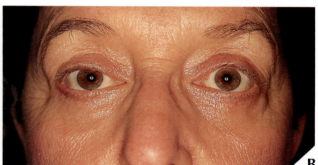

Figure 5.29. (A) Patient 2 months postoperatively with right upper eyelid cicatricial retraction of the mid-lamellar structures (tarsus, orbital septum, and levator aponeurosis). **(B)** Patient 6 months after the release of lid adhesions and a levator recession of the right upper eyelid. Minimal ptosis of the right upper eyelid was deliberately produced. **(C)** Patient 6 months after ptosis correction by tarsomüllerectomy.

usually unilateral, mild to moderate in degree, and associated with a high lid fold, thinning of the upper eyelid, and an upper eyelid excursion greater than 10 mm (Fig. 5.30A,B).

Mechanical ptosis due to postoperative edema is symmetric and transient and usually resolves spontaneously within 48 to 72 hours. A hematoma in the retroseptal space can cause impairment of levator muscle function, maintaining the upper eyelid in a ptotic position. Resorption of the hematoma produces secondary fibrosis of the levator with persistent ptosis. Attempts to create high upper eyelid supratarsal folds involve fixing the skin and muscle edges to the levator aponeurosis. A tractional ptosis is produced if the lid fold is placed too high. The medial and lateral retinaculae become tense and lower the upper lid level (Fig. 5.30C,D). Treatment consists of observation and massage of the upper eyelid. If ptosis persists more than several weeks, removal of the supratarsal fixation sutures is necessary. Ptosis may also occur when adhesions develop between the orbital septum and the levator aponeurosis at a level higher than the original septal origin.[7,9,18]

Severe ptosis with poor levator function and absence of the upper eyelid fold require prompt re-exploration and surgical correction by levator aponeurosis repair, tarsomüllerectomy, or levator resection. Mild ptosis associated with good leva-

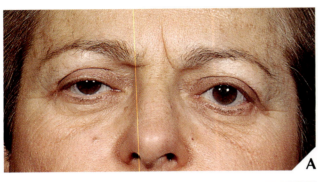
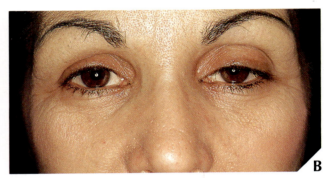
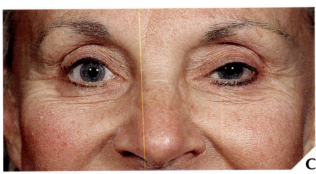
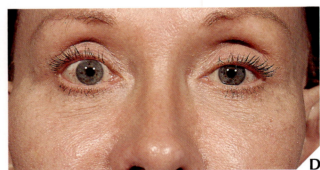

Figure 5.30. (A) Patient who underwent cosmetic blepharoplasty with inadvertent disinsertion of the right levator aponeurosis during orbicularis oculi and retroseptal fat removal resulting in a right upper lid ptosis. (B) Patient following cosmetic blepharoplasty with a left upper lid ptosis from inadvertent levator aponeurosis detachment. (C,D) Patients with left upper eyelid cicatricial ptosis due to adhesions between the levator aponeurosis, orbital septum, and skin.

tor excursion, thinning of the upper eyelid, and a high lid fold should be surgically explored at the earliest possible time. The exploration usually reveals an inadvertently detached or injured levator aponeurosis. Mild degrees of post-blepharoplastic ptosis usually resolve spontaneously and require no more action than reassurance during an observation period. Ptosis that persists longer than 3 months requires surgical exploration and correction.

The most common complication of lower eyelid blepharoplasty is an unnatural distortion of the lower eyelid. This distortion is described as mild eversion of the temporal lid margin, inferiorly displaced lashes, temporal lower lid bowing with scleral show (Fig. 5.31), actual ectropion, or cicatricial lid retraction.

Careful preoperative evaluation of the patient is the most reliable method of reducing the occurrence of these lower eyelid malpositions. Accurate determination of the relationship of the soft tissues to the underlying bony anatomy is essential to determine whether ancillary procedures may be required during blepharoplasty

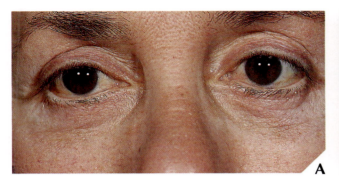

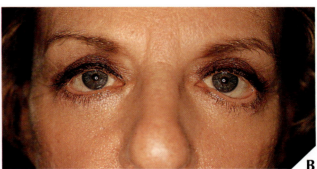

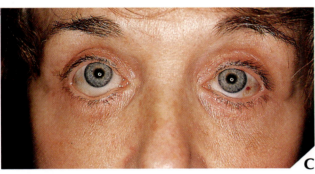

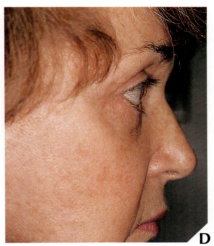

Figure 5.31. Eyelid malpositions following lower eyelid blepharoplasty. **(A)** Patient with bilateral lid margin eversion, rounding of the lateral canthi, and scleral show. **(B)** Patient with lower eyelid horizontal laxity, as well as all the findings shown in **A**. Note the malar hypoplasia. **(C,D)** Patient with marked lower eyelid malpositions and corneal exposure. Note the malar hypoplasia with inadequate bony support to the lower eyelid and ocular globe.

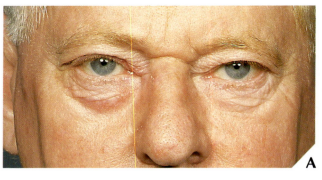

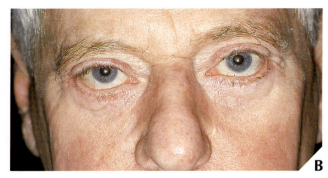

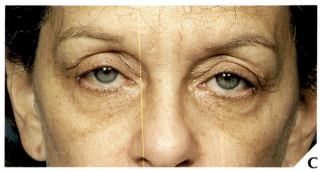

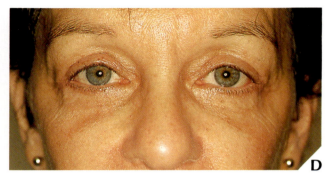

Figure 5.32. (A,C) Preoperative photographs of two patients prone to develop lower eyelid malpositions after lower lid blepharoplasty. They exhibit lower lid laxity and malar hypoplasia. **(B)** The same patient as in **A** 6 months after standard cosmetic blepharoplasty, which resulted in the predictable scleral show, lower eyelid malposition, and rounding of the lateral canthus. **(D)** The same patient as in **C** 6 months after cosmetic four eyelid blepharoplasty with ancillary lateral canthoplasty and horizontal lid shortening.

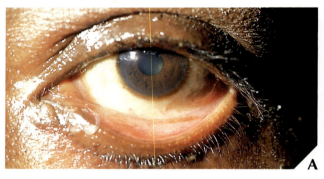

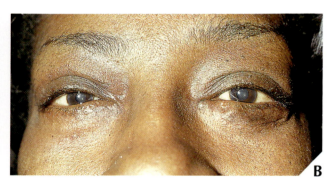

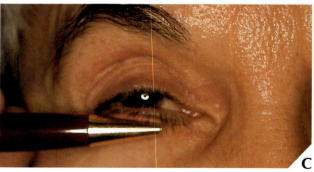

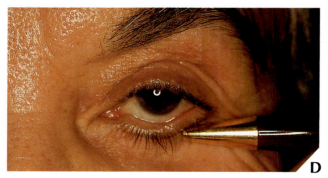

Figure 5.33. (A) Patient with frank ectropion due to excessive skin resection following cosmetic blepharoplasty. **(B)** Same patient 6 months after surgical re-creation of the skin defect, lateral canthal fixation to maintain the defect, and full-thickness skin graft. **(C)** Patient undergoing vertical displacement of the right lower eyelid demonstrates movement of the lid to the mid-pupillary level. **(D)** Same patient undergoing vertical displacement of the left lower eyelid, demonstrating mid-lamellar cicatricial changes preventing movement of the lid (lid retraction).

(Fig. 5.32, see also Fig. 5.10). The causes of lower eyelid malpositions include: (1) excessive skin, fat, or muscle removal, (2) scar contraction, (3) damage or resection of the pretarsal orbicularis oculi muscle, (4) lid edema, (5) mid-lamellar (tarsus, orbital septum, capsulopalpebral fascia) cicatrix, (6) hematoma, and (7) horizontal lid laxity.[12,57] Correction of established ectropion of the lower eyelid due to excessive skin removal requires recreation of the skin defect, lateral canthal fixation to maintain the defect, and full-thickness skin grafting[84,87,88] (Fig. 5.33A,B). Patients with lax lower eyelids, malar hypoplasia, and prominent ocular globes are prone to develop lower eyelid malpositions as the result of cosmetic blepharoplasty[40,75] (see Figs. 5.31 and 5.32). Procedures to tighten the eyelid and elevate the lateral canthus must be combined with cosmetic blepharoplasty in these patients.[21,22,30,56,59,62] The lateral canthalplasty, and its many variations, has proven to be a useful procedure to avoid unfavorable lower eyelid malpositions. In addition, the procedure can be utilized to correct established moderate-to-severe degrees of lower lid and lateral canthal deformities resulting from diverse causes. The most useful types of lateral canthalplasties are the tarsal strip[5,44,51] (Figs. 5.34 and 5.35) and the

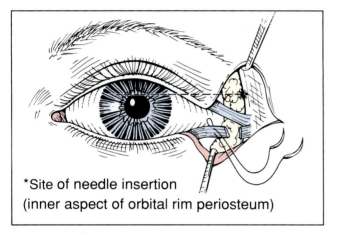

*Site of needle insertion
(inner aspect of orbital rim periosteum)

Figure 5.34. The tarsal strip lateral canthoplasty. The lateral canthus is divided into an intact upper portion and a mobilized lower portion by canthotomy and inferior limb cantholysis. The temporal lid margin, cilia, conjunctiva, skin, and muscle are excised. The tarsal strip can now be positioned onto the superior lateral orbital periosteum with sutures.

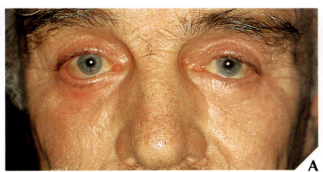

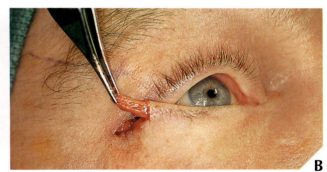

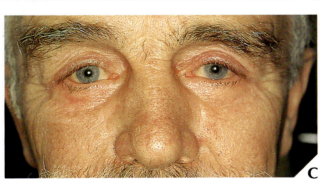

Figure 5.35. (A) Patient exhibiting postblepharoplasty complications of scleral show, temporal bowing, and mild ectropion that is greater on the right side than on the left. (B) The tarsal strip ready for periosteal fixation. (C) Six months after bilateral tarsal strip procedures.

dermal-orbicular pennant[42] (Figs. 5.36 and 5.37). Both of these techniques can be combined with skin, mucosal, fascial, or cartilage grafts to increase the vertical height of the lower eyelid.[61]

Miscellaneous Complications

Excessive fat resection is a most disturbing problem, especially when associated with lower eye-

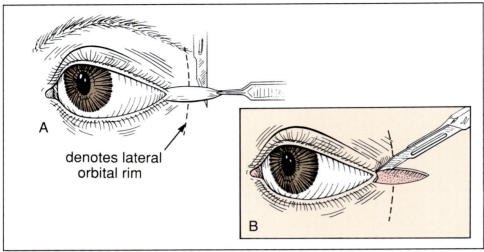

denotes lateral orbital rim

dermis

orbicularis oculi muscle

bone of lateral orbital rim

lower portion of lateral cathal tendon

Figure 5.36. Dermal-orbicular pennant lateral canthoplasty. **(A)** A 1 cm x 0.5 cm ellipse of skin horizontally oriented from the lateral commissure is de-epithelialized. Note that the lateral commissure is left intact and lateral canthotomy is not performed. **(B)** Incision of the superior edge of the de-epithelialized dermal-orbicular pennant is performed with a scalpel. **(C)** The dermal-orbicularis muscle ellipse is elevated and utilized to place traction on the underlying lateral retinaculum structures. **(D)** Scissors lyse the inferior limb of the lateral canthal tendon attachments to Whitnal's tubercle and lateral orbital rim. Lysis of these structures is continued until a mobile lateral canthus and lower eyelid are obtained.

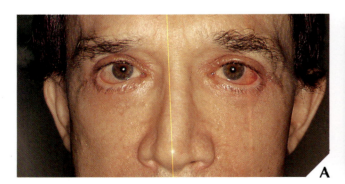

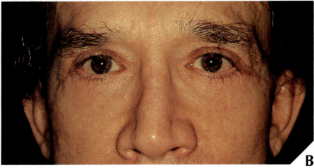

Figure 5.37. (A) Patient with bilateral lower eyelid malposition after blepharoplasty. **(B)** The patient 9 months following bilateral dermal-orbicular pennant lateral canthoplasties.

lid malposition. Autogenous fat pad sliding,[53] fat grafting[23] (Fig. 5.38), and fat injection[78] have been utilized to correct this deformity with variable results. A lateral canthalplasty should be performed at the time of fat augmentation. *Inadequate fat resection* most commonly occurs in the upper and lower medial and lower lateral compartments.[38,64] A small stab incision through the skin, muscle, and septum can be utilized to deliver the residual fat for excision (Fig. 5.39).

Persistent malar bags, or excess skin, can be directly excised and carefully closed to produce

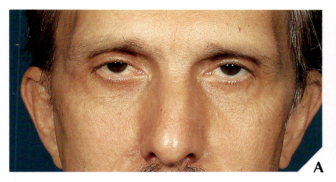

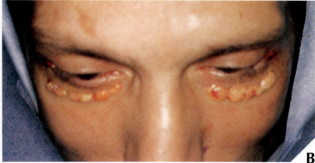

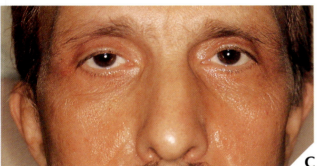

Figure 5.38. (A) Patient with excessive lower lid fat resection with associated lower eyelid malposition. **(B)** The supplementary submental autogenous fat grafts are shown before their placement into a retroseptal position through a lateral canthal incision. Lateral canthoplasties were also performed. **(C)** Patient 1 year postoperatively.

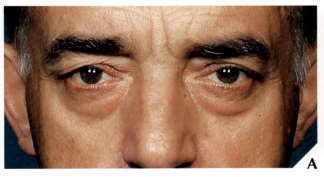

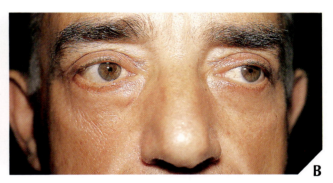

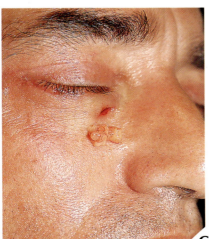

Figure 5.39. (A) Blepharoplastic patient preoperatively. **(B)** Two months postoperatively, inadequate resection of fat from the right lower eyelid medial compartment is evident. **(C)** The fat is removed via a small stab incision through skin, muscle, and orbital septum.

acceptable results (Fig. 5.40). *Epicanthal folds* in the upper medial eyelid result from carrying the incision onto the nasal skin or too close to the medial canthal tendon. Massage and time are the best methods of management (Fig. 5.41). If the deformity persists for more than 9 months, dou-ble opposing Z-plasty or V-to-Y reconstruction may be required.

Chemosis is a milky edema of the subconjunctival tissues. It results from obstruction of the lymphatic drainage channels of the periorbital area (Fig. 5.42). Repositioning the eyelids over the

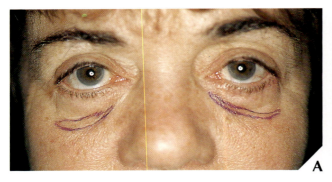

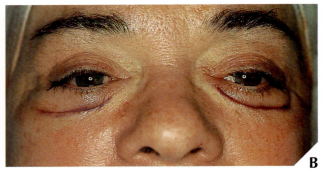

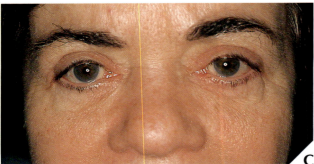

Figure 5.40. (A) Blepharoplastic patient postoperatively with persistent malar excess skin. (B) Immediately after direct excision. (C) A satisfied patient 9 months postoperatively.

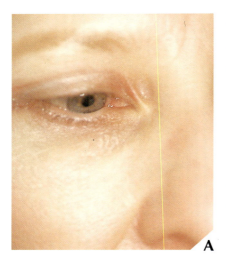

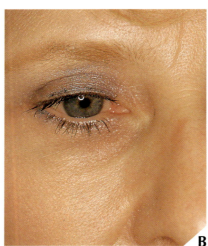

Figure 5.41. (A) Patient 1 month postoperatively with cicatricial right upper eyelid epiblepharon. (B) Three months after massage to the epiblepharon.

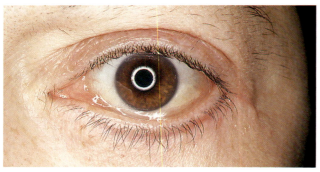

Figure 5.42. Patient with persistent chemosis of the conjunctiva 4 months after blepharoplasty.

chemotic conjunctiva and patching usually resolve the situation. If the chemosis becomes more marked or there is actual incarceration behind the eyelids, temporary suture tarsorrhaphy may be required.

REFERENCES

1. Alfonso E, Levado AJ, Flynn JT: Inferior rectus paresis after secondary blepharoplasty. Br J Ophthalmol 68:535–537, 1984.
2. Allen MV, Cohen IK, Grimson B, et al: Orbital cellulitis secondary to dacryoystitis following blepharoplasty. Ann Ophthalmol 17:498–499, 1985.
3. Anderson, RL: The aponeurotic approach to ptosis surgery. In Bosniak SL, Smith BC (eds): Advances in Ophthalmic Plastic and Reconstructive Surgery. New York, Pergamon Press, 1982.
4. Anderson RL, Dixon RS: Aponeurotic ptosis surgery. Arch Ophthalmol 97:1123, 1979.
5. Anderson RL, Gordy DD: The tarsal strip procedure. Arch Ophthalmol 97:2192, 1979.
6. Anderson RL, Gordy DD: Aponeurotic defects in congenital ptosis. Ophthalmology 86:1493, 1979.
7. Baylis H: Levator injury during blepharoplasty. Arch Ophthalmol 102:570–571, 1984.
8. Baylis HI, Cies WA, Kamin DF: Correction of upper eyelid retraction. Am J Ophthamol 82:790, 1976.
9. Beard C: Ptosis, 3rd ed. CV Mosby, St. Louis, 1981.
10. Bodian M: Lid droop following contralateral ptosis repair. Arch Ophthalmol 100:1122–1124, 1982.
11. Callahan A: Prevention of blindness after blepharoplasty. Ophthalmology 90:1047–1057, 1983.
12. Carraway JH, Mellow CG: The prevention and treatment of lower lid ectropion following blepharoplasty. Plast Reconstr Surg 85:971–981,1990
13. Carrol RP: Blindness following lacrimal nerve block. Ophthalmol Surg 13:812, 1982.
14. Castanares S: Complications in blepharoplasty. Plast Reconstr Surg 5:139, 1978.
15. Caster PL, Tenzel RR, Kowalczak AP: Blepharochalasis syndrome. Am J Ophthalmol 99:424–428, 1985.
16. Collin JR, Beard C, Stern WH, et al: Blepharochalasis. Br J Ophthalmol 63:542–546, 1979.
17. DeMere M, Wood T, Austin W: Eye complications with blepharoplasty or other eyelid surgery. Plast Reconstr Surg 53:634, 1974.
18. Dixon R: The management of thyroid-related upper eyelid retraction. Ophthalmology 89:52, 1982.
19. Doxanas MT, Anderson RL: Clinical Orbital Anatomy. Williams & Wilkins, Baltimore, 1984.
20. Doxanos MT, Anderson RL: Oriental eyelids. An anatomic study. Arch Ophthalmol 102:1232, 1984.
21. Edgerton MT: Causes and prevention of lower lid ectropion following blepharoplasty. Plast Reconstr Surg 49:367, 1972.
22. Edgerton MT, Wolfort FG: The dermal flap canthal lift for lower eyelid support. Plast Reconstr Surg 43, 1969.
23. Ellenbogen R: Free autogenous pearl fat grafts in the face—a preliminary report of a rediscovered technique. Ann Plast Surg 16:3, 1986.
24. Flowers RS: Comments on blepharoplasty—Management of complications and patient dissatisfaction. In Goldwyn RM (ed): The Unfavorable Result in Plastic Surgery, 2nd ed. Little Brown, Boston, 1984.
25. Frueh BR: The mechanistic classification of ptosis. Ophthalmology 87:1019, 1980.
26. Gizzard W, et al: Perforating ocular injuries caused by anaesthesia personnel. Ophthalmology 98:1011–1015, 1991.
27. Gradinger GP: Cosmetic upper blepharoplasty. Clinics in Plastic Surgery, Vol. 15, No. 2. WB Saunders, Philadelphia, 1988.
28. Gradinger GP: Preoperative considerations in blepharoplasty. In Symposium on Problems and Complications in Aesthetic Surgery of the Face, Vol. 23. CV Mosby, St. Louis, 1984.
29. Graham WP, et al: Keratoconjunctivitis sicca symptoms appearing after blepharoplasty. Plast Reconstr Surg 57:57, 1976.
30. Hamako C, Baylis HJ: Lower eyelid retraction after blepharoplasty. Ophthalmology 89: 517–521, 1980.
31. Harley RD, Nelson LB, Flannagan JC, et al: Ocular motility disturbances following cosmetic blepharoplasty. Arch Ophthalmol 104: 542–544, 1986.
32. Hartley JH Jr, Lester JC, Schatten WE: Acute retrobulbar hemorrhage during elective blepharoplasty. Plast Reconstr Surg 52:8, 1973.
33. Hay A, et al: Needle penetration of the globe during retrobulbar and peribulbar injections. Ophthalmology 98:1017–1023, 1991.
34. Hayreh SS, Kolder HE, Weingeist TA: Central retinal artery occlusion and retinal tolerance time. Ophthalmology 87, 1980.
35. Hayworth RS, Lisman RD, Muchnich RS, et al: Diplopia following blepharoplasty. Plast Reconstr Surg 52:8, 1973.
36. Hepler RS, Sugimura GI, Straatsma BR: On the

occurrence of blindness in association with blepharoplasty. Plast Reconstr Surg 57:233–235, 1976.

37. Hinderer UT: Blepharocanthoplasty with eyebrow lift. Plast Reconstr Surg 56:402, 1975.
38. Horton CT, Carraway TA, Podenz AO: Treatment of a lacrimal bulge in blepharoplasty by repositioning the gland. Plast Reconstr Surg 61:701, 1978.
39. Hueston JT, Heinze JB: Successful early relief of blindness occurring after blepharoplasty. Plast Reconstr Surg 59:430–431, 1977.
40. Jelks GW, Jelks EB: The influence of orbital and eyelid anatomy on the palpebral aperture. Clinics in Plastic Surgery, Vol. 18, No. 1, WB Saunders, Philadelphia, 1991.
41. Jelks GW, McCord CD Jr: Dry eye syndrome and other tear film abnormalites. Clinics in Plastic Surgery, Vol. 8, No.4, WB Saunders, Philadelphia, 1981.
42. Jelks GW, Smith B: The reconstruction of the eyelid and associated structures. In McCarthy JG (ed): Plastic Surgery. WB Saunders, Philadelphia, 1990.
43. Jelks GW, Smith B, Bosniak S: The evaluation and management of the eye in facial palsy. Clin Plast Surg 4:397–419, 1979.
44. Jordan DR, Anderson RL: The lateral tarsal strip revisited: The enhanced tarsal strip. Arch Ophthalmol 107:604, 1989.
45. Kelly PW, May DR: Central retinal artery occlusion following cosmetic blepharoplasty. Br J Ophthalmol 64:1980.
46. Kimble JA, Mauris RE, Witherspoon CS, et al: Case report: Globe perforation from peribulbar injection. Arch Ophthalmol 105:749, 1987.
47. Lemoline AN Jr: Discussion of acute retrobulbar hemorrhage during elective blepharoplasty. Plast Reconstr Surg 52:12, 1973.
48. Leone CR Jr, Hand SI Jr: Reconstruction of the medial eyelid. Am J Ophthalmol 87:797, 1979.
49. Levine et al: Complications of blepharoplasty. Ophthalmol Surg 6:53–57, 1975.
50. Lisman RD, Hyde K, Smith B: Complications of blepharoplasty. Clinics in Plastic Surgery, Vol. 15, No. 2, WB Saunders, Philadelphia, 1988.
51. Lisman RD, Rees T, Baker D, et al: Experience with tarsal suspension as a factor in lower lid blepharoplasty. Plast Reconstr Surg 79:897, 1987.
52. Lloyd WC, Leone CR: Transient bilateral blindness following blepharoplasty. Ophthalmol Plast Reconstr Surg 1:29–34, 1985.
53. Loeb R: Fat pad sliding and fat grafting for leveling lid depression. Clinics in Plastic Surgery, Vol. 8, No. 4, WB Saunders, Philadelphia, 1981.
54. MacKinnon SE, Fielding JC, Dellon AL, et al: The incidence and degree of scleral show in the normal population. Plast Reconstr Surg 80:15–20, 1987.
55. Mahaffey PJ, Wallace AF: Blindness following cosmetic blepharoplasty—a review. Br J Plast Surg 39:213–222, 1986.
56. Marsh JL Edgerton MT: Periosteal pennant lateral canthoplasty. Plast Reconstr Surg 64:24, 1979.
57. McCord CD Jr, Shore JW: Avoidance of complications in lower lid blepharoplasty. Ophthalmology 90:1039–1046, 1983.
58. McCord CD Jr: Complications of upper lid blepharoplasty. In Putterman AM (ed): Cosmetic Oculoplastic Surgery. Grune & Stratton, New York, 1982.
59. Montandon DA: A modification of the dermal flap canthal lift for correction of the paralyzed lower lid. Plast Reconstr Surg 61:555, 1978.
60. Morgan SC: Orbital cellulitis and blindness following a blepharoplasty. Plast Reconstr Surg 64:823–826, 1979.
61. Mustardé JC: Repair and Reconstruction in the Orbital Region. Livingstone, Edinburgh, 1969.
62. Neuhaus RW, Baylis HI: Complications of lower eyelid blepharoplasty. In Putterman AM (ed): Cosmetic Oculoplastic Surgery, Grune & Stratton, New York, 1982.
63. Ousterhont DK, Weil RB: The role of the lateral canthal tendon in lower eyelid laxity. Plast Reconstr Surg 69:620, 1982.
64. Owsley JQ Jr: Restoration of the prominent lateral fat pad during upper lid blepharoplasty. Plast Reconstr Surg 65:4, 1980.
65. Patipa M: Levator ptosis in patients undergoing upper lid blepharoplasty. Ann Ophthalmol 16:266–270, 1984.
66. Putterman AM: Ectropion of the lower eyelid secondary to Mueller's muscle-capsulo palpebral fascia detachment. Am J Ophthalmol 85:814, 1978.
67. Quickert MH, Rathbun E: Suture repair of entopion. Arch Ophthalmol 85:304, 1971.
68. Rafety FM: Complications of cosmetic blepharoplasty. Cos Surg 2:17–29, 1983.
69. Rafety FM: Transient total blindness during cosmetic blepharoplasty. Ann Plast Surg 3:373–375, 1979.
70. Rees TD: Correction of ectropion resulting from blepharoplasty. Plast Reconstr Surg 50:1, 1972.
71. Rees TD: Dry eye complications after blepharoplasty. Plast Reconstr Surg 56:375, 1975.
72. Rees TD: Prevention of ectropion by horizontal shortening of the lower lid during blepharoplasty. Ann Plast Surg 11:17, 1983.
73. Rees TD, Craig SM, Fisher Y: Orbital abscess following blepharoplasty. Plast Reconstr Surg 73:126, 1984.

BLEPHAROPLASTY

74. Rees TD, Jelks GW: Blepharoplasty and the dry eye syndrome: Guidelines for surgery? Plast Reconstr Surg 68:249–252, 1981.

75. Rees TD, LaTrenta GS: The role of the Schirmer's test and orbital morphology in predicting dry eye syndrome after blepharoplasty. 82:619–625,1988.

76. Rodriguez RL, Zide BM: Reconstruction of the medial cathus. Clin Plast Surg 15:255, 1988.

77. Schultz RC, Swartz S: Dry eye following blepharoplasty. Plast Reconstr Surg 54:644, 1974.

78. Silkiss RZ, Baylis HI: Autogenous fat grafting by injection. Ophthal Plast Reconstr Surg 3:71–75, 1987.

79. Smith B: "Lazy-T" operation for the correction of ectropion. Arch Ophthalmol, July 1976.

80. Smith B: Postsurgical complications of cosmetic blepharoplasty. Trans Am Acad Ophthalmol Otolaryngol 73:1162–1164, 1967.

81. Smith B, Della Rocca R, Nesi FA, et al: Complications in blepharoplasty. In Smith BC, Della Rocca R, Nesi FA, Lisman RD (eds): Ophthalmic Plastic and Reconstructive Surgery. CV Mosby, St. Louis, 1987.

82. Smith B, Nesi F: The complications of cosmetic blepharoplasty. Trans Am Acad Ophthalmol Otolaryngol 85:726–729, 1978.

83. Smith B, Nesi F: Upper lid loss due to formalin injection. Surg Reconstr, Feb 1979.

84. Stasior OG: Complications of ophthalmic plastic and reconstructive surgery. Trans Am Acad Ophthalmol Otolaryngol 81:550, 1976.

85. Sutcliff I, et al: Bleeding in cosmetic blepharoplasty; an anatomical approach. Ophthal Plast Reconstr Surg 1:107–113, 1985.

86. Tenzel RR: Treatment of lagophthalmos of the lower lid. Arch Ophthalmol 81:366, 1969.

87. Tenzel RR: Complications of blepharoplasty, orbital hematoma, ectropion and scleral show. Clin Plast Surg 7:797–802, 1981.

88. Tenzel RR: Surgical treatment of complications of cosmetic blepharoplasty. Clin Plast Surg 5:517–523, 1978.

89. Tenzel RR, Buffman FV, Miller GR: The use of the lateral canthal sling in ectropion repair. Can J Ophthalmol 12:199, 1977.

90. Waller RP: Eyelid malpositions in Graves' ophthalmopathy. Trans Am Ophthalmol Soc 83:855, 1982.

91. Waller RP: Is blindness a realistic complication in blepharoplasty procedures? Trans Am Acad Ophthalmol Otolaryngol 85:730–734, 1978.

92. Warwick R: Eugene Wolff's Anatomy of the Eye and Orbit, 2nd ed. WB Saunders, Philadelphia, 1976.

93. Weis FA: Surgical treatment of entropion. J Am Coll Surg 21:758:1954.

94. Wesley RE: Tarsal ectopion from detachment of the lower eyelid retractors. Am J Ophthalmol 93:491, 1982.

95. Wesley RE, Pollard ZF, McCord CD Jr: Superior oblique paresis after blepharoplasty. Plast Reconstr Surg 66:283–287, 1980.

96. Whitnall SE: The Anatomy of the Human Orbit, 2nd ed. Oxford University Press, London, 1932.

97. Zide BM, Jelks GW: Surgical Anatomy of the Orbit. Raven Press, New York, 1985.

98. Zide BM, McCarthy JG: The medial canthus revisted—an anatomical basis for canthopexy. Ann Plast Surg 11:1, 1983.

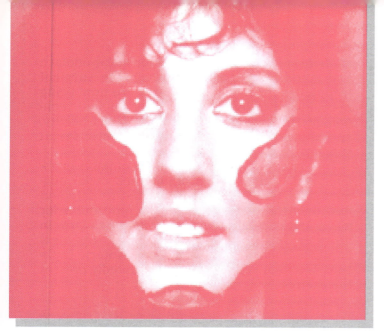

CHIN AND MALAR AUGMENTATION

Edward O. Terino

C H A P T E R

6

Facial aesthetic surgery has made monumental progress in the past 25 years. The most dramatic advance has occurred within the past decade through the development and use of implants in operations for chin and malar augmentation. The number of such operations has increased greatly.

Implants have been more widely used in chin than in malar augmentations (Figs. 6.1 and 6.2). Since chin augmentation has traditionally relied on simpler surgical techniques and the improvement of the facial profile is more readily apparent, its wide acceptance is understandable. Moreover, malar augmentation has been less popular among surgeons because it involves controversial techniques and sometimes produces unacceptable results (Figs. 6.3 and 6.4). Due to an increase in patient demand for malar-midface and mandible surgery, however, the surgical techniques for these procedures are now being re-evaluated in light of the newer implant technology, the changing concepts of facial beauty, and the recent advances in aesthetic facial surgery.

This chapter will discuss the common problems and complications of chin and malar augmentation that have been reported to date and how they can be resolved. As the procedures for malar and chin augmentation continue to grow in number and popularity (Fig. 6.5), and new implants become available, more esoteric problems and their solutions will undoubtedly present themselves.

Figure 6.1 Membership Experience with Malar-Mandible Augmentation*

Facial Implants	No. Performed	Avg. No. per MD
Chin	20,000	67
Malar	3,000	10

*Doctors reporting: 9% (300 of 3200 members)
From ASPRS survey, April 1990.

Figure 6.2 Percentage of Members Who Have Performed Chin and Malar Implants

Total No. of Implant Procedures	Chin	Malar
0 to 10	33	85
< 50	70	98
> 100	30	1
> 500	1.5	0

From ASPRS survey.

Figure 6.3 Quality Comparison of Standard vs. Extended Anatomic Chin Implants

	Type of Implant	
	Standard	Extended-anatomic
Superior	10%	35%
Excellent	45%	22%
Good	35%	35%
Fair	8%	5%
Poor	1%	0%
Totally unsatisfactory	1%	2%

From ASPRS survey.

Figure 6.4 Quality Comparison of Standard vs. Extended Anatomic Malar Implants

	Type of Implant	
	Standard	Extended-anatomic
Superior	8%	20%
Excellent	30%	40%
Good	35%	22%
Fair	15%	10%
Poor	8%	5%
Totally unsatisfactory	5%	2%

From ASPRS survey.

To gather sufficient data on complications with malar and chin augmentation, the author recently conducted a survey among the members of the American Society of Plastic and Reconstructive Surgery (see Figs. 6.1 and 6.2). Of the 3,200 members, 299 (i.e., approximately 9%) responded. The surgeons who did respond probably represent the majority of those who currently perform malar and chin augmentations. The total number of implant procedures reported was approximately 20,000 chin and 3,000 malar (see Fig. 6.1). These statistics clearly indicate that malar and mandible augmentations, through the use of implants, are fast gaining in popularity.

ANATOMIC ZONES OF THE MALAR REGION

A discussion of complications with alloplastic implants must begin with a brief presentation of the significant surgical anatomy of the malar and mandible regions (Fig. 6.6). The anatomy of the

Figure 6.5 Volume Experience Within Past 2 Years

No. of Procedures	Chin	Malar
0 to 50	90%	98%
50 to 100	10%	2%

From ASPRS survey. Note the dramatic increase in procedures. Compare with Figures 6.1 and 6.2

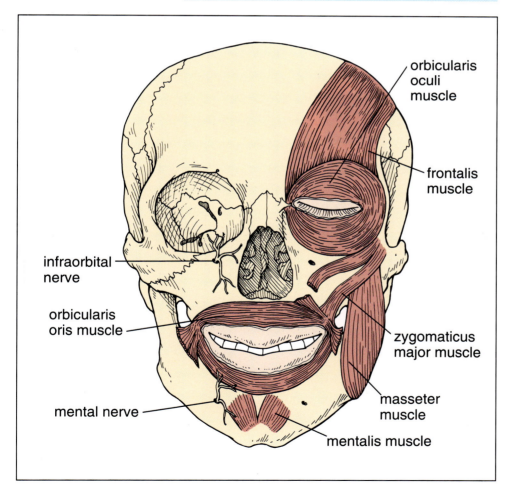

Figure 6.6. Important anatomic landmarks.

orbicularis oculi muscle

frontalis muscle

infraorbital nerve

orbicularis oris muscle

mental nerve

zygomaticus major muscle

masseter muscle

mentalis muscle

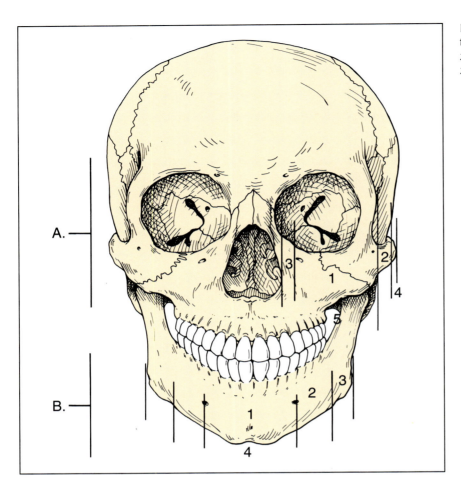

Figure 6.7. Aesthetic zones of the facial skeleton. **(A)** Malar zones 1–5. **(B)** Premandibular zones 1–4.

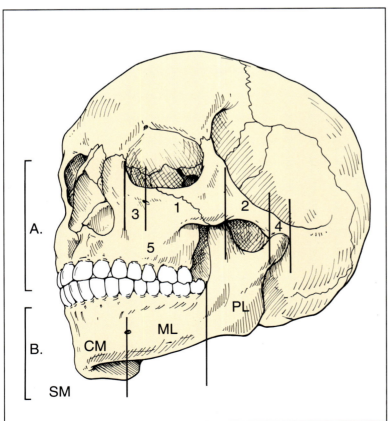

Figure 6.8. Aesthetic zones of the facial skeleton. **(A)** Malar zones. **(B)** Premandibular zones. (CM = central mentum, ML = midlateral zone, PL = posterolateral zone, SM = submandibular zone)

malar area can be divided into five zones (Figs. 6.7 to 6.9).

Zone 1, the largest anatomic area, includes the major portion of the malar bone and the first-third of the zygomatic arch. This region is the primary site for augmentation. The middle-third of the zygomatic arch constitutes zone 2. Simultaneous augmentation of both zones 1 and 2 produces the greatest aesthetic alterations.

The paranasal area medial to the infraorbital nerve is called zone 3. Only occasionally will the surgeon wish to design an implant to augment this area, because increasing the tissue volume in this zone rarely produces significant results.

The posterior-third of the zygomatic arch, or zone 4, is another area of lesser significance. Dissection in this area is very difficult since the bony zygomatic arch is thin and damage to the facial nerve branch of the frontalis muscle superiorly, as well as to branches innervating the orbicularis and zygomaticus muscles inferiorly is possible. Temporomandibular joint dysfunction may also ensue.

Zone 5 consists of the submalar region or space. Implants in this area also modify cheek and midface contour. This zone lies inferior to the anatomic confines of the malar bone and extends down over the fibrous tendon of the masseter muscle as it originates from the inferior aspect of the malar zygomatic arch. When augmented, it provides midface fullness, thereby correcting the atrophy caused by heredity or age. More importantly, malar shell augmentation in the upper malar zones 1 and 2 must extend down into this area to form a lower, more rounded, full cheek (Fig. 6.10). Many different implants exist to augment zones 1, 2, and submalar zone 5.

ANATOMIC ZONES OF THE PREMANDIBLE

Chin implants have traditionally been placed in the central mentum (CM), or zone 1, between the two mental foramina. This area, however, represents only one region of mandibular anatomy that can be augmented. Implants placed only in this

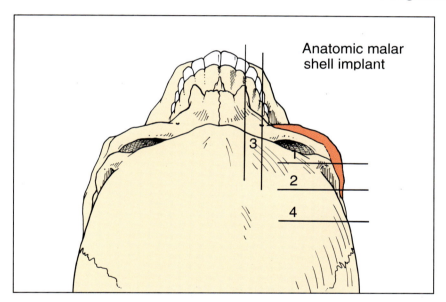

Anatomic malar shell implant

Figure 6.9. Malar augmentation by zone.

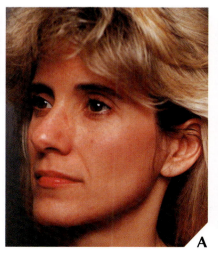
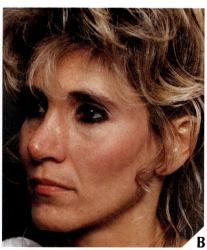

A   B

Figure 6.10. Patient with malar and submalar implants in place, creating a rounder lower cheek and fuller midface. **(A)** Preoperative view. **(B)** Postoperative view.

central segment most often produce an abnormal central protuberance that may be unattractive (Fig. 6.11).

The midlateral zone (ML) of the mandible (zone 2) extends from the CM laterally to the middle half of the horizontal ramus in the area of the oblique line. The simultaneous augmentation of the ML and CM can often create the most natural alloplastic chin-jaw contour. The recently developed extended anatomic contour implants are now being used in this area (Fig. 6.12).

Zone 3 is the posterolateral mandible (PM), which includes the mandibular angle. Augmentation in this zone broadens the face and helps to define the posterior jawline. Current techniques and implants have produced promising results in this area, although further exploration and modifications of the posterior jaw and angle contour are needed (Fig. 6.13).

Zone 4, the submandibular zone (SM), lies beneath the inferior border of the mandible. Augmentation here can lengthen the face from the lower lip to the inferior chin line (Fig. 6.14) and may also help correct a marionette groove, or anteromandibular pre-jowl sulcus.

CHARACTERISTICS OF AN IDEAL FACIAL IMPLANT

The type of implant selected is of paramount importance in determining the outcome of mandible and malar augmentation. Complications resulting from the character of the implant can occur. New, improved implant designs, however, are continually becoming available.

The ideal alloplastic facial implant should have the following features: 1) easily implantable, 2) nonpalpable, 3) readily replaceable, 4) con-

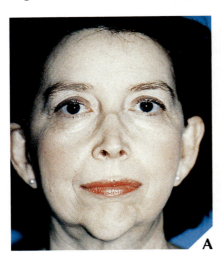
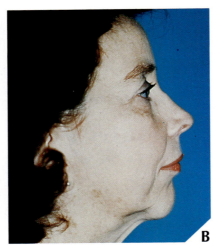
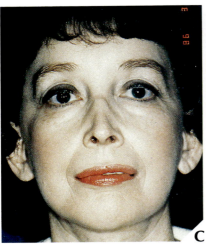
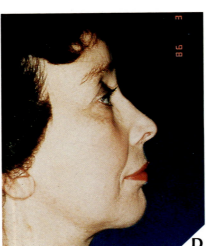

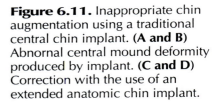

Figure 6.11. Inappropriate chin augmentation using a traditional central chin implant. **(A and B)** Abnormal central mound deformity produced by implant. **(C and D)** Correction with the use of an extended anatomic chin implant.

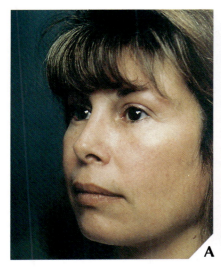 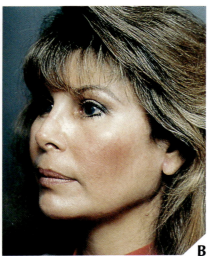

Figure 6.12. Patient with anatomic premandibular implant extending into the midlateral zone. **(A)** Preoperative view. **(B)** Postoperative view.

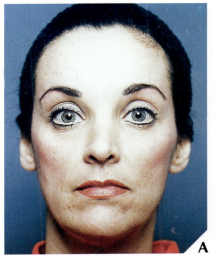 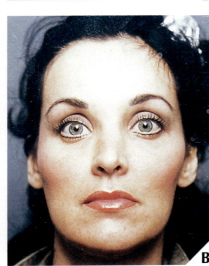

Figure 6.13. Patient with malar shell and lateral mandibular bar implants in place. **(A)** Preoperative view. **(B)** Four months postoperatively .

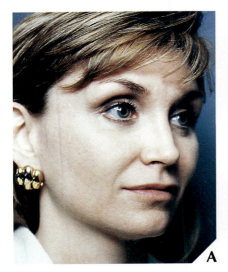 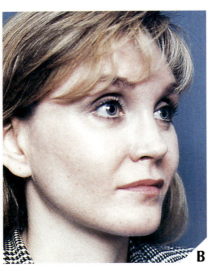

Figure 6.14. Patient with vertical extension implant to augment the submandibular zone. **(A)** Preoperative view. **(B)** Postoperative view.

formable, 5) acceptable to the host, 6) forgivable to infection, and 7) modifiable by the surgeon (Fig. 6.15).

Silicone Implants

To date silicone implants are the implants of choice among plastic surgeons. A smooth silicone implant, when placed directly on bone (Fig. 6.16), will fix securely and rapidly by fibrosis and capsular formation. Moreover, silicone implants can readily be removed and exchanged for another size or shape when necessary.

Furthermore, medium-grade silicone is easily implantable and conformable. It is flexible enough to be inserted through small tissue apertures and soft enough to mold to bony contour. Unlike Proplast, all margins of the silicone implant will remain firmly attached to bone. When these implants are finely tapered, they are minimally, if at all, palpable through the layers of skin. Proplast, on the other hand, may curl at the edges and may even be visible through the soft tissue.

Silicone implants can also be easily shaped, carved, and modified at the operating table or prior to surgery. The surgeon can rapidly alter the implant using sharp scissors, a scalpel, or a dermabrader.

Solid silicone implants can resist surrounding inflammation and even some degrees of infection or purulence without absolute indication for removal. Adequate antibiotic treatment, drainage, and, perhaps, continuous irrigation can sometimes abort impending implant loss.

Proplast and Other Materials

Alloplastic materials that are porous (such as Proplast) or that stabilize to the bone (such as Hydroxyapatite) have not been used by the author. According to the ASPRS survey, their use has been significantly less than that of silicone implants (Fig. 6.17). The porous materials offer an advantage in implant stability. These substances do, however, present special problems. In every series reported, Proplast implantation resulted in

Figure 6.15 Comparison of Qualities of Most Commonly Used Facial Implant Materials

Ideal Characteristics	*Materials*		
	Silastic	*Proplast*	*Other*
Exchangeable	++++	+	−
Conformable	++++	++	++
Modifiable	+++	++++	−
Host acceptable	++++	++	++
Nonpalpable	+++	+	+
Insertable	++++	+++	++

From ASPRS survey. ++++, most ideal; +, least ideal; −, not available.

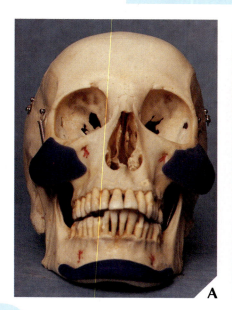 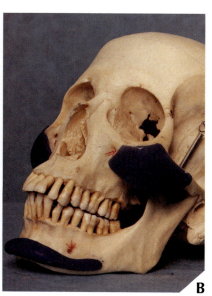

A B

Figure 6.16. Correct positioning of silicone implants. Contoured, smooth implants fix rapidly and securely to bone. **(A)** Frontal view. **(B)** Oblique view.

a significant incidence of infection because of the matrix's propensity for bacterial invasion. The ASPRS survey reveals a high rate of patient dissatisfaction, specifically with external implant contour shape and size. Until precise, predictable techniques for these newer implants evolve, it is more prudent for surgeons to use nonporous, non-adhering implants that encapsulate and fix firmly to the bone, but can be easily removed and replaced to correct size and shape, as required.

MALAR AUGMENTATION

Technical Considerations in Prevention of Complications

The malar space can be approached through four different incisions, all of which are suitable, but each carrying its own risk for malpositioning.

SUBCILIAL BLEPHAROPLASTY

This incision allows the surgeon to accurately visualize the position of the implant. It minimizes contamination, and provides a sturdy inferior cheek shelf on which the implant can rest. The dissection also avoids contact with and visualization of the infraorbital nerve. Despite these merits, this approach is generally avoided by surgeons because of the potential to produce morbid distortions of the eyelid anatomy.

Excessive trauma with bleeding into the lid tissues will stimulate fibrosis and contracture within the middle lamella of the lower lid, which may produce ectropion (Figs. 6.18 and 6.19). Maneuvers that can minimize this outcome are: 1) adequate hemostasis achievable by large volume infiltration of dilute local anesthesia, 2) atraumatic dissection, 3) copious irrigation with antibiotic

Figure 6.17 Volume Comparison of Most Commonly Used Implant Materials.

Material	% of MDs
Silicone	85
Proplast	12
Other	3

From ASPRS survey.

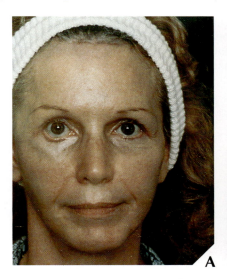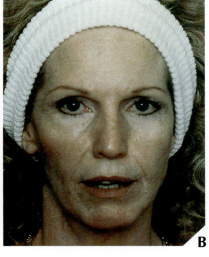

Figure 6.18. Patient 3 months following malar implantation to correct post-traumatic malar-zygomatic arch fracture deformity. A subcilial blepharoplasty approach was used. **(A)** Preoperative view. **(B)** Six months postoperatively. A lateral canthopexy procedure was required.

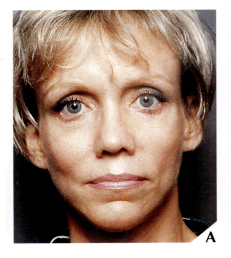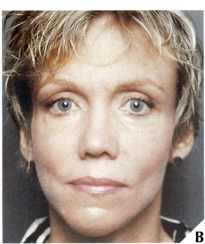

Figure 6.19. Patient with severe bilateral ectropion following subcilial blepharoplasty. **(A)** Two months postoperatively. **(B)** Six months postoperatively before canthopexy reconstruction.

solutions, and 4) percutaneous vacuum drainage, when indicated.

The incision through the periosteum onto the malar bone is performed 4 mm anterior and inferior to the orbital rim in its lateral one third (Fig. 6.20). This prevents retraction of adhesions between bare bone at the rim and the other structures in that area, i.e., the orbicularis muscle, the orbital septum, and the other eyelid depressors. Lateral canthopexy may be used to secure upward stability of the lower eyelid and lateral canthus to help prevent ectropion (Fig. 6.21). Resection of skin and muscle flap should be minimized or avoided because of the additional downward traction on the lower lid produced by volume expansion under the malar-zygomatic tissues by the implant.

INTRAORAL APPROACH

The intraoral approach to malar augmentation is the traditional one and is well described in the literature. Nonetheless, the author believes that this approach offers greater risk of inaccurate placement, hematoma, infection, extrusion and subse-

quent removal of implant. Nonetheless, it is the access route of choice for placement of large malar shell implants and zone 5 submalar implants.

The risk of injuring the infraorbital nerve is a matter of great concern. Dysesthesia or other symptoms of damage may be attributed to either 1) transection of small branches in the lip during incision or 2) direct damage of the major nerve bundle during dissection. This complication should be easily avoidable if the following approach is taken: 1) A mucosa-only vertical incision of 1.5 to 2 cm in length is made over the anterior maxillary buttress above the first molar and 2.5 cm medial to the parotid duct orifice (Fig. 6.22). 2) Blunt muscle penetration with an elevator is accomplished directly onto bone in a vertical direction and at the most inferior aspect of the incision (Fig. 6.23), thereby minimizing damage to branches of the infraorbital nerve. 3) Dissection is then directed obliquely up the malar buttress, onto the malar bone, and over to the zygomatic region (Fig. 6.24). The dissection never extends medially into the territory of the infraor-

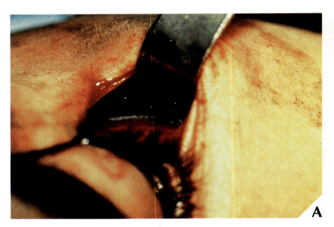
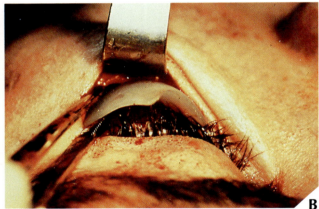

Figure 6.20. (A and B) Subcilial placement of a malar shell implant 4 mm anterior and inferior to the lateral orbital rim.

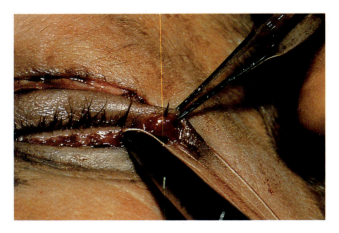

Figure 6.21. Lateral canthopexy to prevent ectropion following malarplasty.

bital nerve and its foramen. These structures are easily identified topographically by palpating the infraorbital notch prior to surgery and drawing a vertical line down the anterior face in the paranasal region with a marking pen.

Another problem with the intraoral approach is that it creates incisional weakness in the muscle floor inferiorly. This appears to increase chances of rotational asymmetries and medial inferior descent of the implant (Fig. 6.25). One method to prevent rotation is early fixation of the implant with a posterior temporal hairline traction suture. This consists of a double-armed, 2-0 Surgibond suture with two 7-inch-long Keith needles that passes through the tail of the implant. The needles are placed from inside the malar

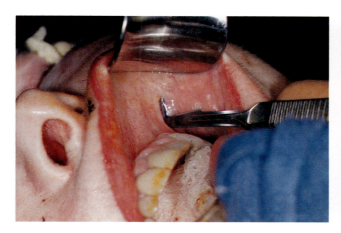

Figure 6.22. The preferred incisional approach to the malar and submalar region—an intraoral and vertical incision.

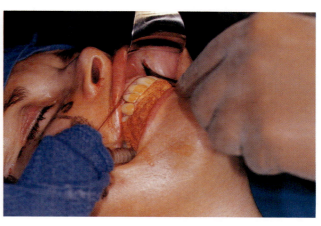

Figure 6.23. An elevator is used to penetrate the muscle bluntly in a vertical direction down to the bone.

Figure 6.24. Dissection is directed obliquely up onto the malar bone to avoid the infraorbital nerve.

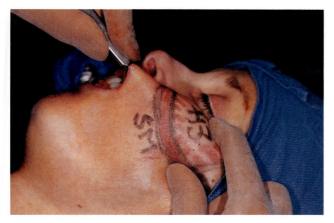

Figure 6.25. Rotation and descent of a malar implant (left side). Implant was inserted through an intraoral approach. **(A)** Preoperative view showing the asymmetry. **(B)** Postoperative correction by elevation and repositioning.

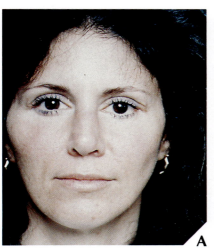

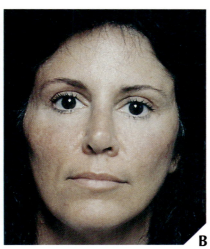

A

B

space backward and out posterior to the tempo-ral hairline (Fig. 6.26). By means of these traction sutures, the implant can then be pulled firmly into its lateral position overlying the zygomatic arch from which it is unlikely to rotate. These sutures are easily removed after 2 to 3 days. Both malar and submalar implants may be fixed by this method.

Anterior stabilization of the implant may be accomplished by securing it into the anterior fibers of the masseter tendon with a 4-0 suture of choice, which will help maintain the medial and inferior position (Fig. 6.27). Finally, a firm, two-lay-ered closure of the muscle pillars and mucosa within the incisional aperture help support the floor of the malar space to prevent implant descent.

RHYTIDECTOMY APPROACH

Creating the malar space directly over zone 1 pre-cludes incidents of morbidity that ordinarily can occur during the other described dissections. Once the rhytidectomy flap is elevated over the malar eminence in zones 1 and 2, there are no underlying anatomic structures over the bone that can be seriously impaired. The roof of the malar space is penetrated through the SMAS and the zygomaticus origins onto the malar bone. By creating an oblique aperture that parallels muscle and facial nerve fibers, there is minimal risk of impairing orbicularis oculi function. The critical maneuver in creating the malar space through a rhytidectomy approach involves elevation along the zygomatic arch into zone 2 to permit implant placement without buckling of the tail. This poste-

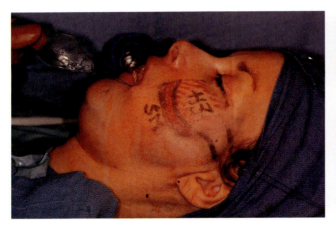

Figure 6.26. A double-armed Surgibond traction suture is placed through the implant to pull it into the malar space. The implant is about to be pulled into the correct position.

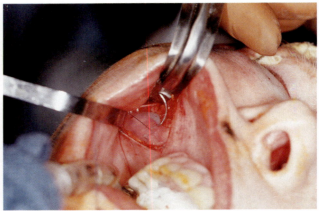

Figure 6.27. Submalar implant being sutured into anterior position through the anterior fibers of the mas-seter tendon.

Figure 6.28 Frequency of Severe Complications Following Chin and Malar Augmentation

	% of Total MD Experience	Author's Experience (%)
Asymmetry or malposition requiring correction	25	1
Cellulitis requiring surgery	15	0.04
Extrusion	20	0
Nerve symptoms requiring surgery	2	0
Permanent nerve dysfunction		
Anesthesia	4	0.02
Hypesthesias	5	0.02
Paresthesias	2	0

From ASPRS survey.

Figure 6.29 Frequency of Most Common Complications With Malar Implants

	% of MDs
Asymmetries	25
Malposition	35
Hematoma/ seroma/infections	15
Extrusion	15
Nerve dysfunction	8
Sensory	3
Motor	5
Ectropion (subcilial route)	2

From ASPRS survey.

rior dissection is very necessary, and usually not difficult to perform.

Rhytidectomy offers two advantages over the other approaches: 1) it is a sterile entry wound that is readily accessible, and 2) it offers a reasonable opportunity for accurate placement, accompanied by direct palpation and observation. Although the approach is not frequently used by the author, it should be seriously considered by all surgeons undertaking malarplasty. It should provide a high degree of placement accuracy and facial symmetry.

TEMPORAL-ZYGOMATIC APPROACH

The author's experience with the temporal-zygomatic approach, either preauricularly or through coronoplasty, is at this time limited. The ASPRS questionnaire indicated limited experience by other surgeons as well. Craniofacial subperiosteal facelifting, as recently reported in the literature, has not been performed by the author. Although this method of malar implant insertion may be excellent, the frequent incidence of frontalis nerve damage, often permanent, represents a significant deterrent to the surgeon. Further experience and studies by plastic surgeons are necessary, and presumably will be forthcoming, before this approach can be advocated.

Complications

The ASPRS survey revealed the following complications from malar augmentation, in order of importance and frequency (Figs. 6.28 and 6.29): 1) patient and/or doctor dissatisfaction; 2) asymmetries; 3) malposition; 4) hematoma, seroma, and infection and removal; 5) infraorbital nerve dysfunction (intraoral route); 6) zygomaticus lip elevation dysfunction (intraoral route); and 7) lower eyelid ectropion (subcilial route).

Although the data from the survey did not show the exact number of occurrences for each complication, it did reveal what percent of the respondents had encountered each complication.

PATIENT DISSATISFACTION

Patient dissatisfaction is the most common complication to arise after aesthetic malar augmentations. The results of the ASPRS survey reveal that patients' disappointment with the size, shape, or contour of their cheek or jawline is equal to, if not greater than, their dissatisfaction about asymmetry. Nearly 30% of the surgeons reported these complaints following malar augmentation as compared to 20 to 25% for asymmetry.

Patient dissatisfaction may stem from inappropriate size or shape of the implant (Fig. 6.30) or from incorrect positioning at the time of surgery. Techniques for ideal placement of implants have been controversial, and specific guidelines have been essentially nonexistent.

Implant Choice

Patients have precise visual images of the cheek contour and malar-zygomatic prominence that they would like to emulate. Detailed discussions with the patient will reveal the subtleties and nuances of their expectations regarding shape. These expectations must be clearly and mutually understood prior to surgery. Then, the surgeon must determine whether the improvement requested can be attained by enhancing the upper lateral malar zygomatic region (producing a sharper, high-angular appearance) or by augmenting the submalar region (producing a fuller lower cheek) (see Fig. 6.10). This decision is the most important consideration in achieving an outcome in keeping with the patient's specifications. Thus, the augmentation that produces the results that most closely approximate the patient's desired image depends first and foremost on the

Figure 6.30. Patient with early anatomic malar implants that were too small and too lateral in design. The implants produced an artificial effect.

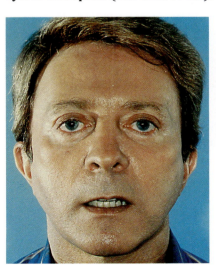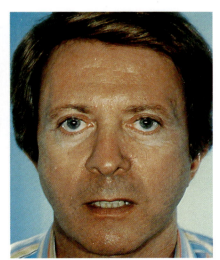

choice and placement of the implants. Because implants are available in varying sizes and shapes, both styles of facial contour—angular or full—can now be produced.

Submalar implants augment lower cheek fullness by 4 to 6 mm (depending on the implant thickness) by adding volume to the canine fossa along the medial and inferior aspects of the patient's natural bony malar-zygomatic eminence. They are best used to augment midfacial malar cheek contour medially and inferiorly in patients who have adequate upper malar-zygo-

matic volume. Malar shell implants augment the volume posteriorly in zone 2 (by creating a superolateral zygomatic high arch) or inferomedially in zone 1 and zone 5 (creating a low, round, and full cheek).

Implant Placement
The merit of the subcutaneous versus the subperiosteal location for implants is still being debated. Placement directly on bare bone produces maximum fixation and immobilization while subcutaneous placement frequently results in insta-

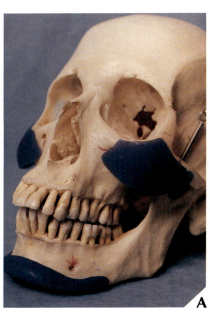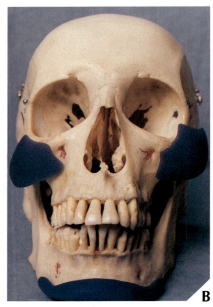

Figure 6.31. Complications with malar augmentation. **(A)** Left implant encroaching on the infraorbital nerve. **(B)** Implant rotating into orbit.

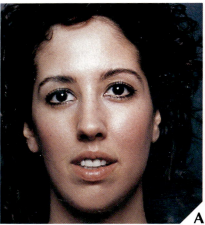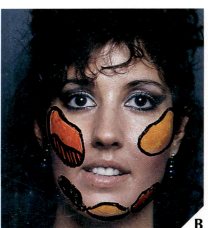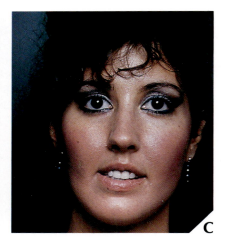

Figure 6.32. Significant facial asymmetry. **(A)** Preoperative view. **(B)** Design showing proposed size and placement of implants **(C)** Correction using malar and lateral mandibular implants that are differently sized and shaped and a unilateral submuscular implant.

bility. Removal of an implant from a subcutaneous space and replantation on bone will correct the latter problem.

Neither porous ingrowth nor internal scar fixation through fenestrations is necessary.

The correction of a malpositioned implant often requires repositioning and replacement (Fig. 6.31). It is prudent, therefore, for the surgeon to practice technical approaches that allow exchange of implants. Meticulous attention to the choice of implant, as well as its placement, will minimize patient dissatisfaction.

ASYMMETRIES

Asymmetry in faces occurs universally and naturally. After augmentation surgery, patients may first notice asymmetric facial areas even though the asymmetry had been there all along! This common reaction can result in obsessive behavior on the part of the patient, followed by blame directed at the surgeon. Pre-existing asymmetries are very difficult to handle (Fig. 6.32).

In managing patients with asymmetries, there are two essential steps to be taken from the onset: 1) there must be an accurate perception and an acceptance of the asymmetry by the patient, and 2) there must be an open discussion between the surgeon and patient regarding the asymmetry, including documentation through photographs and chart data. Patient anxiety and disappointment following surgery can be significantly allayed by reminding them visually of their preoperative asymmetry.

Presently, there is no fail-proof method for evaluating and correcting facial asymmetry totally by cosmetic malar-mandible augmentation. Although computer-imaging and C-MAX technology can provide explicit methods for delineating facial bone defects, they can create only semi-accurate reconstructive models. Advances in this area of computerized technology are being made rapidly, and soon the technology will be able to assist aesthetic plastic surgeons in analyzing implant size and shape, as well as facial contour and form.

The new anatomically shaped malar shell implants and malar-submalar implants can correct a great majority of facial asymmetries. These implants are larger than previous design and fill the entire malar space and cheek region, including the submalar portion (Fig. 6.33). The means for improving or correcting asymmetry at the present time are rather complex and sophisticated, requiring the use of implants of different sizes

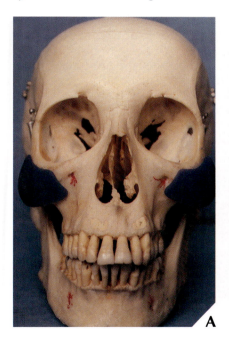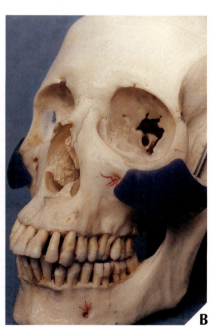

Figure 6.33. New malar shell implants in correct positions. **(A)** Frontal view. **(B)** Oblique view.

and shapes, placed in different positions (Fig. 6.34). Either self-carved or custom-manufactured implants can have identical contours but have slightly larger or smaller projections. Such implants can be used to the surgeon's advantage in correcting asymmetry.

For example, a common facial variation is that of one side being flatter than the other, including the malar-zygomatic architecture, the lateral mandibular contour, and the soft tissue. This flatness is often accompanied by a raised eyebrow and orbit, and a more angular malar-zygomatic eminence, with the opposite, corresponding anatomic elements being lower and fuller. In these patients, an implant with a round contour, significant projection, and increased vertical height may be used and would be placed in a slightly lower position on the high, flat side. The implant choice, then, for the lower, fuller side would be shorter and less prominent. A slightly higher placement on the full side can help compensate as well by creating a higher malar-zygomatic prominence. Needless to say, success in executing this augmentation requires keen perception and surgical judgment on the part of the surgeon and honest communication between patient and surgeon.

Another useful technique to help correct postoperative asymmetry is the manipulation of an implant within the first 2 to 3 weeks by the surgeon and/or the patient. During this period, capsular fibrosis has not yet solidified to the point of implant immobility. Steady pressure, either upward or downward, can manipulate a slightly displaced implant into its proper position. Repeated pressure of this type by the patient, with frequent re-examinations and manipulations by the surgeon, can alter, improve, and resolve early postoperative asymmetries. This method of treatment can only be attempted with a smooth, nonfixed, nonfenestrated, and nonporous implant material, such as Silastic. The small, but real risk of injury from this form of manipulation is the potential stimulation of a hematoma or seroma.

Perhaps the most important principle for the surgeon to remember is that minor asymmetries have a natural tendency to adjust and correct themselves over a 6-month postoperative period as the fibroblastic, collagenous, capsular healing process around the implants relaxes and softens the contour.

Unfortunately, no method presently exists for precise correction of facial asymmetries or for correlation of the patient's needs and requests with accurate implant selection. As previously mentioned, C-MAX and computer-imaging technology will most likely contribute greatly to the elimination of these shortcomings in facial augmentation in the next 5 years.

EXTRUSION, INFECTION, AND REMOVAL

The third most common category of complications found in the ASPRS survey is infection, extrusion, and removal. These problems were experienced by 15 to 25% of the reporting surgeons although the statistical incidence of occurrence is low: in the author's individual series it is 0.04% (see Fig. 6.28).

What are the relevant factors producing these results? Again, the implant material is a significant element. All the reported series of intraorally placed implants, including the data from the ASPRS survey, reveal the highest incidence of infection, extrusion, and necessary removal when

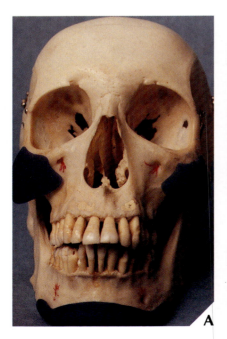 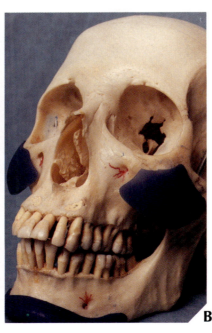

Figure 6.34. Skull with malar shell implants in different positions for correction of asymmetry. **(A)** Frontal view. **(B)** Oblique view.

Proplast is used. This porous material permits access of tissue, blood, and bacteria, a deadly combination for contamination and proliferation. Even sterile atraumatic technique cannot prevent infection in this material. There are no data indicating methods by which infections from Proplast can be predictably and significantly diminished or abolished.

Implants of smooth Silastic have a low infection rate and can be salvaged in the face of contamination, inflammation, cellulitis, and even gross purulence. For these reasons, the author prefers to use them. There are case reports of adequate resolution of infection when prompt, traditional regimens of antibiotics, warm compresses, rest, and drainage or irrigation were instituted. Sound surgical judgment, combined with judicious courage, close surveillance, and prompt intervention are required for the successful management of inflammatory wound pathology.

Inflammation, cellulitis, and infection from Proplast warrants immediate implant removal. Midface infection is a significant hazard that surgeons dare not risk. Cellulitis and inflammation from a Silastic implant may be treated more expectantly; the recorded reports demonstrate control and ultimate cure (Fig. 6.35). Frequent causative contaminants are skin organisms, such as *Staphylococcus aureus*, which are often sensitive to penicillin and the cephalosporins. Duricef, 500 mg twice daily for 5 days in acute inflammation and impending infection may provide great relief. Additionally, 2 or 3 weeks of less-potent antibiotic suppression are indicated if subsidence occurs. When indicated and prudent, a several-day course of intravenous antibiotics may be attempted. If rapid improvement of an inflammatory process does not occur, immediate measures must be taken to drain the area adequately or to remove the prosthesis, even when Silastic is in place.

Another remedy that has been reported and that resolves Silastic implant infection is spontaneous or deliberate drainage of a malar implant abscess through the intraoral incision, in addition to systemic antibiotic therapy. A preventive measure during the primary surgery is also possible. A small, percutaneous catheter suction drainage system can be created from the implant cavity through the temple region during malar implant placement as prophylaxis against accumulation of blood.

NERVE DAMAGE

Damage to facial nerves incurred from malar or chin augmentation represents the most detrimental of the medical complications. Fortunately, such injury is extremely rare and, when it occurs, is usually transient.

The ASPRS survey revealed that approximately 8% of surgeons reported nerve complication in patients following malar augmentation surgeries (see Fig. 6.29). Understandably, nerve symptoms and dysfunction arouse the greatest concern among patients. Disturbance to sensation or motor function are two of the most frightening results of facial surgery. These results create the greatest anxiety for surgeons as well.

In malar augmentation, the infraorbital nerve is the primary sensory nerve of concern. Its position, however, relative to the dissection and placement of the implant, is quite protected. Only occasionally, when augmentation of the paranasolabial malar, or zone 3, is desired, is it necessary to extend the dissection into the region of the infraorbital nerve. Nevertheless, disturbances of infraorbital nerve function have been significant in number, according to the ASPRS survey. If the necessary precautions are taken, as described earlier, occurrences should be rare and controllable.

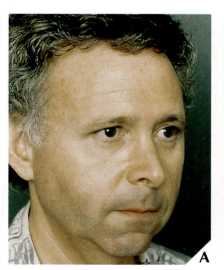 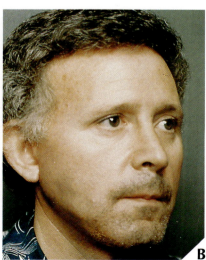

Figure 6.35. Patient who recovered completely from a premandibular implant abscess and cutaneous fistula. Treatment consisted of percutaneous drainage, antibiotics, implant removal, irrigation, and implant replacement. **(A)** Postoperative view. **(B)** After healing.

Disturbances of facial nerve function are even more frightening because they involve motor dysfunction that can result in animated asymmetries or, even worse, total functional deficits. These results are only possible when dissections penetrate the region of the seventh nerve and its branches. They are more likely to occur when the dissection does not stay directly on the bone. Invasion or trauma of the subcutaneous tissues and muscle planes may directly damage motor nerves and muscle tissues. Similarly, dissections posterior along the zygomatic arch into zone 4 that extend superior or inferior to the arch may inadvertently lead into the parotid gland, the facial nerve branches, or the facial musculature.

Obviously, damage to these structures can result in nerve disorders and, perhaps, parotid fistulas.

The author's series contains two patients who experienced temporary and partial paralysis of frontalis and orbicularis oculae function (Fig. 6.36). The conditions completely disappeared after several weeks. Two additional patients suffered transient disturbance of orbicularis oris function following intraoral placement of malar implants (Fig. 6.37).

Secondary operations for malar augmentation carry even greater risk for nerve and muscle damage. In the author's experience, over 30% and perhaps closer to 50%, of secondary procedures were associated with some manifestation of nerve

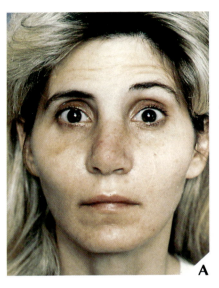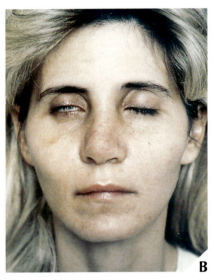

Figure 6.36. Patient with partial and temporary paresis of orbicularis and frontalis function immediately following malar augmentation. **(A)** Elevation of brow. **(B)** Closure of eyes.

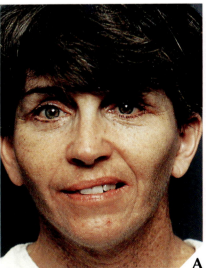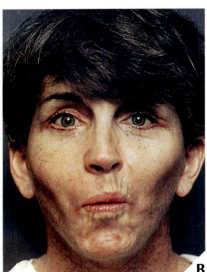

Figure 6.37. Patient displaying nasolabial paresis and orbicularis dysfunction 6 months following malar and submalar augmentation. **(A)** Smiling. **(B)** Whistling.

and/or muscle symptoms. Although the actual number of afflicted patients was few, the significance of these complications was appreciable. During the removal of porous implants with tissue ingrowth, the surgical dissection can easily disrupt the surrounding tissues containing nerve and muscle. Silastic implants that are fenestrated or Dacron-backed are equally hazardous in this regard. Dissections into and through the capsule surrounding an implant, particularly when it is necessary to expand the space to accommodate a larger or differently shaped implant, also predisposes the area to muscle or nerve damage.

The author has observed this development on two occasions. In one case, the patient was referred, having had five previous malar operations by the intraoral route. These had resulted in three infections, requiring implant removal, as well as bilateral ectropion that had been reconstructed by an oculoplastic surgeon. There was also partial, but permanent damage to the lip elevator muscles. This produced asymmetric nasolabial function—a "crooked smile" (see Fig. 6.37). In addition, sensation was diminished in the infraorbital nerve distribution, even after several postoperative years. Implant removal followed by accurate replacement resulted in some alleviation of nerve and muscle dysfunction and aesthetic dissatisfaction was abated. In the second patient, a secondary malarplasty was necessary to replace fenestrated Silastic implants. The trans- and peri-prosthetic encapsulation fibrosis neces-sitated excessively traumatic removal and space expansion (Fig. 6.38). Prolonged nasolabial paresis and unilateral ectropion requiring secondary canthopexy ensued.

Orbicularis oculi dysfunction has been noted in several other cases. It can occur from dissection by any route. The manifestation has been temporary (see Fig. 6.36). This complication is due to the posterior dissection along the zygomatic arch in the territory of the facial nerve branches where elevation of the tissue must sometimes be done with force.

Subcilial blepharoplasty produces much less nerve morbidity than any other route, for the following reasons: 1) the infraorbital nerve can be easily visualized to avoid it, if desired; and 2) the dissection does not need to go into the region of the infraorbital nerve and foramen and therefore should not disturb its function.

HEMATOMA AND SEROMA
Hematoma and seroma are not infrequent occurrences following malar and chin augmentation. In fact, they are so common that they may even be considered a standard postoperative condition. However, they can have dangerous implications. When dissection is accomplished through the intraoral route (or possibly other route), an accumulation of blood encourages growth of bacterial contamination, subsequent cellulitis, and possible infection. Also, hematoma and seroma can imitate early (and sometimes late) postoperative asym-

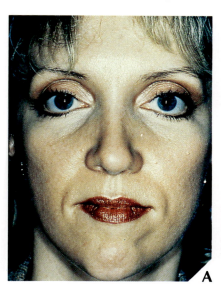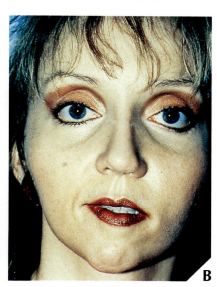

A   B

Figure 6.38. Secondary malar augmentation resulting in ectropion requiring canthopexy. Transient nasolabial paresis also occurred. **(A)** Preoperative view. **(B)** Postoperative view before canthopexy.

metries (Fig. 6.39). This manifestation can make diagnosis and analysis of implant position difficult and confusing to the physician, as well as alarming to the patient. Hematoma and seroma may also result in excessive fibrosis, producing capsular or other soft tissue contour defects, conditions that plastic surgeons have encountered following breast augmentation.

The author's initial experience with malar augmentation through the intraoral approach resulted in a significant incidence of hematoma and seroma. Therefore, this route was temporarily abandoned for subcilial blepharoplasty. Difficult visualization and dissection with excessive bleeding have been the *sine qua non* of the intraoral approach, especially when operations are performed under local standby anesthesia. Although the patients are well sedated, they frequently have an elevated blood pressure and become agitated and/or apprehensive during the intraoral surgical manipulations.

Etiology

Factors causing hematoma and/or seroma formation are numerous: traumatic dissection leading to excessive bleeding during and following surgery, 2) inadequate anesthesia techniques, both locally and systemically, that do not properly control blood pressure and vasoconstriction, 3) early postoperative blood pressure elevation, nausea, vomiting, agitation, urinary retention, etc., 4) trauma to the operative site immediately following surgery, possibly even caused by excessive mastication activity, and 5) secondary procedures that necessitate lysis of capsular adhesions to and through implants and require dissection to expand the malar space (Fig. 6.40).

Hematoma in the postoperative period may be difficult to assess unless it is large. There is always considerable swelling in the first few days following these operative procedures. The exact degree of swelling indicating hematoma is subjective, but usually the swelling is exceptional and obvious. Moderate or minimal hematomas are hard to diagnose. They may simply appear as excessive postoperative swelling with asymmetry. Most of these resolve adequately without treatment or sequelae within 10 to 14 days postoperatively.

On the other hand, a great degree of swelling may occur with hemorrhage into the sclera and other tissues about the orbital region. This is particularly true when the subcilial blepharoplasty approach is used. Large hematomas may also produce symptoms relating to the temporomandibular joint.

Methods of Treatment

As in any surgery, a large hematoma, recognized early, should be evacuated. Copious irrigation with an antibiotic solution (50,000 units of bacitracin in 1l of saline) until the irrigant color is clear is advisable during all implant surgery. Preoperatively, the implants are kept in the bacitracin solution until needed. Attempts are made to avoid touching external skin surfaces with the sterile implants during insertion. The intraoral mucosa is thoroughly prepped with Betadine just as surface skin is prepared for an external operative approach.

Untreated hematomas may result in 1) excessive capsule formation, 2) malposition of the implant, and 3) infection. Seromas may ensue within 10 to 14 days. Percutaneous aspiration of

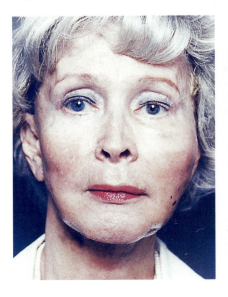 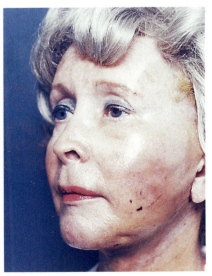

Figure 6.39. Hematoma on left side causing early postoperative asymmetry.

liquefied hematomas or seromas, 2 to 4 weeks postoperatively, should be performed to minimize the possibility of capsular fibrosis and infection. Repeated aspirations can be avoided by effective continuous drainage. This can be instituted by placing a No.-16G Angiocath percutaneously into the submalar space and attaching it to a Vacutainer or rhytidectomy Hemovac system for 48 to 72 hours. Antibiotic coverage is mandatory (Fig. 6.41).

When cellulitis or visible purulence occurs, vigorous treatment with potent antibiotics is indicated, possibly including intravenous administration with bedrest for 24 to 48 hours. Should the process progress, instead of significantly regress, immediate open drainage of the intraoral wound should be accomplished. Once again, when resolution does not occur rapidly, the implant should promptly be removed. Secondary implantation can be planned for 6 to 12 months later. Skin pathogens, such as *Staphylococcus aureus,* are fre-

quent causative agents of such infections. Although it may be possible to use continuous antibiotic irrigation of the space to save an implant, there are no published reports of this treatment, and it has not yet been attempted by the author.

Another solution to this problem, which may be attempted cautiously, is to remove the implant, thoroughly irrigate the cavity with Betadine solution, and resterilize and reinsert the implant, leaving the intraoral buccal wound open to drain. This course of action is probably not advisable unless the infection occurs late in the postoperative period, after the first 4 to 6 weeks. At that time, a protective capsular fibrosis will have formed around the implant.

Delayed seroma has been observed in one or two cases. This is treated either by repeated aspirations or by continuous suction. Culture and sensitivities of the fluid are mandatory. Sometimes a small growth of organisms is present. With long-

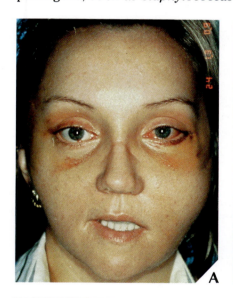

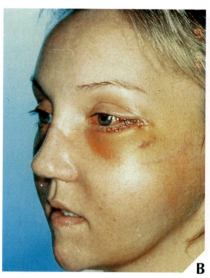

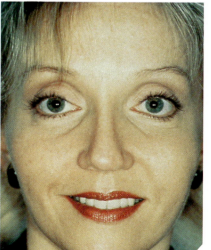

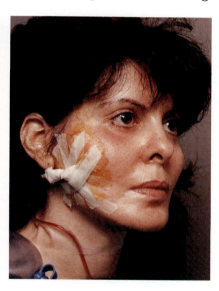

Figure 6.40. (A and B) Large hematoma occurring after secondary malar augmentation and space expansion. **(C)** Resolution of hematoma.

Figure 6.41. Patient 4 months after secondary malar augmentation with suppurative abscess. The abscess was drained percutaneously with a Hemovac system.

term antibiotic therapy, the clinical inflammation around Silastic implants may permanently resolve.

Prevention Through Anesthesia and Surgical Techniques

Intraoperative and postoperative control of bleeding is critical in preventing hematoma. The following techniques adopted by the author seem to have minimized the incidence of hematomas and seromas to an almost negligible statistic: 1) Control of the patient's blood pressure to a level of 90 to 100 mm Hg systolic during the intra- and postoperative period. This is best accomplished under general anesthesia. 2) Routine administration of Tenormin, 25 mg p.o., on the morning of surgery and p.r.n. again in the postoperative period for agitated patients with elevated blood pressure and pulse. This successfully stabilizes the blood pressure and pulse in most patients. Bradycardia in the range of 45 to 60 beats per minute is customary and does not create a problem. The stabilizing effect of Tenormin lasts as long as 24 hours. 3) Large-volume (50 to 75 cc) infiltration of dilute lidocaine solution (0.2%) with an adrenaline concentration of 1/600,000 is injected extensively into the anatomic malar or mandible area subperiosteally and into the tissues surrounding the upper and lower borders of the malar bone and mandible. This maneuver will minimize bleeding during dissection. 4) Adequate fiberoptic techniques and gentle elevation of soft tissues while staying directly on the bony plane also avoids excessive trauma and bleeding. 5) Copious irrigation with antibiotic solution during and at the end of the procedure helps eliminate blood product (Fig. 6.42). This also assists in minimizing the potential for bacterial contamination.

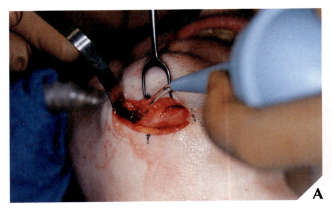
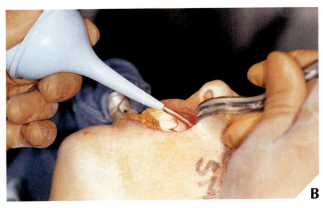

Figure 6.42. Copious irrigation with antibiotic solution helps eliminate blood and minimize infection. **(A)** Irrigation during submental chin augmentation. **(B)** Irrigation during intraoral malar augmentation.

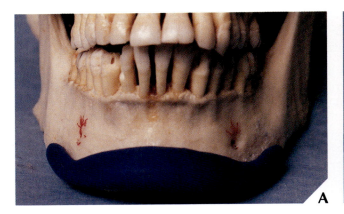
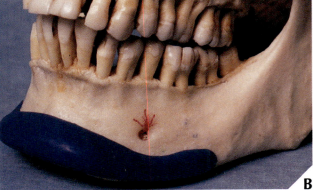

Figure 6.43. Extended anatomic chin implants fit the mandibular contour. **(A)** Frontal view. **(B)** Oblique view.

6) Although percutaneous Vacutainer or Hemovac drainage has not been routinely used by the author, it may be advisable, particularly in secondary procedures where additional bleeding may occur.

The author does *not* use compression bandages postoperatively. Nevertheless, it is certainly sound theoretically to do so initially for 24 to 48 hours. Prevention of postoperative bleeding and hematoma formation is worth a pound of cure. Prevention is largely determined by proper intraoperative surgical technique, as well as by methods of anesthesia.

MANDIBLE AUGMENTATION

Technical Considerations in Prevention of Complications

Augmentation of the mandible for aesthetic reasons has existed for 30 years. The improvement of the nasomentum profile through mentoplasty is well accepted and well understood by plastic surgeons. New implants, developed within the last 5 to 10 years, have extended central chin implants into much larger onlay premandible implants that simulate normal anatomy. Such implants can alter the shape and size of the mid-lateral and posterior mandible, as well as the central segment (Fig. 6.43). Of the respondents to the ASPRS survey, 43% reported experience with extended Silastic chin implants (Figs. 6.44 to 6.46). Thirty percent used them exclusively. Comments from the group revealed a growing satisfaction with the chin contour produced by the new extended anatomic chin implants (Fig. 6.46). Whether or not the surgeon approaches the premandible from the submental or intraoral route, the principles for placement of alloplastic implants are the same: 1) cover muscle and soft tissue adequately; 2) maintain the dissection directly on bone; 3) dissect only along the lower border of the mandible to avoid the mental nerve; 4) assure accurate placement by appropriate manipulation and visualization; 5) minimize bleeding; and 6) secure closure with a strong muscle layer.

Figure 6.44 Volume Experience with Extended Anatomic Chin and Malar Implants.

| No. of Patients | % of MDs | | % of Utilization | % of MDs | |
	Chin	Malar		Chin	Malar
0 to 10	68	87	0 to 10	45	30
<50	93	97.1	50 to 90	20	10
50 to 100	6	–	90 to 100	35	60
>100	2.1	1.1			

From ASPRS survey.

Figure 6.45 Experience With Extended Anatomic Facial Implants

	Total No. Used	No. of MDs	Avg. No. Implants Per MD
Chin	1800	140	13
Malar	1300	90	15

From ASPRS survey.

Figure 6.46 Comparison of Most Common Type of Chin Implants

Type	% of MDs
Central	55
Extended–anatomic	40
Self-carved	3
Fixed with fenestration	1
Fixed with backing	1

From ASPRS survey.

SURGICAL PROCEDURES

A 2-cm submental incision is made transversely down to the bone (Fig. 6.47). Elevation of the soft tissue and muscle pad occurs directly on the bony plane.

In the intraoral approach, in order to prevent ptosis, incision placement is vertical. A transverse 2-cm incision is made through mucosa only, and the mentalis muscles are divided vertically through their midline raphe to avoid transection of the muscle bellies. This aperture affords access directly downward onto bone. The customary muscle-transecting incisions not only lead to inadequate closure but may cause weakness and laxity of the mentalis muscle, producing a potential for ptosis and a centrally drooping chin deformity. These problems can be avoided by using the vertical entrance wound.

Dissection with a blunt spatula elevator inferior to the foramen will avoid the risk of nerve damage. The muscular attachments are elevated from the most inferior border of the mandible (Fig. 6.48). Hugging this lower margin, particularly beneath the mental nerve, prevents damage to this important structure. A tight area of periosteum just beneath the mental foramen must be released. The mental nerve and foramen are situated between 2.5 to 3.5 cm lateral to the midline, just beneath the first or second premolar, and 8 to 15 mm up from the lower border of the mandible.

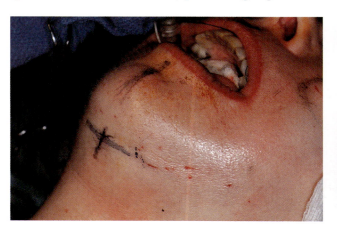

Figure 6.47. The submental approach to mandibular augmentation. A 2-cm transverse incision is used.

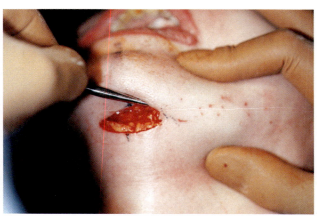

Figure 6.48. Dissection maintained directly on bone.

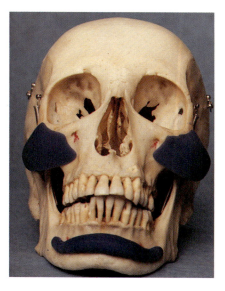

Figure 6.49. Complication with the extended anatomic implant. Incorrect placement producing mental nerve compression.

Figure 6.50 Frequency of Complications With Chin Implants

Asymmetries	20%
Malposition	20%
Hematoma/seroma/infection	15%
Mobility	15%
Extrusion	20%
Nerve dysfunction	10%
Sensory	9%
Motor	1%

From ASPRS survey.

Anatomic variations locating the nerve and foramen 1.5 to 4.5 cm from the midline have been reported in as high as 20 to 30% of cases. Multiple or, most commonly, double mental nerves and foramina are also possible. The direction of the foramen is superior, directing the nerve upwards into the lower lip.

Although the nerve and its sheath are quite durable and resistant to avulsion injury, traction injuries during surgery are common and produce transient postoperative dysesthesia and hypesthesia. Total loss of sensation is rare. It may indicate that implant misplacement is compressing the mental nerve (Fig. 6.49). When this symptom is noted, prompt re-exploration within the first 2 weeks postoperatively is indicated. Mental nerve complications are discussed again later in the chapter.

When using small extended chin implants, it is not necessary to visualize the mental nerve and foramen, although for the security and comfort level of the surgeon, this procedure may be advisable. In inserting large extended chin and mandible implants, however, direct observation of the mental nerve and foramen is definitely indicated.

Complications

The reported complications of extended chin-mandible augmentation are similar to those found in malar augmentation. These consist of: 1) surgeon and patient dissatisfaction with the implant size, shape, or contour; 2) asymmetries and malpositioning; 3) hematoma, infection, or extrusion, necessitating implant removal; and 4) symptoms relating to dysfunction of the mental nerve following implantation (Fig. 6.50). Bone resorption is also a commonly reported complication, which is discussed later in the chapter.

SURGEON AND PATIENT DISSATISFACTION

Beside cephalometrics, the only practical means to assess the size and shape of the implant needed is by using the well-known zero-meridian, popularized by Mario-Gonzales Ulloa. This system relies heavily on the surgeon's individual experience and artistic judgment. The traditional, centrally placed implants are small and often create an abnormal, central chin mound with a visible, unnatural, and unattractive lateral depression (see Fig. 6.11), known as the geniomandibular sulcus. By today's standards, this contour defect is frequently unacceptable to both the surgeon and the patient. The geniomandibular sulcus, or marionette groove, deformity also develops during aging into a jowl and is corrected only by four-layer reconstruction. These techniques must address the skin, subcutaneous fat, SMAS, and finally, skeletal plane. Mandibular implants inserted at the time of rhytidectomy minimize or prevent this deformity (Fig. 6.51).

Centrally placed implants also tend to rotate. Rotational or lateral displacement of even a few

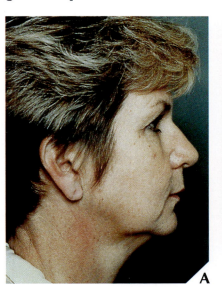 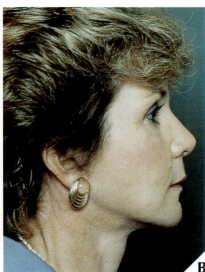

Figure 6.51. Improvement of the anteromandibular pre-jowl sulcus with a premandibular implant at the time of rhytidectomy.
(A) Preoperative view.
(B) Postoperative view.

millimeters can create noticeable asymmetry in the augmented chin (Fig. 6.52).

IMPLANT SELECTION

At present, there are no complete guidelines for choosing implant size and shape for the patient.

Many young men ask for a bold, square jawline. In these cases, the junction between the central mentum and midlateral mandible may need to be augmented 8 to 10 mm, with further posterolateral augmentation of 3 to 5 mm on each side. One large implant can accomplish both of these goals. Either one central or three (two additional and one lateral) intraoral incisions may be used. Another alternative is to use three implants, a central extended one along the chin line and two posterolateral ones (one on either side) to create the same effect.

There are also isolated mandibular implants for the ML and PL zones that create the illusion of a wider, stronger lower facial segment. Finally, the author has designed a vertical wrap-around implant that extends beneath the mandibular border into the SM zone to enhance the vertical length from the lower lip to the submentum by 3 to 4 mm. Again, very specific and repeated preoperative conversations should take place to understand precisely the visual result expected by the patient. Patients tend to be very discerning about the jawline desired (e.g., pointed, rounded, more square, broader, more defined, etc.). Alteration of available extended implants by the above-described techniques, as well as the use of calipers during surgery to monitor precision, gives the surgeon the best opportunity for success.

The currently available, extended implants lie laterally and beneath the mental nerve sufficiently to prevent encroachment upon the mental foramen. These implants supply volume to the anterolateral jawline, as well as to the central chin. Certain implants will augment midlateral deficiencies (in the ML zone), as their primary function and will provide only 2 or 3 mm of central projection if enhancement of the central chin mound is not indicated.

IMPLANT PLACEMENT

Subperiosteal dissection is used in all chin augmentations, regardless of the implant selected. Implants placed supraperiosteally or subcutaneously may become unstable and rotate asymmetrically. Implants placed directly on bone will become securely fixed. In some instances, the posterolateral limb of the extended anatomic implant may be slightly mobile during palpation and may slip around the lower mandibular margin (Fig. 6.53). This is caused by dissecting too far below the mandibular border, thereby creating a mandibular tunnel that is too large. This occurs infrequently, however, and usually does not produce an aesthetic defect. Correction is necessary only at the patient's request. To stabilize the implant, it should be removed and reinserted directly on bone after secondary elevation of the periosteum laterally.

Another infrequent occurrence is folding or buckling of the lateral extension limb. Again,

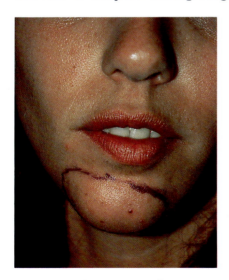

Figure 6.52. Patient with external chin deformity due to rotation of central implant.

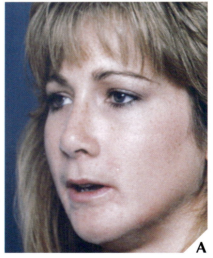

Figure 6.53. Slippage of lateral limb of extended mandibular implant. **(A)** Preoperative view. **(B)**

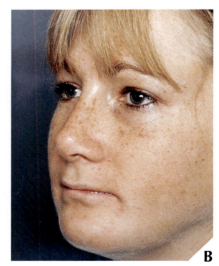

Postoperative view displaying abnormal mandibular curve.

removal and replacement or in situ correction and realignment with an elevator will easily remedy this complication.

According to ASPS survey, contour abnormalities along the lateral margins occurred infrequently when extended mandible implants were used. Such complications are due solely to the inadequate techniques for refining and tapering the lateral lines of currently available implants (Fig. 6.54). Computer-generated designs and production molds that will be available should remedy this problem by providing the needed precision. Presently, to avoid contour abnormalities, the surgeon may hand carve the tails of the implant to 1 to 2 mm. Calipers are essential for choosing proper facial implants. In self-carving, the surgeon may achieve better precision by using either scissors or a conventional Dermabrader with a special coarse rotational tip.

HEMATOMA AND INFECTION

Hematoma and infection are uncommon occurrences with alloplastic chin and mandible implants. In the ASPRS survey, this complication was experienced by only 10 to 20% of the responding surgeons (se Fig. 6.50). The control of bleeding by local and systemic anesthesia assists in preventing hematoma. Accurate dissection directly on bone, without extending dissection into the muscle planes, also minimizes this possibility. Copious irrigation with antibiotic solution is used to flush out undesirable blood. Patients who develop postoperative blood pressure elevation, agitation, nausea, vomiting, etc., are managed by the anesthetic approach previously described.

Persistent swelling after chin-mandible augmentation is normal for several weeks. It appears that nearly all patients who undergo chin-mandible implants experience moderate pain and discomfort, in contradistinction to malar augmentation, which is followed by a minimum of pain.

Cellulitis is customarily managed by proper antibiotics, expectant waiting, and frequent, close observation. Unless prompt resolution occurs, removal of the implant is indicated. Gross infection accompanied by purulence usually mandates immediate implant removal.

Such infections are quite uncommon with smooth Silastic implants. Porous materials, such as Proplast and Dacron-backed implants, encourage the ingrowth of bacterial contamination. The incidence of infection with these materials in considerably greater. In fact, the difference is so great that in the author's opinion, their use should be prohibited. If infection should occur around Silastic implants, it can be resolved with adequate drainage and antibiotic techniques, as described previously. Infections of porous implants are nearly impossible to suppress.

SEROMA

Postoperative seroma in chin-mandible implants is unusual, but may occur 10 to 21 days following surgery. Percutaneous needle aspiration is indicated. Gram-stain and bacterial culture of the aspirated fluid dictates antibiotic coverage.

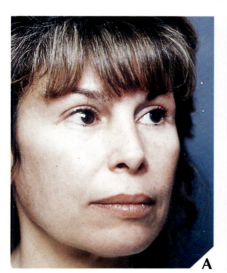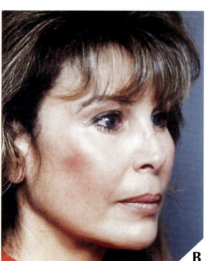

Figure 6.54. Patient with malar and mandibular augmentations with slight lateral prominance of implant in the ML zone. **(A)** Preoperative view. **(B)** Postoperative view displaying slight lateral deformity.

EXTRUSION

Extrusion of chin-mandible implants should rarely occur. It can be prevented by creating a comfortable space for the implant, as well as providing adequate soft tissue coverage (Fig. 6.55).

Extrusion can occur following traumatic displacement of the implant or inadequate healing of the overlying soft tissue. The latter may develop from ischemic tissue damage or wound tension during insertion. Even the largest extended chin-mandible implants should not produce problematic wound healing or extrusion. The causes of these complications are technical and can be avoided by accurate use of the surgical procedures herein described.

MENTAL AND FACIAL NERVE DYSFUNCTION

When alloplastic chin augmentation is performed, the complication of greatest concern to the surgeon is nerve dysfunction. Aberrations of physical shape, size, or position of implants can, in most cases, be altered or corrected. Nerve dys-function, however, may have an element of permanence. It is always a concern because of its crippling effect on the patient's movement and sensation.

In premandibular implantation, mental nerve damage is possible. Damage to the marginal mandibular branch of the facial nerve resulting in permanent disruption of normal lower lip function (Fig. 6.56) is also possible, although the author has never observed this complication, nor was it reported in the ASPRS survey. Such consequences of surgery can be devastating to patients. The primary consideration in preventing nerve injury is to dissect directly on the bone, not into soft tissue. The anatomy of the marginal mandibular branch of the facial nerve and the mental nerve must be well known. The surgeon should follow the orthopedic dictum that the bony plane is safe. Elevation of the tissues from the bone should rarely, if ever, create nerve damage. The premise was confirmed in the ASPRS survey, which revealed a low incidence of permanent nerve dysfunction (see Fig. 6.44).

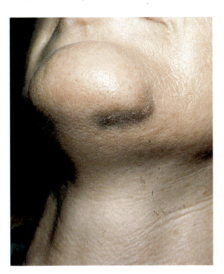
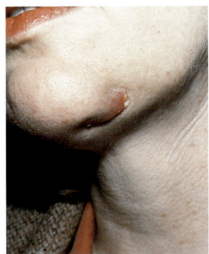

Figure 6.55. Patient with extrusion of implant 3 months postoperatively (etiology unknown). (Courtesy of John Osborne, M.D.)

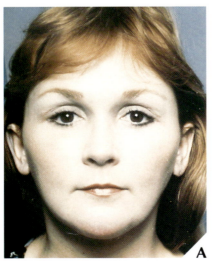
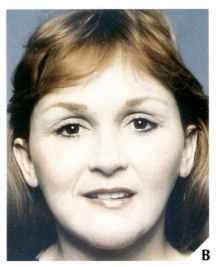

Figure 6.56. Patient with transient marginal mandibular nerve paresis 2 weeks following chin augmentation. **(A)** Face in repose. **(B)** Animated face demonstrating nerve dysfunction.

The mental nerve is encased in a strong perineural sheath. The mental foramen directs the nerve in a superior direction, keeping it highly protected from the assaults of the surgeon's instrument. By maintaining the surgical dissection along the inferior aspect of the mandible, the nerves are avoided. The marginal branch of the facial nerve, which animates the lower lip, resides in the soft tissues above the bony plane and should not be injured unless there is severe traction or direct injury.

Nonetheless, traumatic damage to the mental nerve is reported consistently. A significant percentage of patients temporarily experience numbness and hypesthesia in greater or lesser areas of the lower lip. These symptoms are probably caused by traction of the mental nerve and stretching of its fibers during the manipulation needed to insert extended chin implants. These results are almost nonexistent when the dissection and insertion of these implants into the soft tissue tunnel is done gently. Such an approach is facilitated by directly visualizing the nerve, using proper instruments, such as narrow retractors and lighted fiberoptics (Fig. 6.57). Implants can and should be inserted accurately and with minimal trauma to the tissues (Fig. 6.58).

In some instances, nerve symptoms may result from implant malposition, with infringement on the mental nerve and foramen territory. This can be avoided by accurate placement. Secondary correction involves repositioning or, ideally, substituting an extended contour implant, which is less likely to become unstable.

SECONDARY MALAR-MIDFACE AND CHIN-MANDIBLE AUGMENTATION

Secondary chin augmentation involves the same principles as primary chin augmentation. As previously discussed, fenestrated, cloth-backing, or porous implants, such as Proplast, make secondary dissections difficult.

During implant removal, the following principles should be followed: 1) Expand the tissues surrounding the implant and beneath the periosteum with a large volume of local anesthesia; 30 to 50 cc of dilute Lidocaine (0.1%) with epinephrine (1/400,000) are injected beneath the implant into bone, as well as into the surrounding soft tissue where the elevator dissection may traumatize tissues. 2) Elevate the implant from the bone by secondary subperiosteal dissection; at the same time this dissection should be extended to completely create the floor of the implant space. 3) Open the implant capsule and dissect directly upon the implant itself, especially when dealing with Proplast and fenestrated Silastic implants. In other words, to avoid nerve or muscle damage, *only dissect within the capsule and directly on the surface of the implant.* A gentle scissor-spreading dissection directly on the implant will generally release it from either tissue ingrowth or the adhesions that bridge through the fenestration. 4) Apply traction on the implant with a straight clamp during the extraction process to visualize the implant, allowing the surgeon

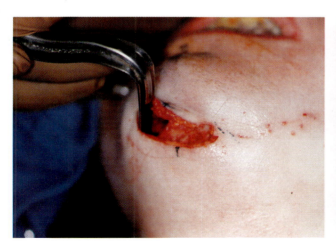

Figure 6.57. Fiberoptic retractors facilitate visualization of the mental nerve.

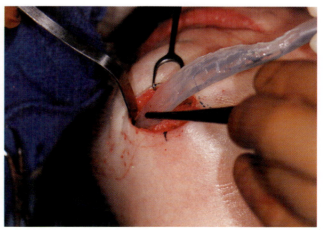

Figure 6.58. Implants should be placed accurately and with minimal trauma.

to remove it in its entirety without leaving fractured fragments. 5) The extraction forces must be gentle to prevent damage to the mental nerve. If removal is traumatic and involves dissection into the surrounding soft tissues, significant chin deformities may result (H. Kawamoto, personal communication, 1990).

Adequate expansion of the space to accommodate a new implant is accomplished with a dissection procedure identical to that used for any other implant. The incidence of nerve damage, hypesthesia, and paresthesia are increased with secondary augmentation; however, when they occur their symptoms and longevity should be minimal.

Patients occasionally will develop, in the central chin mound region, peculiar muscle adhesions that may become visible during facial animation, such as smiling, talking, whistling, etc. This occurrence is rare and usually minimal, and mostly resolves itself during healing, softening, and attenuation of the capsule, which normally occurs over a prolonged time period.

BONE EROSION AND RESORPTION

No discussion of alloplastic face implants would be complete without addressing the topic of bone erosion. Although many investigators have extensively reviewed this subject, it is noteworthy that very few cases of dental damage have been cited. This was also found to be true in the ASPRS survey. Bone erosion was not specifically mentioned as a complication in the comments and data provided by the 300 responding surgeons.

One fact is irrefutable, however. For unknown reasons, bone erosion exists in a significant percentage of patients with facial implants. Whether the erosion occurs more frequently from subperiosteal placement or supraperiosteal has never been established in investigators' studies.

Bone erosion does exist in mandible augmentation, even when extended anatomic implants are used. In cases observed by the author, the degree of erosion appears to be minimized, however, with the use of extended implants. Perhaps this is because the soft tissue pressure forces are distributed over a broader anatomic surface area.

Bone erosion has also been observed occasionally in patients with malar implants that were inserted 8 to 15 years previously. The process has been noted with both Proplast and Silastic implants. It does not seem that malar bone erosion presents a significant problem, unless it becomes severe enough to produce a gross contour deformity if an implant were permanently removed. This seems unlikely.

Bone erosion with small centrally placed chin implants is not unusual, and can be significant. The erosion is oval or square, depending on the shape of the implant, and it may be as deep as five to 8 mm. It presents a problem for surgical correction when it interferes with the positioning of a new implant. An osteotome or a power tool may be necessary to contour the resultant bone irregularities that are preventing a new implant from resting symmetrically and securely upon the bone (Fig. 6.59). Another option is to fill the bony excavation with autogenous tissue, such as temporalis fascia or galea. Bone wax may also be used.

Bone erosion from alloplastic facial implants apparently does not cause significant medical problems, for the statistics do not show any resulting dental complications, such as root impingement or abscess. Instead, thousands of successful augmentations have been performed over the past 30 years without such data being

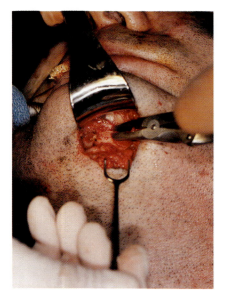

Figure 6.59.
Bone erosion in a patient postoperatively. Correction of an osseous deformity is necessary to allow accurate positioning of a new implant.

presented. In fact, reported series of dental complications are notably non-existent.

When an atrophic mandible is augmented, there is concern about erosion weakening the structural integrity of the bone. This theoretical complication has also not been frequently reported as a problem. Nevertheless, it should be considered when dealing with the older patient or a patient with frequent dental problems. Mandibular resorption with aging occurs from the tooth socket down toward the mental foramen, whereas implants are located on the bone inferior to the tooth roots. This part of the mandibular architecture remains sturdy throughout life.

There are a few reported cases of dental infections posing a threat to alloplastic implants, but in very few of these cases was removal of the implant necessary. Concern is always present, however, when dental infections of the mandible of maxilla arise. These infections should be treated even more intensively with antibiotics in the presence of malar or mandible implants. All facial implant patients should be placed on prophylactic antibiotic coverage 12 to 24 hours prior to any dental procedure, even cleaning.

To conclude, bone erosion in patients with facial implants presents a potential hazard more than a real one, but it should always be considered by the surgeon.

CONCLUSION

Malar and mandibular augmentation surgery made remarkable advances through the 1970s and 1980s and is continuing to do so today. The procedures have won acceptance by both physicians and patients. In the future, computerized technology will provide the surgeon with accurate correlation between facial image and implant design, as well as the means for precise production and selection of implants. At the present time, postsurgical complications are not rare, but they do not occur in statistically or prohibitively high numbers. New materials and improved techniques resulting from the increased experience of physicians will provide more accurate diagnoses and performance, thereby dramatically reducing the incidence of complications and patient dissatisfaction.

ACKOWLEDGEMENT

I would like to gratefully acknowledge the superb assistance of my father, Anthony and Dr. Sekhar in creating this manuscript.

BIBLIOGRAPHY

Binder WJ, Kamer FM, Parkes ML: Mentoplasty—a clinical analysis of alloplastic implants. Laryngoscope 91:383, 1981.

Courtiss E: Complication in aesthetic malar augmentation—discussion. Plast Reconstr Surg 71:648, 1983.

Dan JJ, Epker BN: Proplast genioplasty: a retrospective study with treatment recommendations. Ang Orthod 47(3):173, 1977.

Gonzales-Ulloa M: Building out the malar prominences as an addition to rhytidectomy. Plast Reconstr Surg 53:293, 1974

Gonzales-Ulloa, M: Planning for the integral correction of the human profile. J Int Coll Surg 36:3, 1961.

Hinderer UT: Malar implants for improvement of the facial appearance. Plast Reconstr Surg 56:157, 1975.

Hoffman S: Loss of a silastic chin implant following a dental infection. Ann Plast Surgery 7(6):484, 1981.

Jabaley M, Hoopes J, Cochran T: Transoral silastic augmentation of the malar region: Br J Plast Surg 27:98, 1974.

Kent JN, Westfall RL, Carlton DM: Chin and zygomaticomaxillary augmentation with Proplast: long-term follow-up J Oral Surg 39:912, 1981.

Lilla JA, Vistenes LM, Jobe RP: The long term effects of hard alloplastic implants when put on bone. Plast Reconstr Surg 58:14, 1976.

McKenzie ML: Mandibular reconstruction using silicone: fifteen-year follow-up. Plast Reconstr Surg 74(4):531, 1984.

Millard RD: Augmentation mentoplasty. Surg Clin North Am 51:333, 1971.

Robinson M, Shuken R: Bone resorption under plastic chin implants. J Oral Surg 27:116, 1969.

Schultz, RC: Reconstruction of facial deformities with alloplastic material. Ann Plast Surg 7(6):434, 1981.

Whitaker LA: Aesthetic augmentation of the malar midface structures. Plast Reconstr Surg 80(3):387, 1987.

Wilkinson TS: Complications in aesthetic malar augmentation. Plast Reconstr Surg 71(5):643, 1983.

Wolfe SA: Chin advancement as an aid in correction of deformities of the mental and submental regions. Plast Reconstr Surg 67(5):624, 1981.

Zarem HA: Silastic implants in plastic surgery. Surg Clin North Am 48:129, 1968.

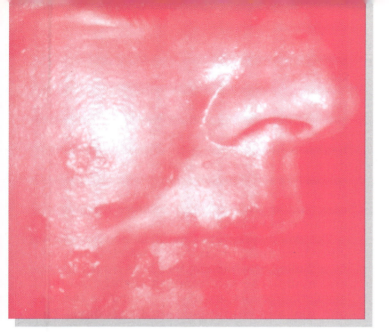

CHEMICAL FACE PEELS

Clyde Litton
Edward H. Szachowicz II

C H A P T E R 7

HISTORY OF CHEMICAL FACE PEELING

Several early reports exist of the use of a superficial skin exfoliant without the use of tapes or an adhesive mask.[1,10,21] However, Urkov[27] in 1946 appears to be the first medical practitioner to combine the use of a phenol peel with adhesive dressing for facial skin irregularities. Brown et al.[5] authored the first scholarly account of the phenol face peel, replete with details of formulas, technique, and a histologic review of phenol-induced skin changes. In 1962, Litton[16] presented the technique to plastic surgeons in the United States and added studies of serum phenol levels after the phenol peel. Since that time, facial plastic surgeons have successfully used the technique of chemoexfoliation on thousands of patients.

SKIN PEELING AGENTS AND FORMULAS

Superficial Chemical Peeling

Superficial chemical peel solutions (Fig. 7.1) create a wound limited to the upper layers of the skin (stratum granulosum or upper papillary dermis). Agents typically found in this category include 10 to 35% trichloroacetic acid (TCA), Jessner's solution (Fig. 7.2), resorcin (Unna's paste, Fig. 7.3), alpha-hydroxy acids (glycolic or lactic acids), azelaic acid, and topical retinoic acids.

These mild exfoliating chemicals are used to rejuvenate actinically damaged facial skin and to treat acne vulgaris, pigmentary disturbances (melasma, berloque dermatitis, postinflammatory pigmentary changes), fine wrinkling and superficial scarring.

Although many patients would obtain more benefit from deep chemical peeling or dermabrasion, light chemical peeling may be a rewarding option for patients who are limited by general health or are unwilling to undergo the longer duration of recovery associated with deep chemical peeling and dermabrasion. These "light peels" are simple to perform, require little postoperative care, and, if properly used, produce minimal significant complications.

The skin responds to superficial peeling with an immediate flush, or erythema, which is followed by a dulling or whitening that lasts from 1 to several hours. The skin remains slightly red until exfoliation occurs, usually beginning on the second day and continuing for 3 to 5 days. The degree of peeling is equivalent to that occurring after a mild sunburn, with the skin usually healing enough for a repeat peel after 1 week. Occasionally, in sensitive individuals, the redness and crusting may last up to 3 weeks; however, gradual progressive improvement is usual in these patients also. Deep-pigmented patients may have some brownish crusting during the initial series of peels, when a large amount of pigment is exfoliated.

Medium-Depth Chemical Peeling

TCA as a peeling solution can produce a relatively deep cutaneous burn without serious systemic toxicity. TCA peels are often preferred for the elderly patient, thus avoiding the myocardial toxicity inherent with phenol peel solutions.

Figure 7.1.
Superficial Chemical Peeling Agents

Very Light

Resorcin	Alpha hydroxy acids
Jessner's solution	TCA 10–20% (superficial)
CO_2	Modified Unna's paste
Retin-A	Azelaic acid
5-FU	

Light

TCA 35% (unoccluded, single or multiple frost)

Figure 7.2.
Jessner's Solution

Resorcinol	14	gm
Salicylic acid	14	gm
Lactic acid	14	cc
Q.S. ethanol	100	cc

Figure 7.3.
Letessier's Modification of Unna's Paste

Resorcin	40	gm
Zinc oxide	10	gm
Ceyessatite	2	gm
Benzoin axungia	28	gm

Penetration of the epidermis by the TCA peeling solution can be altered by many variables (Fig. 7.4). Topical retinoic acid (Retin-A) may be used for several months prior to the TCA peel to enhance the results of chemical peeling. Superficial peeling agents (solid CO_2, liquid nitrogen, salicylic or lactic acid) may also be used prior to the TCA peel to disrupt the epidermal barrier, thereby achieving greater depth of penetration into the skin. Furthermore, additional ingredients (Fig. 7.5) may be added to the milder TCA peel solutions (e.g., 35%) that increase penetration into the skin without increasing the concentration of the TCA (methyl salicylate and DMSO). The penetration of TCA into the skin will continue with repeated applications of the peel solution to the skin, and a deep peel can result if a medium-strength solution is reapplied several times.

Generally, light or superficial peels are performed with TCA concentrations ranging from 10 to 25%. Deep TCA peeling can be performed with TCA concentrations of 35 to 50%. Moreover, different concentrations may be used during the deep TCA peeling. Concentrations of TCA as high as 45 to 50% may be applied to the thicker skin of the forehead and cheeks, 35% to the thinner skin of the eyelids, and 25% to the skin of the neck, since it contains fewer adnexal appendages.

The medium-depth TCA peel solutions produce a white frost of the skin, which may last for 20 to 30 minutes and be replaced by erythema. In 2 to 3 days the skin of the face becomes dry and cracked, and moisturizers are begun along with frequent washing of the peeled skin to remove the sloughing skin and serum. Re-epithelialization usually occurs within 7 to 9 days.

Deep Chemical Peeling
PHENOL-OCCLUDED OR UNOCCLUDED
The chemical compositions of the phenol peeling agents create a turbid emulsion that must be thoroughly stirred with the applicator each time the solution is used. The mixture will remain potent for a period of 3 to 6 months and will turn dark brown with age. Croton oil is added in minute amounts as a skin irritant to cause more inflammation, vesication and secondary collagen formation. A soap (glycerin or Septisol) acts as a surfactant to lower surface tension and as an emulsifier to aid in the penetration of the waxes and cholesterol esters on the skin and pore surfaces.

Phenol (C_6H_5OH), also known as carbolic acid, is an aromatic hydrocarbon derived from coal tar. Topically, phenol in high concentrations is a protein precipitant, causing extremely rapid, irreversible denaturation and coagulation of the surface keratin. This layer of keratocoagulation consists of surface keratin proteins bound to the phenol, creating large molecules, and thus forming a protective eschar, which may act as a barrier to further phenol absorption.[22]

PATIENT SELECTION
The therapeutic indications for chemical face peel include multiple actinic and seborrheic keratoses, superficial basal cell malignancies, lentigo maligna, lentigines, and melasma (discoloration of the skin secondary to pregnancy). Cosmetic indications include atrophic changes in the skin due to excessive actinic exposure (Chataigne, sailor's, or farmer's skin), fine rhytides of the face (especially the perioral ridges or grooves; forehead,

---

Figure 7.4.
Penetration Variables in TCA Peels

1. Concentration of TCA
2. Additional ingredients to increase penetration (methyl salicylate, DMSO)
3. Technique of application
4. Prepeel skin preparation (degreasing)
5. Sebaceous gland density and activity
6. Application of prepeel keratolytic agents and solutions (solid CO_2, liquid nitrogen, salicylic or lactic acid)

Figure 7.5.
Medium-Depth Chemical Peeling Agents

TCA
TCA + CO_2
TCA + Jessner's
TCA + methyl salicylate + DMSO

periorbital, and glabellar rhytides), superficial acne scarring, benign pigmentation abnormalities, and excessive skin that cannot be removed by other surgical means.

We believe the phenol peel is not indicated as treatment for invasive malignant lesions, telangiectasia, nevoid lesions (including port-wine stains, hemangiomas, neurofibromatosis, and café-au-lait spots), pre-existing blotchy pigmentation, or enlarged pores. Patients with an active facial herpes simplex infection, hepatorenal disease, unstable cardiac disease, and a known sensitivity to phenol are also not candidates for this procedure.

Treatment of areas other than the face (i.e., the neck below the level of the thyroid cartilage, forearms, and hands) may lead to unpredictable scarring. Fair-complected patients with fine wrinkles are the best candidates. Thick, oily skin with large pores produces a less favorable result.

TECHNIQUE
The patient should be clearly informed about potential sequelae that may result from any pre-existing skin defects, (i.e., excessive pore size on the nose and paranasal regions, abnormal pigmentation, telangiectasia, nevi, etc.). A patient history should be gathered with special attention to any liver, kidney, or cardiac disease. A previous sensitivity to phenol is especially important. A preoperative electrocardiogram and urinalysis are part of our usual evaluation. Screening liver function tests are included if suggested by the history.

A nonflammable skin degreaser (Freon Skin Degreaser) is used to thoroughly cleanse lipids from the areas to be peeled; lipids form a barrier to the penetration of the phenol and a nonuniform peel may result if not removed. A well-ventilated room is essential.

Cardiac arrhythmias are infrequent if the full-face peel is extended over the period of 1 hour, and if no greater than 50% of the face is treated within a 30-minute period.[26]

The patient will experience a stinging sensation and the skin will immediately turn white (frost) as the phenol solution causes keratolysis and keratocoagulation of the epidermis. The denaturation of the keratin protein prevents further penetration and absorption of the phenol.

Extreme caution must be exercised when peeling in the periorbital region, as phenol causes immediate clouding of the cornea. Copious eye irrigations should be performed if phenol comes in contact with the conjunctiva or the cornea. Tears should be wicked away with dry cotton-tipped applicators during the procedure, as tears can mix with the adjacent phenol and run back into the eye or run down the cheek, diluting the phenol solution and resulting in postoperative streaking. The solution is extended over the eyebrows and into the hair of the forehead and temple. The lips should be treated to just beyond the vermillion border.

We usually extend the peel inferiorly below the mandibular margin into the shadow area of the inframandibular region, thus disguising the transition line. Feathering the demarcation line of the phenol peel is not very effective as the keratocoagulation is an "all-or-none" phenomenon. However, by ending the taping at the mandibular margin, the depth of the peel in the inframandibular region will not be as great. Tape, when applied over the treated areas, will ensure a maximal chemical reaction within the skin by minimizing phenol evaporation. Usually two or three layers of tape are applied with care to avoid causing folds or irregularities in the skin, which would cause aberrations postoperatively. After the application

Figure 7.6.
Local Pigmentary Alterations

1. Demarcation lines
2. Hyperpigmentation
3. Hypopigmentation
4. Phenol bleaching
5. Blotchy pigmentation
6. Darkening of existing nevi

Figure 7.7.
Sun-Reactive Skin Types

Skin color (unexposed skin)	Skin type	Sunburn	Tan
White	I	Yes	No
	II	Yes	Mininal
	III	Yes	Yes
Brown	IV	No	Yes
	V	No	Yes
Black	VI	No	Yes

of the tape mask, the patient will again experience a stinging sensation, which will last for 4 to 6 hours.

The patient should be carefully monitored for approximately 1 to 2 hours postoperatively and supplied with generous analgesics (we use Demerol tablets) for the first postoperative day. We can only stress that the patient needs to be instructed to self-medicate before the need arises during this period or else he or she will be left with a distinctly unpleasant recollection of this time.

Forty-eight hours after the tape mask is removed, Vaseline petroleum ointment is gently applied to the face by the patient, softening the eschar. The patient is advised not to remove the crust aggressively, as premature separation of the eschar is the primary cause of localized scarring due to injury to the newly forming epidermis. The eschar will soften and slough with repeated applications of the ointment.

LOCAL SEQUELAE

Abnormal Pigmentation

The most common local complication after any chemical face peeling is abnormal pigmentation (Fig. 7.6). These local pigmentary changes include depigmentation, hypopigmentation, hyperpigmentation, blotchy pigmentation, and darkening of existing nevi. Fewer of these pigmentary abnormalities occur in patients with lighter skin (Fitzpatrick Skin Types I to III, Fig. 7.7). In 1981, when Litton and Trinidad surveyed 588 plastic surgeons using phenol, two out of three surgeons reported pigmentary problems, usually in patients with skin of a lighter color.[18]

A line of demarcation between peeled and unpeeled skin is more evident in people with Type IV skin. Type V (i.e., Asians, Latin, and Indian) skin can develop the most diffuse pigmentary changes with any peeling or wounding agent of the skin, but these changes are more apt to occur with phenol formulas. Type VI skin (i.e., blacks) can also be peeled with phenolic agents, but the skin may be hyperpigmented for as long as 18 to 24 months postpeel.[4]

The histologic changes in peeled skin include a thinning of the epidermis, encompassing a more regular distribution of melanocytes in the basilar cells. These melanocytes now produce many fine melanin pigment granules dispersed in a uniform pattern, eliminating lentigines, freckles, and so-called skin spots, which together represent an uneven distribution of melanin granules in the epidermis. The phenol bleaching, or pink-colored skin, that remains after chemosurgery is caused by hypopigmentation, which allows visibility of the underlying capillary bed, thus producing this color. In some instances, the pink-colored skin may persist for several years. The amount of hypopigmentation after a phenol peel is proportional to the quantity of phenol applied (Figs. 7.8 and 7.9). Deep TCA peels in Types IV to VI skin will usually produce less hypopigmentation than phenol peels. While frequently performed for physician and patient assurance, test spot peels provide no guarantee of the healing of the remaining portion of facial skin.

Hypopigmentation is very common and produces a demarcation between the untreated and treated areas, most noticeable along the angle of

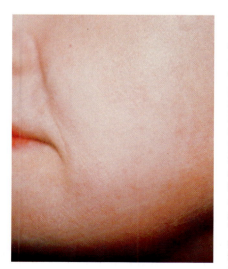

Figure 7.8 Hypopigmentation, which is more common with phenol peel formulas, may not always be homogenous. This patient has uneven return of skin pigmentation in the central cheek and upper lip. The contrast is easily camouflaged in patients with lighter skin.

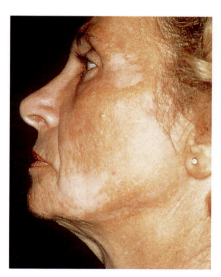

Figure 7.9. Blotchy hypopigmentation as a result of a phenol face peel is very noticeable in patients with darker skin.

the jaw (Figs. 7.10 and 7.11). Camouflaging of the junction between peeled and nonpeeled regions with a phenol solution has been attempted with a very dry applicator and/or application under the jawline using a zig-zag pattern. When only a circumoral phenol peel is being done, the solution can be extended to, and slightly beyond, the nasolabial fold (approximately 5 mm). The lower eyelids should be peeled inferiorly to the infraorbital rims and laterally onto the temple to eradicate the "smile" lines.

Hyperpigmentation is more common with TCA peels, usually due to ultraviolet light exposure, resulting in blotchy pigmentation mostly over the upper cheek area. Pre-existing areas of hyperpigmentation may become more apparent after the peel, resulting from the hypopigmented areas outlining the darker region. Applications of a bleaching formula containing steroids should be started as soon as the abnormal pigmentation is noted. Hyperpigmentation, especially in patients with Type V skin, can be minimized by applying a bleaching solution prophylactically to the peeled skin immediately, or as soon as possible after epithelialization (a combination of 0.1% retinoic acid, 4% hydroquinone gel, and steroid cream no stronger than 0.1% triamcinolone).[4,7]

Hyperpigmentation can also result from a phenol peel, and may be due to exogenous estrogens, pregnancy within 6 months postpeel, photosensi-tizing drugs, phenothiazines, and benzodiazepines. These medications may need to be discontinued before the patient's hyperpigmentation resolves or responds to therapy (application of a bleaching agent or reapplication of phenol over the persistent hyperpigmented areas).[6]

Patients are advised to wear a sunscreening ointment, avoid unnecessary sun exposure and be patient for a period of 6 to 18 months, awaiting the return of normal pigmentation. They should also be reminded that reflected light from glass (as occurs inside a car), water, sand, and other light colored surfaces can stimulate irregularities in pigmentation.

In resistant cases, the use of 5% hydroquinone in Vehicle/N can be topically applied to hyperpigmented areas. We have also found that using salicylic acid and resorcinol has produced some beneficial lightening, when applied as a light peeling solution with a minimum of 3 months between peeling procedures.[18] When only a bleaching effect is needed, 20% TCA may be used; however, the use of 50% TCA has been associated with hypertrophic scarring.

Blotchy or even streaked pigmentation is the manifestation of differences in the depth of the peel caused by one or more of the following factors: faulty technique, failure to cleanse the skin properly, inadequate stirring of the phenol solution during application, nonuniform application of

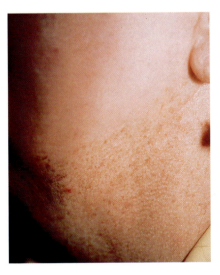

Figure 7.10. A line of demarcation between peeled skin and unpeeled skin is more evident in heavily pigmented, freckled skin. Hypopigmentation of the skin is a common sequela of phenol peel formulas.

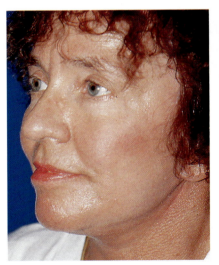

Figure 7.11. This patient with heavily pigmented skin underwent a phenol peel 6 months after a facelift. An attempt was made to hide the transition line between peeled and unpeeled skin in the shadow zone beneath the mandibular margin. Note the homogenous hypopigmentation of the facial skin compared to the unpeeled neck skin.

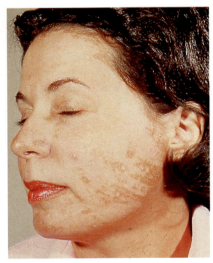

Figure 7.12. Streaked pigmentation across the cheek of this patient may have resulted from 1) failure to degrease the skin properly prior to the peel, 2) inadequate stirring of the phenol emulsion during the peel, or 3) an unevenly applied tape mask. This patient was later repeeled and healed with homogenous pigmentation.

the solution to the skin, or an unevenly applied tape mask (Fig. 7.12). Repeeling of the involved areas with phenol or TCA should be considered 3 to 4 months following the initial peel.

Pigmented nevi may appear darker following a phenol peel in contrast to the surrounding hypopigmented skin. Every nevus on the face should be documented and large or very obvious nevi should be removed prior to the peel. A nevus that appears darker following a peel may be lightened by the application of liquid nitrogen.

Persistent Erythema

Postinflammatory erythema is seen in all patients following a chemical peel, with severe erythema lasting up to 14 days. After the second week, if there are areas of persistent erythema alongside generalized healing, the residual erythema in these areas may indicate incipient scar formation. It may be appropriate to treat these areas with a fluorinated steroid cream or, if necessary, systemic steroids.[6]

The bright erythema seen early postpeel typically disappears in 4 to 8 weeks but may disturbingly persist up to 20 weeks (Figs. 7.13 to 7.15). Early postpeel, the erythema can be associated with pruritus and dermatographism. Postpeel pruritus can be severe and excoriation with possible scarring can result. To minimize itching and burning in the immediate postpeel interval, Hydroxyzine (25 to 50 mg P.O. at night) and, if needed, Diphenylhydramine (25 mg at night) are recommended.

Collins[6] states that the resolution of the erythema and pruritus may be hastened by the administration of systemic steroids (1.5 ml IM of Celestone Soluspan); topical steroids, although effective, might accentuate or produce telangiectasia.

Spira et al[24] described an unusual patient with recurrent episodes of malar and cheek erythema continuing for more than 2 years after a rhytidectomy followed by a full face phenol peel. It has been suggested that the ingestion of alcoholic beverages may be associated with a temporary increase in erythema.

Telangiectasia

Telangiectasias are vascular dilatations of small or terminal vessels located intradermally; they are not usually affected by the chemical peel. However, the subsequent thinner, clearer skin of the postpeel patient may make pre-existing telangiectasias more apparent. We recommend that electrocoagulation (with an insulated platinum wire) of the feeder vessels be done prior to the chemical peel, as telangiectasias are difficult to handle postpeel without noticeable scarring.

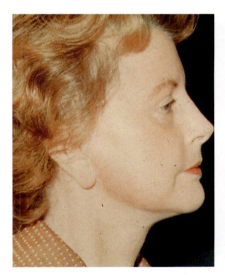

Figure 7.13. Postinflammatory erythema is common in the first 6 to 8 weeks postpeel and is classified as persistent if the duration extends beyond 8 weeks. This patient with light skin manifests some residual erythema on the cheek, adjacent to the mandibular line, at 6 weeks.

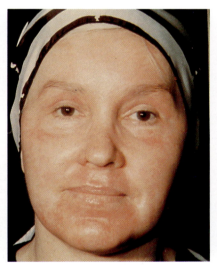

Figure 7.14. The region of the upper cheek and lower eyelids is often the last region to have the erythema resolve. This patient also continues to have redness in the perioral region.

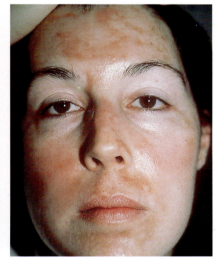

Figure 7.15. The erythema may be blotchy and irregular early postpeel. Postpeel pruritus can be severe, and the patient may need to be medicated to prevent excoriation.

Cutaneous pulse laser therapy may be a new modality that may prove beneficial for treatment of telangiectasia.

Milia

Milia, or inclusion cysts, appear 4 to 6 weeks postpeel and may result when dermal debris or ointment cause temporary blockage of the pilosebaceous unit. Fine milia clear spontaneously; resolution may be hastened by gentle abrasion (Buf Puff), sharp incision with the edge of a fine needle, or application of retinoic acid. Pretreatment with retinoic acid can reduce the occurrence of milia after face peeling.

Skin Pore Prominence

The orifices of the pilosebaceous glands of the nose and paranasal regions may increase in size whenever the procedure involves the deep dermis, whether by chemical peeling or dermabrasion. Because the orifice of these glands enlarges as they descend into the deeper layers of the skin, a larger ductal opening is exposed with the loss of the upper dermis. To avoid this negative sequela, if the indication for the chemical face peel is abnormal pigmentation (not deep rhytides), the peel should be superficial and not occluded with tape. Peel no deeper than necessary to treat the patient's problem.

The skin pores will also appear more prominent when not masked by other textural and pigmentary problems of the untreated skin.

COMPLICATIONS

A complication is a condition occurring during the peeling that may adversely affect the expected outcome. When discussing a chemical peel with patients, they should be informed of sequelae as well as possible complications. Complications may occur despite reasonable precautions and meticulous technique. Awareness is the key to rapid recognition of possible complications, followed by appropriate treatment to minimize the severity of the problem.

Cardiac Arrhythmias

TCA is not absorbed through the skin and is nontoxic to the internal organs.[6] However, phenol is readily absorbed and can be cardiotoxic (Fig. 7.16), hepatotoxic, and nephrotoxic. Dilution with a solvent, such as water or alcohol, may actually increase the amount of phenol absorbed, as coag-

---

Figure 7.16.
Cardiac Toxicity from Phenol

Prepeel Evaluation

1. Arrhythmias occur more frequently in patients with a previous history or current problem of cardiac disease
2. Toxicity may be enhanced in presence of kidney or liver disease

Technique

1. Continuous cardiac monitoring
2. Apply phenol to small facial units while allowing 10- to 15-min intervals between units; duration of procedure 60 min or greater
3. Absorption depends more on total area of skin treated than concentration of solution
4. Intravenous hydration and diuresis before and during the phenol peel

Treatment

Common types of arrhythmias from phenol: premature ventricular contractions, bigeminy, paroxysmal, atrial and ventricular tachycardia,[26] with progression to atrial fibrillation in severe cases[11]

1. Stop phenol application if arrhythmias appear
2. Deliver nasal oxygen
3. Ventricular arrhythmias - Lidocaine
4. Supraventricular arrhythmias - Propranolol
5. Resume peeling only after normal sinus rhythm has been established for 15 min, then extend the peel interval between facial units by an additional 15 min (McCollough & Langston)

ulation of the dermal proteins may not occur, thus allowing even more phenol to enter the circulation. As phenol is absorbed through the skin, it penetrates all the tissues extremely rapidly; the severity of the intoxication is in direct relation to the concentration of free (unconjugated) phenol in the blood and tissues.[7] The liver, kidney, gastrointestinal tract, lungs and red blood cells all have some ability to detoxify circulating phenols by conjugation with sulfates and glucuronides (60 to 80% of the dose).

Signs of systemic toxicity include initial central nervous system stimulation (tremors, hyperreflexia, hypertension) followed by central nervous system depression (respiratory failure, hypotension, and cardiac arrhythmias).

Deaths as a result of phenol chemosurgery are decidedly rare. In our own three surveys of plastic surgeons and in a review of the literature, thousands of cases of phenol facial peels have been done with only one mention of a fatal complication.[20]

METABOLISM OF PHENOL

The mammalian body has pre-existing mechanisms for the removal of phenol by conjugation, oxidation, and direct excretion. Deichmann and Witherup[8] state that the extent of absorption of phenol from the skin appeared to be determined primarily by the magnitude of the skin exposed and secondarily by the concentration of the solution. The nonabsorbed phenol can be oxidized to carbon dioxide and water; small quantities are oxidized to catechol and quinol.[22] Free, unconjugated phenol can be directly excreted in the urine; this usually occurs when the serum level of free phenol is high. Wexler et al[28] have demonstrated that the excretion of free phenol during a chemical peel can be facilitated by a forced diuresis (a fluid infusion combined with a diuretic); alkalinization of the urine will further increase the renal tubular excretion of this weak acid.[1] In 1973, Litton et al[17] reported three cases of cardiac arrhythmias in a survey of 493 plastic surgeons who performed phenol face peels. Truppman and Ellenby[26] analyzed 43 consecutive patients with continuous cardiac monitoring throughout the phenol chemosurgical procedure. Ten of 43 patients (23%) developed some form of arrhythmias. The incidence of arrhythmias was highly correlated with: 1) duration of the procedure, and 2) size of the area covered with the phenol solution. All 10 of the 43 patients who developed the arrhythmias did so within 30 minutes of the start of the procedure and, in all 10, 50% or more of the surface area of the face had been painted with the phenol solution by the onset of the disturbance. No arrhythmias occurred in any patient whose chemical peel spanned 60 minutes or more, or when the treated areas involved less than 50% of the face.

In a follow-up survey, Litton and Trinidad[18] reported that 13% of the 588 plastic surgeons responding who used phenol for face peels encountered some type of cardiac arrhythmias in their patients (however, only 51% used continuous cardiac monitoring). These authors hypothesized the sequence of events leading to the disturbances resulted from the rapid absorption of phenol into the bloodstream, with a direct toxic effect on the sensitive myocardium producing tachycardia (atrial and ventricular), premature ventricular contractions, and, if not treated adequately, ventricular fibrillation and cardiac arrest.

Serum phenol levels drawn at the end of the procedure followed an incremental elevation as additional surface area of the face and neck was included. Gross[11] found that serum phenol levels varied dramatically among patients, but were higher than the initial studies by Litton, as reported earlier.[16] No relationship could be formulated between serum phenol level and the appearance of cardiac arrhythmias. The duration of the arrhythmias ranged from 2 to 19 minutes and appears to closely match the time necessary for the detoxification of the phenol to below the individual patient's arrhythmia threshold.

Wexler et al.[28] demonstrated a significant reduction in ventricular arrhythmias during the topical application of phenol in rabbits concurrently prepared with a fluid load and furosemide to promote a brisk diuresis. Importantly, no arrhythmias occurred in animals undergoing a gradual application of the phenol face peeling solution (i.e., over 20 to 30 minutes).

Considering the many reports of phenol cardiotoxicity which are emerging,[15] it is clear that continuous cardiac monitoring and the slow application of the phenol solution are essential. There is no known antidote after the phenol is absorbed into the bloodstream.

If arrhythmias do occur, the application of phenol should stop immediately. Most mild arrhythmias will then spontaneously revert before treatment can be administered. Nasal oxygen should be delivered along with intravenous administration of Lidocaine for ventricular arrhythmias, or propranolol for supraventricular arrhythmias. If arrhythmias persist, removal of the remaining phenol should be considered. Soap and copious amounts of water or olive oil are used to remove any remaining phenol from the skin surface. Alcohol should be avoided as it may facilitate the absorption of more phenol.

Scarring

Scarring is the second most-reported complication (21% of the surgeons in our survey reported some type of resulting scar[18]) following chemical face peeling, which is most frequently performed for the rhytides of the circumoral region. Therefore, the lip, chin, and perioral regions are the most frequently reported sites of scarring, the scarring usually presenting within the first 3 months (Figs. 7.17 to 7.25). However, the concavi-

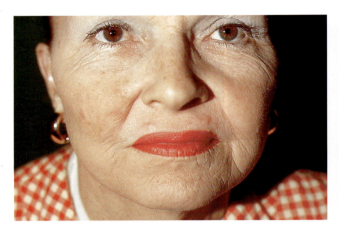

Figure 7.17. Scarring following a chemical peel is most frequently found in the lip, chin, and perioral regions. The scarring may be limited to specific foci, as in this patient with two separate scars in the central portion of the white skin of the upper lip on the right and left sides.

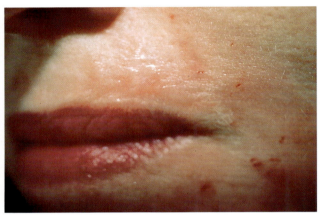

Figure 7.18. Scarring can also present as a broad planar surface of subdermal fibrosis, as seen in this patient's upper lip. Electrolysis of facial hair may effect the outcome of a chemical peel or dermabrasion. Electrolysis destroys skin appendages, which contribute to the regeneration of the upper layers of the skin after removal via a peel or dermabrasion.

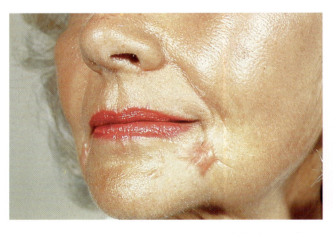

Figure 7.19. Hypertrophic scarring of the lower lip, causing distortion of the oral commissure. This is matched by scarring on the opposite side, as well as a small locus of scar near the chin.

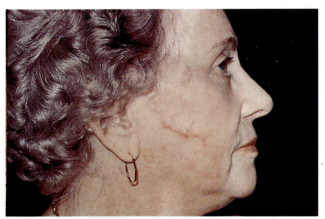

Figure 7.20. Even regions of the face that have thicker skin may have deep dermal injuries resulting in scarring. Note the hypertrophic scar of the central cheek.

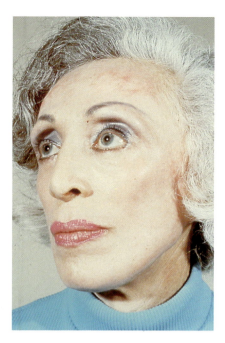

Figure 7.21. An irregular scar across the central forehead region. Dermal injury despite thicker skin is seen once again.

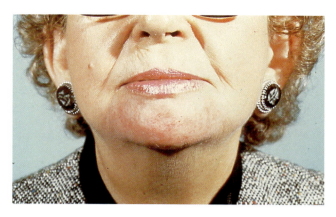

Figure 7.22. Scarring over the chin. When using the tape occlusion technique, the chin and mandible are by far the most mobile structures beneath the tape. The overlying skin in these regions may undergo shearing forces under the tape during the wound and healing phases of the peel. Furthermore, as with any technique, bacterial contamination from saliva may be a factor in unfavorable healing in the chin region.

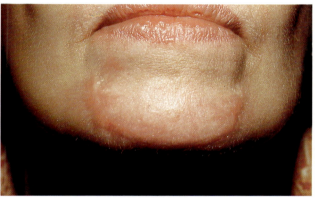

Figure 7.23. Scarring of the chin similar to that seen in Figure 7.22.

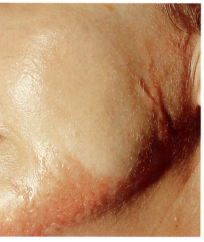

Figure 7.24. Extensive scarring, which may occur at the margin of the mandible. When using the tape occlusion method, caution must be taken not to tape below the mandibular line.

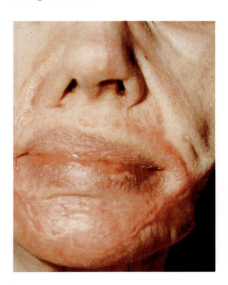

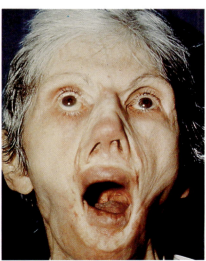

Figure 7.25. This patient underwent a face peel by a lay practitioner in Mexico City. This extreme case demonstrates the dense, hypertrophic scarring that may occur with uncontrolled deep dermal wounding. Note blanching of the scar with mouth opening and the severe distortion of the base of the nose.

ties of the neck and suprasternal regions have a known propensity to develop hypertrophic scars, and these have also been reported with TCA[2,6](Fig. 7.26).

Spira et al.[24] caution against insulting the skin by peeling and undermining the same area simultaneously. These authors reported that the only scars in their series of patients resulted from perioral peels combined with an extended surgical rhytidectomy. The only full-thickness loss of skin occurred in one patient who underwent a chemical peel of the forehead immediately following a browlift procedure (Fig. 7.27). We also recommend that 6 months elapse before chemosurgery is used as an adjunct to blepharoplasty in order to avoid ectropion and scarring (Fig. 7.28).

After chemical peeling and dermabrasion, the mid-to-deep layers of the dermis are exposed and are very susceptible to injury from either mechanical or infectious insults until complete epithelialization occurs. Baker and Gordon[3] feel that limiting the movement of the patient's facial structures (i.e., all nutritions and other fluids through a straw and minimal talking) may be helpful in preserving the integrity of the dermis during healing and may prevent unfavorable scarring. Furthermore, tape, if used, should not be applied in a constricting fashion, which may lead to tissue necrosis with subsequent facial edema or may cause mechanical shear forces on the skin (Figs. 7.29 and 7.30). No tape is applied to the skin of the inferior border of the mandible. These authors suggest that, when a limited perioral peel is performed, taping should be done only around

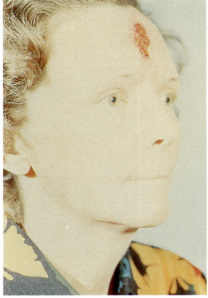

Figure 7.26. Deep chemical peel extended onto the skin of the neck. As the neck skin in females has few adnexal skin appendages with which to regenerate skin, severe scarring has resulted.

Figure 7.27. Caution should be exercised when insulting the skin by chemical peel and undermining the same region simultaneously. This patient experienced a slough of skin when she underwent a chemical peel of the forehead immediately following a browlift procedure.

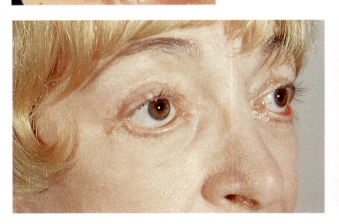

Figure 7.28. Ectropion can result when blepharoplasty is soon followed by a chemical peel. When a chemical peel is planned to remove the fine lines after blepharoplasty, only a conservative amount of skin resection should be undertaken. This condition eventually resolved without any additional treatment.

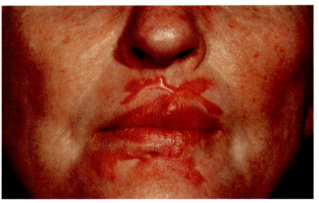

Figure 7.29. Caution must be exercised in postpeel taping to ensure that the circumferential tape is not constricting. Postpeel swelling may cause a constriction in the blood supply. The patient has scarring of the lower lip, which is more typically seen in the central portion of the white skin of the upper lip.

the vermillion ridge to eliminate vertical rhytides and to avoid local skin tensions with more extensive taping.

Szachowicz and Wright[25] have compared the healing after phenol peels to the healing that occurs following freeze injuries to the skin. Freeze-induced injuries heal with much less contraction or hypertrophic scarring, presumably because the freeze injury in these wounds preserves the integrity of the collagen matrix in the dermis. The body replaces the damaged, but intact, matrix gradually, and the myofibroblasts are stimulated to a lesser degree than when a burn injury destroys the collagen matrix. Therefore, the goal for wound healing after a chemical peel is rapid epithelialization with minimal trauma to the remaining dermis by mechanical trauma or infection. These authors reported on two patients who had delayed healing (epithelialization) for up to 6 weeks after a chemical peel, this subsequently healed by conservative treatment, with inapparent scarring.

Concentrations of 50% (or greater) TCA induce deep peeling of the skin; extra caution should be exercised to avoid scarring. Taping is not recommended if TCA is used in these concentrations.

Isotretinoin (Accutane), which is used to treat cystic acne, should be stopped for at least 6 to 12 months before any medium-depth or deep peeling is considered, to prevent the possibility of uncontrolled scarring.[4] Deep face peeling has been reported after facial skin irradiation;[29] however, diminished or absent skin appendages may impair epidermal regeneration and delay wound healing.

Any resultant hypertrophic or contractual scarring should be treated conservatively with intralesional steroids; early scar revision is usually unwarranted (Figs. 7.31 and 7.32).

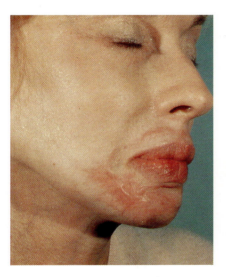

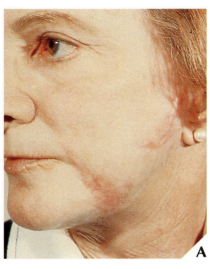

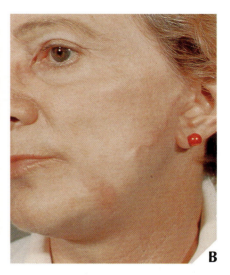

Figure 7.30. Lower lip, as well as upper lip, scarring in patient with constricting postpeel taping.

Figure 7.31. Conservative management with intralesional steroids and tincture of time prove beneficial in the treatment of significant scarring. Note flattening of the scars in the cheek and oral commissure in this patient after 6 months of treatment (**B**).

Figure 7.32. Improvement in scarring over 2 months of conservative management. Note lightening of the pigmentation, resolving of the erythema, and flattening of the contour irregularities (**B**).

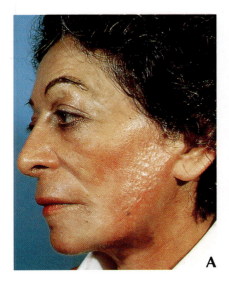

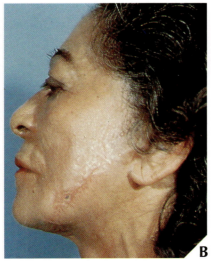

Infection

Phenol and, to some degree, TCA are antiseptics, and infection following a chemical peel is rare. However, an infection can cause rapid and extensive damage to the exposed dermis with subsequent scarring. Meticulous care postpeel is the best preventative measure, followed by rapid recognition and treatment of any infection.

The classic description of the phenol face peel uses an occlusive tape mask that is removed after 48 hours.[16] Then thymol iodide powder is applied to dry the skin and provide topical antibacterial activity until epithelialization takes place.

Since epithelialization occurs more rapidly when the wound is not allowed to dry,[12] we now recommend the use of the occlusive ointments after the slough of the superficial skin layers. These ointments should be completely cleansed away several times per day as serum weeps from the dermis until epithelialization occurs. Crusts should not be allowed to form as bacteria will grow beneath their surface.

Occlusive ointments may promote folliculitis, which may become secondarily infected with *Streptococcus* or *Staphylococcus* and should be treated with penicillinase-resistant antibiotics.

Pseudomonas infections[4] are rapidly progressive and may occur from improper care during healing, or when the patient becomes inoculated from animal contact or acquires a nosocomial infection. The infection is readily treated with oral ciprofloxacin and meticulous wound care (Fig. 7.33).

A recurrence of a facial herpes simplex infection may be activated by the chemical peel and is usually heralded by the onset of unusual and unexpected postpeel pain[4] (Figs. 7.34 and 7.35). Rapaport and Kamer[23] describe four patients who had an exacerbation of facial herpes simplex after phenol chemical peels and none of the patients had residual scarring. Patients with a history of frequent recurrence of herpetic lesions can be prophylactically treated with 200 mg of acyclovir (Zovirax) three times daily 24 hours before the peel and for 4 to 5 days postpeel. An active herpetic outbreak should be treated with therapeutic doses of 400 mg of acyclovir five times daily.

Toxic shock syndrome has been reported in three patients following a staphylococcal infection after a phenol peel.[9,19] The signs of a local

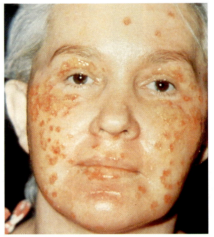

Figure 7.34. Herpes simplex infections should be suspected in patients who experience unexpected postpeel pain. Treatment generally consists of topical and oral acyclovir. Occasionally, scarring may result from the viral infection.

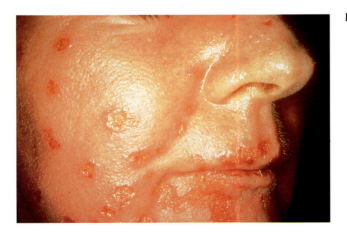

Figure 7.33. A florid *Pseudomonas* infection of the dermis following a chemical peel secondary to improper post-peel care at home. This patient resolved with aggressive management.

Figure 7.35. Herpes simplex infection postpeel.

wound infection are usually minimal or absent, although *Staphylococcus aureus* can usually be grown on cultures. Toxic shock syndrome is a severe toxin-mediated multisystem disease characterized by an acute onset of high fever, hypotension, scarlatiniform rash and desquamation of the skin (especially on the hands and soles of feet), vomiting, diarrhea, and laboratory evidence of multiorgan dysfunction. The typical incubation period of the disease in patients is 2 days postpeel. Aggressively supportive treatment is necessary and anti-staphylococcal agents are used.

HIV-positive patients may be at greater risk for secondary infection postpeel and may have delayed wound healing.[4] Care must also be exercised in the immediate postpeel phase to use generalized wound precautions against the theoretical transmission of the disease.

Systemic Complications

Klein and Little[13] believe that the exposure to either the phenol or the ether (degreaser) vapors precipitated symptoms of laryngeal edema (stridor, hoarseness, and tachypnea) in three patients who were chronic smokers. Brody[4] reported that laryngeal edema occurred in approximately 1.2% of his series of peels and proposed the cause to be a hypersensitivity reaction in the larynx already chronically irritated by cigarette smoke. Pretreatment of chronic smokers with antihistamines may help avoid this condition.

Theoretically, hepatic and renal injury can occur as phenol is detoxified in the liver and excreted through the kidneys. However, no hepatorenal complications from a phenol peel of the face have thus far been reported.

Psychologic disturbances may be caused in those people with claustrophobia who are to have an occlusive tape mask applied postpeel. Furthermore, patients should be psychologically prepared for the appearance of their face for the first few days postpeel, as a properly informed patient is easier to manage.

ACKNOWLEDGMENT

The authors wish to gratefully acknowledge Drs. Thomas Baker, George Brennan, Harold J. Brody, and Howard L. Gordon for their contribution of patient photographs. Because of their expertise in chemical peeling, they have been consulted on patients with poor outcomes and have generously shared their experience with us.

REFERENCES

1. Ayres S III: Dermal changes following application of chemical cauterants to aging skin. Arch Dermatol 82:578, 1960.
2. Ayres S III: Superficial chemosurgery. Arch Dermatol 89:395, 1964.
3. Baker TJ, Gordon HL: Chemical face peeling. Goldwyn RE, (ed): The Unfavorable Result in Plastic Surgery. Little, Brown, Boston, 1972.
4. Brody HJ: Complications of chemical peeling. J Dermatol Surg Oncol 15:1010, 1989.
5. Brown AM, Kaplan LM, Brown ME: Phenol-induced histological skin changes: hazards, technique, and uses. Br J Plast Surg 13:158, 1960.
6. Collins PS: The chemical peel. Clin Dermatol 5:57, 1987.
7. Deichmann WB: Phenol studies V. The distribution, detoxification, and excretion of phenol in the mammalian body. Arch Biochem 3:345, 1944.
8. Deichmann WB, Witherup S: Phenol studies VI. The acute and comparative toxicity of phenol and o-, m-, and p-cresols for experimental animals. J Pharmacol Exp Ther 80:233, 1944.
9. Dmytryshyn JR, Gribble MJ, Kassen BO: Chemical face peel complicated by toxic shock syndrome. Arch Otolaryngol 109:170, 1983.
10. Eller JJ, Wolff S: Skin peeling and scarification. JAMA 116:934, 1941.
11. Gross BG: Cardiac arrhythmias during phenol face peeling. Plast Reconstr Surg 73:590, 1984.
12. Hinman CD, Maiback H: Effect of air exposure and occlusion on experimental human skin wounds. Nature 100:377, 1963.
13. Klein DR, Little JH: Laryngeal edema as a complication of chemical peel. Plast Reconstr Surg 71:419, 1983.
14. Kligman AM: A new formula for depigmenting human skin. Arch Dermatol 3:40, 1975.
15. Koopman CF Jr: Phenol toxicity during face peels. Otolaryngol Head Neck Surg 90:383, 1982.
16. Litton C: Chemical face lifting. Plast Reconstr Surg 29:371, 1962.
17. Litton C, Fournier P, Capinpin A: A survey of chemical peeling of the face. Plast Reconstr Surg 51:645, 1973.
18. Litton C, Trinidad G: Complications of chemical face peeling as evaluated by a questionnaire. Plast Reconstr Surg 67:738, 1981.
19. LoVerme WE, Drapkin MS, Courtiss EH, Wilson RM: Toxic shock syndrome after chemical face

peel. Plast Reconstr Surg 80:115, 1987.

20. Lotter AM: Human pigment factors relative to chemical face peeling. Ann Plast Surg 3:231, 1979.

21. McKee G, Karp F: The treatment of post-acne scars with phenol. Br J Dermatol 64:456, 1952.

22. Pardoe R, Minnami RT, Sato RM, Schlesinger SL: Phenol burns. Burns 3:29, 1976.

23. Rapaport MJ, Kamer F: Exacerbation of facial herpes simplex after phenolic face peels. J Dermatol Surg Oncol 10:57, 1984.

24. Spira M, Gerow FJ, Hardy SB: Complications of chemical peeling. Plast Reconstr Surg 54:397, 1974.

25. Szachowicz EH II, Wright WK: Delayed healing after chemical peels. Fac Plast Surg 6:8, 1989.

26. Truppman ES, Ellenby JD: Major electrocardio graphic changes during chemical face peeling. Plast Reconstr Surg 63:44, 1979.

27. Urkov JC: Surface defects of skin: treatment by controlled exfoliation. Ill Med J 89:75, 1946.

28. Wexler MR, Halon DA, Teitelbaum A, Tadjer G, Peled IJ: The prevention of cardiac arrhythmias produced in an animal model by the topical application of a phenol preparation in common use for face peeling. Plast Reconstr Surg 73:595, 1984.

29. Wolfe SA: Chemical face peeling following therapeutic irradiation. Plast Reconstr Surg 69:859, 1982.

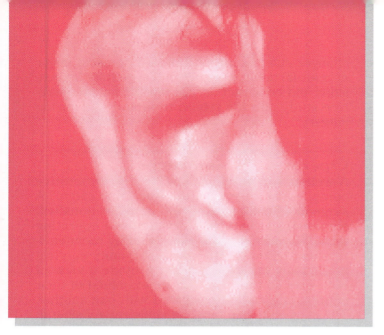

OTOPLASTY

David W. Furnas

CHAPTER 8

Few operations in plastic surgery give greater satisfaction than an otoplasty in a child with conspicuously prominent ears and, fortunately, few operations are as free of complications. Because of its vigorous blood supply, the ear is resistant to wound infections and to surgically induced ischemia. However, the ear is not without vulnerabilities. Among these are the exposed position of the auricle, the thinness of its skin-subcutaneous cover, the delicate, convoluted shape, and the avascularity of the underlying auricular cartilages.

When they occur, surgical complications can be deeply disappointing to the child, the family, and the surgeon. Methods of preventing or dealing with such problems are the subject of this chapter. Topics include pre- and intraoperative steps for prevention of complications, the recognition and treatment of complications of a general nature, and the recognition and treatment of complications specific to otoplasty.

PREVENTION OF COMPLICATIONS

Preoperative Steps

Prevention of complications begins during the initial examination. Detailed evaluation and measurement of the deficiencies of the ears are carried out, with special attention to the character of the cartilage components. Standardized 35-mm photographs of the face and close-up photos of the ears are taken. At the same time a series of Polaroid close-up photos is made and marked with measurements and points of interest. These photos are placed on view during the initial examination to enhance the surgeon's ability to see subtle asymmetries and discrepancies. The photos are valuable for display during surgery where they aid in distinguishing intrinsic features from changes due to surgery. If the ears present major or unusual deformities, we obtain geltrate impressions and construct acrylic models for preoperative study and for sterilization and use during surgery.

Operating Room Steps

A well-known surgical "law" is: "Postoperative complications begin in the operating room!" A surgeon who wants to avoid complications will emphasize attention to detail at the operating table. He must see that the operating room environment lends itself to highest-quality surgical craftsmanship. Drapes must provide a view of both ears so that they can be examined in their entirety and can be compared with one another. The eyes and nose must be sufficiently visible to place the ears in context. The sterile towel around the head must be placed so it will not affect the position of the ears (either before or after the ears have been repositioned). Sterile tapes secure the towel to the forehead and neck. (If towel clips alone are used, the towel will loosen after the head has shifted a few times.) A sterile shower cap secured with sterile tapes is a convenient substitute for a head towel (Fig. 8.1).

Loupes and a coaxial headlamp capture the delicate auricular anatomy for viewing from any angle. A fine-tipped bipolar cautery forceps provides maximum hemostasis with minimum damage to cartilage. Intravenous antibiotics are commenced before making the incisions in order to minimize the chance of stray bacteria establishing residence in the wound.

The specific consistency, thickness, and flexibility of the auricular cartilage of each individual patient is important, and the operative plan must take each feature into account. An otoplasty is, in reality, not an entity, but any of a number of combinations of maneuvers dealing with the antihelix,

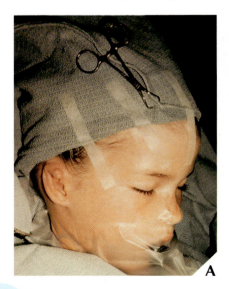 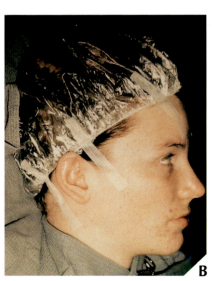

Figure 8.1. Draping with ample view of ears and facial features. **(A)** Head drape with Steri-Strips. Endotracheal tube covered with clear plastic. **(B)** Sterile shower cap substitutes for a head drape.

the concha, the upper pole, the lobe, etc. The surgeon must have an adequate surgical repertoire from which to choose, and he must mentally audition the most promising maneuvers while he is examining and re-examining the patient. At surgery, he must think through the biomechanical and aesthetic consequences of each surgical move, anticipating any negative effects. Critical evaluation continues with each step as it is performed. Sutures that fail to fulfill their mission are removed and replaced.

Dilute Marcaine (bupivacaine) with epinephrine is infiltrated in the operative area at the end of the procedure to minimize postoperative discomfort, restlessness, and movement.

For dressings, we mold Vaseline gauze into the postauricular sulcus and into the anterior interstices of each ear. The ears are then padded with soft cotton or knit gauze fluffs, and the head is wrapped with a turban of soft knit gauze. Preplaced vertical gauze strips are then tied tightly, lifting the turban upward from the eyes (mastoid dressing). Instructions are given for the patient to maintain a head-higher-than-heart position at all times during the early postoperative period, and antiemetic suppositories are made available.

COMPLICATIONS OF A GENERAL NATURE: RECOGNITION AND TREATMENT

Certain complications of otoplasty, such as bleeding, infection, and hypertrophic scars, are common to operative procedures performed elsewhere on the body. Other complications are specific to otoplasty alone. The general complications are discussed first.

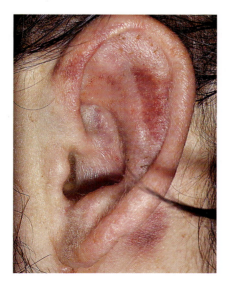

Pain and Tenderness

Excessive pain or tenderness of the ear on the first or second postoperative day suggests the possibility of a hematoma,[3] and the ear is promptly exposed to confirm or deny this suspicion (see discussion on bleeding/hematoma). Pain or tenderness a few days later is suggestive of infection (see discussion on infection).

Occasionally, transient pain is associated with the regeneration of sensory branches of the greater auricular nerve or other sensory nerves that have been transected in the course of surgery. We have heard anecdotal reports of severe, persistent pain of sensory nerve origin, but have not encountered this in practice. Serial injections of bupivacaine should help break up this cycle.

Bleeding and Hematoma Formation

Early recognition of bleeding and hematoma formation is essential to avoid such problems as pressure necrosis and infection. If the wound bleeds to the extent that even a small spot of blood is visible on the dressing, or if pain is a significant complaint, immediate attention is needed (Fig. 8.2). The dressing is removed and the wound inspected. Steps for drainage and hemostasis are instigated in a timely fashion if needed.

Bleeding may result from the "rebound effect" when locally injected epinephrine has been metabolized. While performing hemostasis, the surgeon must maintain a mental image of the large, abundant vessels, which are masked by vasoconstriction. He must thoroughly coagulate even the smallest-appearing vessels with a fine-tip bipolar electrocautery. This will almost eliminate

Figure 8.2. Bleeding. Early diagnosis and prompt treatment of bleeding afford a good prognosis. (Reproduced with permission from Elliott RA Jr: Complications in the treatment of prominent ears. Clin Plast Surg 5:479–490, 1978.)

the possibility of postoperative bleeding or hematoma.

Rarely, bleeding may result from other causes, such as occult coagulopathy, postoperative trauma, or undetermined causes. One of our patients developed simultaneous hematomas in both ears without discernible cause. Bilateral wound drainage was performed and uneventful healing took place.

Infection

Pain, tenderness, inflammation, and swelling are suggestive of wound infection. Once the provisional diagnosis of infection has been made, prompt antibiotic treatment is initiated to avoid involvement of cartilage.

We routinely administer intravenous cefazolin or other antibiotics during surgery to eliminate chance bacterial intruders. Of the two postoperative infections that have occurred in our otoplasty series in the past decade, neither had received intravenous intraoperative antibiotics.

The first patient, a 30-year-old man, underwent a bilateral otoplasty before the use of intraopera-

tive antibiotics had become routine. Persistent edema of the left pinna was recorded but was not appreciated as a sign of incipient infection. The inflammatory signs increased slowly until the entire ear was red and tender, and acute chondritis was diagnosed (Fig. 8.3). Because of the risk of cartilage necrosis and major ear deformity,[16] the patient was hospitalized and placed on intravenous antibiotics. In 1 week, the signs of infection had disappeared, but this was not the end of the story.

Three years later the patient had an episode of recurrent chondritis of his ear. Several weeks previously he had developed an abscess of the left posterior scalp, which was lanced by a friend. The abscess healed completely, but 3 weeks after the lancing, a florid auricular chondritis developed. Since the permanent sutures and scar tissue of the otoplasty were a site of minimum resistance, they served as a nidus for reinfection from a shower of blood- or lymph-borne bacteria. The patient was again treated successfully with intravenous antibiotic, and has had no further problems.

The second patient was a 12-year-old girl in whom otoplasty for prominent ears was carried

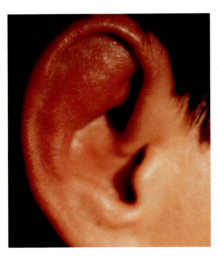

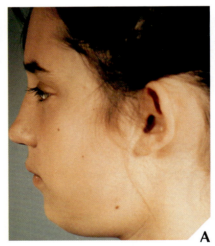

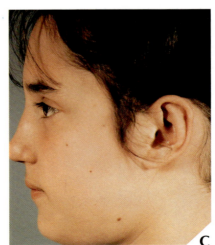

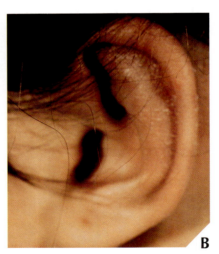

Figure 8.3. Chondritis following otoplasty. Patient was treated with hospitalization and IV antibiotics. A second episode of chondritis occurred 3 years later, which again responded to treatment.

Figure 8.4. Postoperative infection with minimal signs (asymmetric swelling and serous drainage with positive culture for *Staphylococcus aureus*). **(A)** Preoperative. **(B)** Receding edema of right ear 11 days postoperatively during treatment with oral ciprofloxin. **(C)** Postoperative appearance.

out under local anesthesia. In our preoperative discussions with this child, we had promised not to use an intravenous needle and, therefore, we gave no intravenous antibiotics. On examination the day after surgery, the left ear was more swollen than the right. This was attributed to lengthier surgery of the left ear, but after 6 days the swelling persisted and some serous wound drainage was noted. Cultures were taken and cephalexin was given orally. When the sensitivity results were obtained, oral ciprofloxin was substituted for the cephalexin. In 10 days, all signs of infection disappeared and the ultimate outcome of the otoplasty was not compromised (Fig. 8.4).

Allergic Response

Itching of the ears early in the postoperative period suggests an allergic response to allergens, such as iodophors or bacitracin, or an inflammatory response to irritants (Fig. 8.5). The dressing is removed and the ears are inspected. Careful cleansing is carried out (including shampooing if needed). Systemic antihistamines and moist dressings are useful.

Scars and Keloids

Of the exposed facial features, the external ear is the one most prone to unfavorable wound responses. Hypertrophic scarring in the lower half of the postauricular wound is not uncommon. We have seen keloids at this site in five patients, one of which was associated with an extruded suture (Fig. 8.6). Intralesional injection of triamcinolone and application of pressure and massage controlled the process in three cases. In the other two cases, the keloids persisted, and collaboration with the radiotherapy department was obtained (Fig. 8.7). Surgical excision of the keloids and concomitant injections of triamcinolone were followed by 1200 rads of radiation. The radiotherapist delivered the therapy to the wounds in two doses, 600 rads on the day of surgery and 600 rads 1 week later. These steps eliminated the keloids.

Colchicine, penicillamine, and BAPN (beta-amino-propyl nitrile) have provided limited resolution of severe keloids.[15] Methods of treatment of keloids have been reviewed by Rockwell and Cohen.[17]

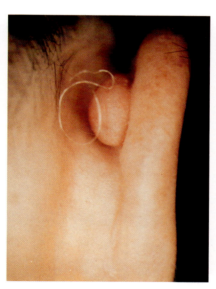

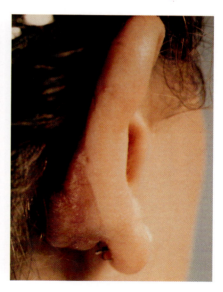

Figure 8.5. Allergic reaction with edema. (Reproduced with permission from Elliott RA Jr: Complications in the treatment of prominent ears. Clin Plast Surg 5:479–490, 1978.)

Figure 8.6. Keloid of postauricular wound with extruded nylon suture 7 years postoperatively. This keloid diminished greatly after the suture was removed.

Figure 8.7. Keloid of postauricular wound after uncomplicated otoplasty. Surgical excision with an injection of triamcinolone and radiation (1200 rads) controlled the keloid.

Psychological Considerations

MacGregor has documented the psychological benefits that are part of every well-selected, well-performed otoplasty.[12] Psychological complications are a negligible risk for surgery in a normal child with clearly prominent ears. However, the surgeon must be cautious in his selection of adult patients and should bear in mind Gorney's cautionary words about procedures on the "Single Immature Male who is Overexpectant and Narcissistic" (SIMON syndrome).[11]

One patient, a 25-year-old man from the Middle East, requested surgical improvement of his earlobes (Fig. 8.8). He had a previous reduction of both earlobes followed by several touch-up procedures. These procedures had been performed with a high degree of finesse by a surgeon in the patient's native land. The earlobes appeared normal and aesthetically acceptable. Nonetheless, the patient was obsessed with the idea that his earlobes were seriously out of proportion with his face. This persistent notion interfered with his interpersonal relationships and his daily living. We advised against further surgery.

COMPLICATIONS SPECIFIC TO OTOPLASTIES

Problems Encountered During Surgery

The wide variety of otoplasty techniques described in the international literature attests to the diversity of maneuvers that can shape or position cartilage. Each maneuver is more effective in some types of cartilage than in others, and each maneuver puts into play side effects that may later appear as early or late complications.

When suture techniques are employed for shaping the auricular cartilage, the character of the cartilage plays an important role in the types of complications that may occur. The surgeon must take this into account during surgery. Certain maneuvers are designed to make heavy, stiff cartilage more compliant, and other maneuvers are designed to gain control over light, floppy cartilage. These maneuvers may be directed at an overdeveloped concha, an underdeveloped antihelix, or another anatomical problem.

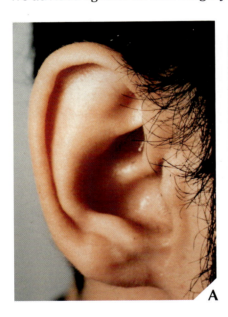 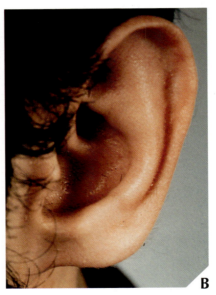

A   B

Figure 8.8. Psychological fixation on shape of earlobes. Patient had previous reduction of both earlobes followed by touch-up procedures. He was obsessed with the idea that he needed further improvement of the earlobes. (**A**) Right earlobe. (**B**) Left earlobe.

HEAVY, STIFF CARTILAGE

If the auricular cartilage is excessively heavy and stiff, the suture force needed to reposition the cartilage may exceed the tolerance of the cartilage for suture erosion. Over a short or long period, the sutures can cut through the cartilage, allowing the ear to drift toward its original position if preventive steps are not taken.

Modifying the Stiff Concha

Reduction of the conchal cartilage by direct excision, from either an anterior or a posterior approach, diminishes the tension needed on the sutures.

From an anterior approach, conchal reduction is done the same way as taking an elliptical skin-cartilage graft. Conchal reduction performed in this manner usually leaves an excellent conchal contour with a pale, fine scar. However, in one of our patients the scar was conspicuous because the linear shape of the scar contrasted with the gentle slope of the concha (Fig. 8.9). The relationship of the scar placement to the conchal contour must be carefully contemplated before using this approach.

Excision of a crescent of cartilage from the posterior part of the conchal floor and the adjoining conchal wall can also be carried out through an incision on the posterior surface of the ear. However, if a large crescent of cartilage is removed, a skin fold or groove may be visible on the anterior surface. Nonetheless, removal of a conservative section of conchal cartilage may enhance the effectiveness of the concha-mastoid sutures in a wide, stiff concha sufficiently to balance the drawback of a groove at the junction of the posterior conchal wall and the conchal floor.

The posterior surface of the conchal floor and the adjacent posterior conchal wall can be thinned with a looped ribbon blade[2] (Fig. 8.10). Total concentration of effort, high-power loupes, and a headlamp are essential when thinning cartilage with the ribbon blade in order to have complete control of the depth of the cuts and to avoid nicks or gouges.

Scoring or rasping of the cartilage on the anterior surface of the concha is another useful maneuver in conchal setback.

Modifying the Heavy Antihelix

The antihelix that is heavy, stiff, and resistent to folding can be approached anteriorly or posteriorly. Scoring or abrading the cartilage of the crest of the superior crus and the antihelix root encourages enhancement of the fold[19] and reduces the force on the sutures. An unmounted diamond burr employed as a hand-held rasp is a useful tool for abrading the cartilage (see Fig. 8.14B).

Although subcutaneous tunnels are our usual access to the cartilage crest of the antihelix, complete "degloving" of the skin of the pinna can provide a direct view of the anterior surface of the scapha-antihelix area and permits very accurate

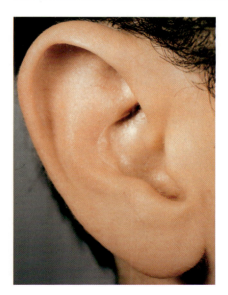
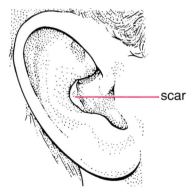

scar

Figure 8.9. Visible scar from anterior conchal cartilage excision in patient who had deep conchae.

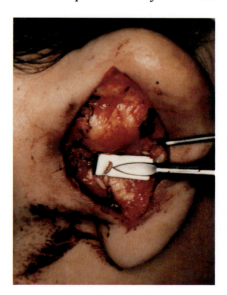

Figure 8.10. Thinning of posterior surface of concha with a ribbon blade (Brody technique).

scoring or abrasion. This approach has provided excellent results when I have employed it. However, detachment of the blood supply from both the anterior and posterior surfaces of the cartilage is a step I prefer to avoid, fearing that, in the rare event of an infection, the devascularized cartilage could possibly be at special risk.

Alternately, the posterior surface of the cartilage of the antihelix can be weakened and the superficial layers of the cartilage trimmed away with a looped blade, taking very thin layers and including a swath 5 to 6 mm wide (see Fig. 8.10). Thinning should be just sufficient that, with mild tension, the sutures will carry the antihelix into a well-rounded curve. The surgeon must be acutely aware that, if the cartilage is thinned excessively, or if the strip which is thinned is too narrow, a narrow fold or a sharp edge can occur, which will spoil the aesthetics of the ear and be difficult or impossible to correct (Figs. 8.11 and 8.12).

SOFT, FLOPPY CARTILAGE

A few times I have encountered prominent ears with soft, floppy auricular cartilage that is overresponsive to mattress sutures. More often than not, these ears have a "third crus" (Figs. 8.13 to 8.15). Normally only the transverse vector of the mattress suture displaces the cartilage, enhancing the longitudinal fold along the crest of the antihelix. However, in soft floppy cartilage, the longitudinal vector also displaces the cartilage, causing buckling of the folded crest. Diminishing the width of the bite of the mattress sutures and placing them closer together helps counteract this

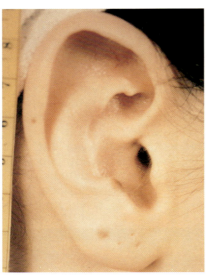

Figure 8.11. Sharp edges and irregularities of cartilage following otoplasty (technique of otoplasty unknown).

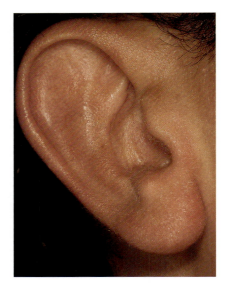

Figure 8.12. Sharp cartilage ridge from excessive thinning and tight sutures. (Reproduced with permission from Elliott RA Jr: Complications in the treatment of prominent ears. Clin Plast Surg 5:479-490, 1978.)

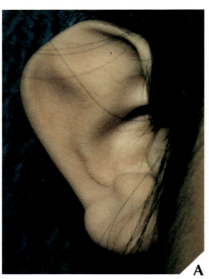

A

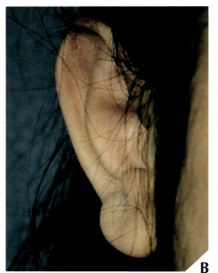

B

Figure 8.13. Soft, floppy cartilage. **(A)** Prominent ears and third crus in patient with floppy, soft auricular cartilage. Conventional placement of mattress sutures caused unwanted buckling; these sutures were removed. **(B)** Correction of ear prominence and third crus with closely placed Mustardé sutures and concha-mastoid sutures. About twice the usual number of sutures were used. Sutures were removed and replaced if buckling appeared.

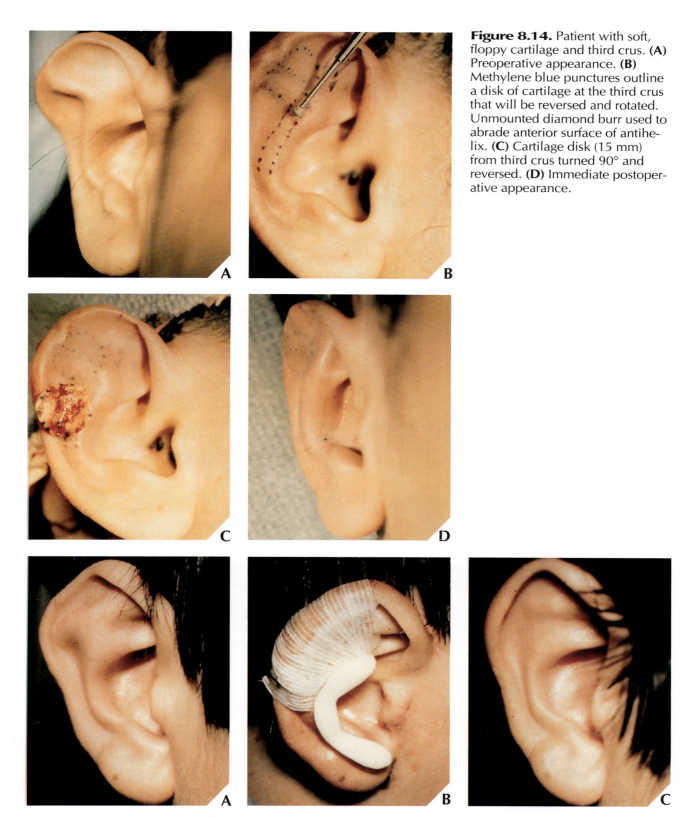

Figure 8.14. Patient with soft, floppy cartilage and third crus. **(A)** Preoperative appearance. **(B)** Methylene blue punctures outline a disk of cartilage at the third crus that will be reversed and rotated. Unmounted diamond burr used to abrade anterior surface of antihelix. **(C)** Cartilage disk (15 mm) from third crus turned 90° and reversed. **(D)** Immediate postoperative appearance.

Figure 8.15. Postoperative molding of ear with soft acrylic. **(A)** Boy with soft, floppy, prominent auricular pinnae (each with a third crus). **(B)** Molding the ear with bone wax covered with Steri-Strips after suture otoplasty and Stenstrom scoring. (The visible C-shaped bone wax on top of the tape is for demonstration only.) The bone wax was available in the operating room; it was soon replaced in the office by a Tru-Soft acrylic mold. **(C)** Appearance 15 months later.

effect. Stenstrom scoring or abrasion is also helpful. Postoperative molding with soft acrylic and Steri-Strips may be helpful (Fig. 8.15B). (This technique is widely used in Japan during the neonatal period for correction of auricular deformities in infants.[13])

OTHER INTRAOPERATIVE PROBLEMS

Several other potential intraoperative problems require the surgeon's attention. Among these are excessive postauricular soft tissue, a tendency for the auditory canal to distort, and development of prominence of the earlobes.

Enhancing Conchal Setback by Soft Tissue Excision (Elliott Maneuver)

Excision of the auricularis posterior muscle and other postauricular soft tissues clears a pocket that accommodates the conchal setback;[4] the sutures pass directly from conchal cartilage to mastoid or sternomastoid fascia. The need for trimming the conchal cartilage is diminished.

Prevention of Distortion of the Auditory Canal

Placement of concha-mastoid sutures too far forward in the mastoid fascia (or too far posterior on the concha) can cause excessive rotation of the concha and narrowing of the auditory canal. The canal is carefully observed as the sutures are tightened,[8,9] and the canal is re-evaluated just before closing the skin.

Prominent Earlobes

For "flyaway earlobes"[6] that become excessively prominent when the pinna is repositioned, I favor the following procedure. A tiny incision is made on the anterior surface of the upper third of the earlobe with a #11 or #65 blade. The edges of the skin are undermined for several millimeters to prevent dimpling. A 6-0 Prolene suture is inserted through the incision, avoiding the superficial layers, engaging the needle in some of the deeper fibrofatty tissue of the earlobe and continuing subcutaneously toward the concha. The needle is retrieved through the postauricular incision, and then it is engaged in an anchorage point in the conchal cartilage. The suture is then passed in the opposite direction, engaging some more fibrofatty tissue of the lobe and emerging from the tiny earlobe incision without catching any of the superficial tissues. The suture is tightened and tied, bringing the lobe medially to the desired position. One or two more sutures are placed as needed to adjust the lobe correctly.[10] These steps are reminiscent of Ely's technique of performing a Stenstrom-type otoplasty through small incisions.[5]

Early Postoperative Changes in Shape or Position

EARLY RELAPSE FROM SUTURE EROSION

I recently treated the partial relapse of a suture otoplasty that occurred a few days after surgery. I had taken too small a bite of conchal cartilage with a key suture and the suture eroded through the cartilage, releasing the pinna. Under local anesthesia, the wound was opened and another suture was placed with a larger bite, correcting the problem.

IRREGULARITIES IN CONTOUR

An otoplasty that shows pleasing, symmetric contours at the completion of surgery can sometimes shift, buckle, or curl from extrinsic pressures (e.g., displaced dressings or misdirected pressure during sleep) or from intrinsic biomechanical effects. Such irregularities can often be corrected in the early postoperative period by maintaining the desired shape with Steri-Strips and molds made from soft acrylic (see Fig. 8.15B) (see discussion on the soft, floppy cartilage.)

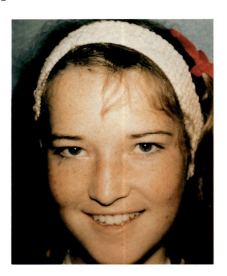

Figure 8.16. Postoperative use of elastic headband. An athletic sweatband is placed to minimize tension on sutures of a suture otoplasty.

HIDDEN HELIX

If prominent ears are over-corrected, the helix will not be seen on frontal view.[18] Even though this is a common finding in normal ears, it is considered unaesthetic in an otoplasty. A slightly hidden helix is acceptable immediately postoperatively as it will emerge into view some months after surgery.

If the antihelix fold is too tight or the conchal setback is excessive, these problems can be corrected, to a certain extent, by a period of very careful manipulation and massage designed to cause carefully controlled erosion and loosening of the sutures. (The risk of complete erosion through the cartilage with release of the sutures and relapse must be borne in mind.) The patient and parents are instructed in the conduct of the massage and manipulation and in careful daily observation of the ears.

UNDESIRED ANGLE OF PROJECTION

The use of an elastic headband, with or without a polyfoam postauricular wedge, is helpful in increasing or decreasing the angle of projection during the early postoperative period (Fig. 8.16).[7] Early recognition and prompt, persistent treatment are important. To diminish the angle of projection, elastic headbands with sufficient elasticity to hold the ears flatter are used. To increase the angle of projection, postauricular wedges are placed and held with tapes and/or a loose headband.

The patient and parents are instructed in careful daily observation of the ears and adjustment of the headband and wedges, according to the response of the ears.

Late Complications

Certain complications do not appear until long after surgery, even though they are a direct consequence of surgical maneuvers. Late relapse, suture exposure, and undesirable shape, such as sharp ridges and irregularities of the cartilage of the pinna, fall into this category.

LATE RELAPSE OF PROMINENT EARS

A small amount of postoperative settling is anticipated when using the suture technique in otoplasty. If the patient is carefully evaluated, the otoplasty maneuvers are carefully selected, and the operation is performed with craftsmanship, the need for correction of a frank relapse will be rare.

To correct a late relapse, we repeat the suture otoplasty (Fig. 8.17). Broad chondral anchorage

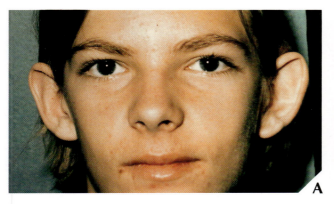
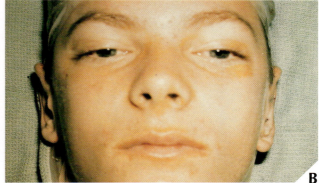
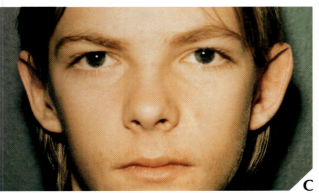
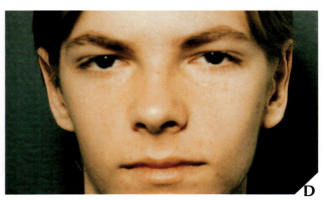

Figure 8.17. Relapse of suture otoplasty. **(A)** Prominent ears preoperatively. **(B)** Appearance immediately after suture otoplasty. **(C)** Drift of ears six months postoperatively. **(D)** Final appearance of ears 1 year after correction of drift with repeat suture otoplasty, Stenstrom cartilage scoring, and postoperative use of headband.

points are used. The concha may be thinned or trimmed posteriorly to facilitate the setback. Sufficient conservatism is exercised in the antihelix maneuvers to avoid inviting the complication of an excessively sharp antihelix fold. Then, for 6 to 12 months, an elastic headband (tennis sweat band) is placed over the ears to minimize the strain of the sutures on the chondral anchorage points (see Fig. 8.16). It is used 24 hours a day at first; then the time periods are gradually modified, using the headband at night and in private.

SUTURE EXPOSURE
The monofilament, nonabsorbable sutures used for suture otoplasties can bridge and erode through the thin postauricular skin (Fig. 8.18). This complication is usually seen many months or years after the original otoplasty. If the sutures have been present 9 months or more, it is unlikely that they are needed for maintenance of the new position. Therefore, they are removed. We have not observed a chondritis as a result of suture exposure, but probably a small risk is present.

Polyfilament sutures have less tendency to erode mechanically but greater tendency to serve as a nidus for infection. Although the period of absorption of recently developed synthetic, absorbable polymer sutures extends for many months, tensile strength may be lost early. Therefore, we still use nonabsorbable material for the key otoplasty sutures.

SHARP RIDGES AND IRREGULARITIES OF THE CARTILAGE
Major post-otoplasty deformities are rare, but probably the most frequent of these is a sharp ridge with irregularities of the cartilage of the antihelix and elsewhere on the pinna (see Figs. 8.11 and 8.12). Causes are diverse. They may result from Luckett-type incisions (completely through the antihelix crest), from excessive thinning or scoring of the cartilage (either posteriorly or anteriorly), or from scarring and wound contraction following skin and/or cartilage necrosis associated with hematomas, infection, or accidents with pressure dressings, etc. Correction is extremely difficult at best, and each case must be individualized for evaluation and treatment (if any).

TELEPHONE DEFORMITY AND REVERSE TELEPHONE DEFORMITY
In the "telephone deformity" (Fig. 8.19), the central portion of the ear appears to have been compressed (as if by a telephone) due to excessive

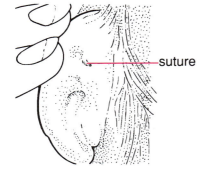

Figure 8.18. Nylon Mustardé scapha-concha suture eroding through the skin.

—suture

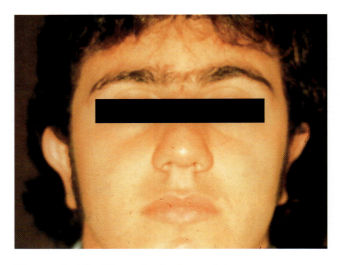

Figure 8.19. Bilateral telephone deformity. (Reproduced with permission from Elliott RA Jr: Complications in the treatment of prominent ears. Clin Plast Surg 5:479–490, 1978.)

conchal reduction or inadequate correction of the upper and lower poles. In the "reverse telephone deformity," the concha projects excessively, while the helix, the lower pole, and the upper pole project insufficiently. These deformities have been cited with a frequency disproportionate to their incidence, but the graphic names have assured perpetuation. They represent but two points on a wide spectrum of possible postoperative deformities. The incidence of such deformities has diminished in recent years as surgeons have adopted more conservative and refined otoplasty techniques.

INCIDENCE OF COMPLICATIONS

In a series of 292 patients, Baker and Converse[1] noted the following complications: hematoma, 0.8%; localized cellulitis, 1.2%; chondritis, 0.7%; hypertrophic scars, 0.7%; telephone deformity, 3%; recurrence after Mustardé technique,[14] 4.3%. Keloids occurred in 11% of black patients (one bilateral) and 2.1% of Caucasian patients.

REFERENCES

1. Baker DC, Converse JM: Correction of protruding ears: A 20 year retrospective. Aesthet Plast Surg 3:29, 1979.
2. Brody GS: Use of disposable razor band to carve cartilage. Plast Reconstr Surg 44:307, 1969.
3. Elliott RA: Complications in the treatment of prominent ears. Clin Plast Surg 5:479, 1978.
4. Elliott RA: Otoplasty: A combined approach. Clin Plast Surg 17:373, 1990.
5. Ely JF: Small incision otoplaty for prominent ears. Aesth Plast Surg 12:63, 1988.
6. Feldman J: Editor's note in Furnas DW: Suture Otoplasty Update. Perspect Plast Surg 4:136, 1990.
7. Furnas DW: Complications of surgery of the external ear. Clin Plast Surg 17:305, 1990.
8. Furnas DW: Correction of prominent ears by concha-mastoid sutures. Plast Reconstr Surg 42:189, 1968.
9. Furnas DW: Plastic and reconstructive surgery of the external ear. Adv Plast Reconstr Surg 5:153, 1989.
10. Furnas DW: Suture otoplasty update. Perspect Plast Surg 4:136, 1990.
11. Gorney, M: Personal communication, 1991.
12. MacGregor FC: Ear deformities: Social and psychological implications. Clin Plast Surg 5:347, 1978.
13. Matsuo K, Hayashi R, Kiyono M, et al: Nonsurgical correction of congenital auricular deformities. Clin Plast Surg 17:383, 1990.
14. Mustardé JC: The correction of prominent ears using simple mattress sutures. Brit J Plast Surg 16:170, 1963.
15. Peacock EE: Wound repair. In Biological and Pharmacological Control of Scar Tissue, 3rd Ed. WB Saunders, Philadelphia, 1984.
16. Reynaud JP, Gary-Bobo A, Mateu J, et al: Chodrites post-operatoires de l'oreille extreme: Two cases from a series of 200 patients (387 otoplasties). Ann Chir Plast Esthet 31:170, 1986.
17. Rockwell WB, Cohen IK, Ehrlich HP: Keloids and hypertrophic scars: A comprehensive review. Plast Reconstr Surg 84:827, 1989.
18. Spira M: Reduction otoplasty. In Goldwyn RM (ed.): The Unfavorable Result in Plastic Surgery:Avoidance and Treatment. Boston, Little,Brown, 1984.
19. Stenstrom SJ, Heftner J: The Stenstrom otoplasty. Clin Plast Surg 5:465, 1978.

AUGMENTATION MAMMAPLASTY

James L. Baker, Jr.

Augmentation mammaplasty is one of the most sought-after cosmetic procedures in the United States. It is estimated that over two million women have safely undergone the operation to date. Despite improvements in technique and implant design since the first implantation of a silicone gel prosthesis in 1963 (by Chronin and colleagues), complications do occur, as with every surgical procedure (Fig. 9.1).

The following presentation discusses silicone prostheses, both the gel and inflatable kinds, as well as textured silicone surfaces. Polyurethane-coated gel prostheses present their own set of complications which are not discussed in this chapter.

HISTORICAL BACKGROUND

The first recorded attempt to enlarge the female breast was reported in 1895 by Czerny who transplanted a lipoma from a patient's thigh to the retromammary space to fill out a breast defect resulting from removal of a large fibroadenoma. Various other attempts at breast enlargement were performed early on, including percutaneous injection of liquid paraffin and insertion of glass balls and polyvinyl alcohol-formaldehyde (Ivalon) sponges into the breast. Later the sponges were coated with polyethylene or polyurethane. Fibrous ingrowth, fluid accumulation, and postoperative infection were common occurrences from these coatings. In an attempt to reduce the high complication rates, the polyether (Etheron) sponge implant was produced and introduced into the market in the early 1960's. While this lowered the rate of postoperative complications, excessive contracture of the material led to undesirable shrinkage and a reduction in breast volume, approaching that of the preoperative state. This characteristic of the material ultimately led to the implant's demise (Fig. 9.2).

Although terrifying complications had been reported from the use of other injectable materials early in the century, silicone injections to augment small breasts were performed by some physicians in the 1950's and early 1960's. It should be noted that the manufacturer of liquid-injectable, medical-grade silicone (Dow Corning) never advised or advocated this use of injectable silicone. The material was readily available, however, during this time and found its way into the

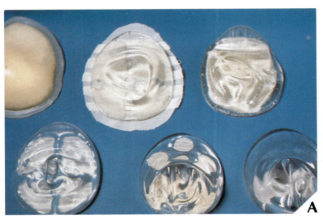 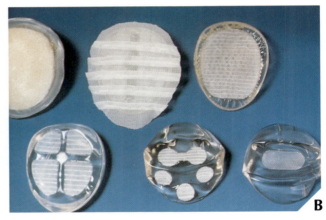

Figure 9.1. (A) Evolution of the breast implant (from top left to bottom right). The original implants were made of two halves and glued at their edges after they were filled with gel. **(B)** Posterior surface of implants.

Note the extensive use of Dacron, employed until the late 1960's, when it was finally removed from the implant (see bottom right). (Courtesy of Dow Corning)

breasts of many women and men alike. In patients with multiple injections, medical-grade silicone can be seen on x-ray dispersed throughout the breast parenchyma, producing multiple, firm, painful nodules and obscuring breast parenchyma from tissue examination (Fig. 9.3). Commercial-grade silicone adulterated with petrochemical bases was commonly used in Asia for breast augmentation. It was frequently introduced through a small stab incision and was given in multiple, large-dose cannula injections. This approach frequently led to granulomata formation, nodularity, inflammation, infection, migration along fascial planes, embolism, and

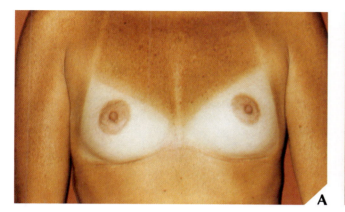

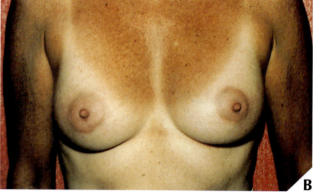

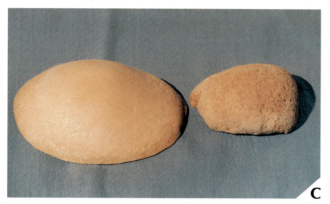

Figure 9.2. **(A)** Patient with Pangman sponge prostheses after shrinkage of the sponges occurred. **(B)** Postoperative view after removal of the sponges and replacement with silicone gel prostheses. **(C)** The Pangman sponge—the preoperative shape on the left and postoperative shrinkage on the right. (**C,** courtesy of Dow Corning)

Figure 9.3. Xerogram showing dispersion of injected silicone throughout the breast parenchyma.

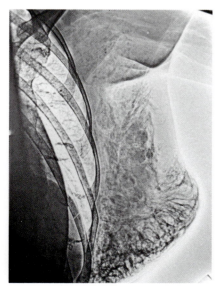

death. Radical treatment is indicated for removal of the contaminated tissue. In Figure 9.4, the patient's breasts were injected in Vietnam by a non-physician utilizing the cannula technique. It was necessary to perform a subcutaneous mastectomy on this patient (Fig. 9.4A). Two of her girlfriends underwent the same procedure, one of whom died of massive embolism immediately following the procedure, the other lost both breasts due to ensuing infection. A two-stage procedure was performed on this patient, and, after several months (Fig. 9.4E), the patient was returned to surgery where bilateral gel prostheses were placed in the subpectoral position (Fig. 9.4F).

In another case, massive silicone injection was performed by a non-physician on a transsexual (Fig. 9.5). Severe pain, discomfort, and subcuta-

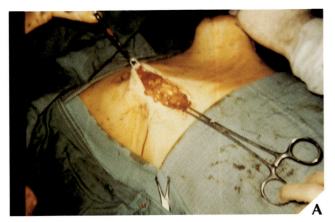

Figure 9.4. (A) Subcutaneous mastectomy for removal of silicone injection into breast parenchyma. **(B)** Tissue specimen following removal from the breast. **(C)** Cut surface of the breast parenchyma. Note the free silicone (on black background) removed from specimen. **(D)** Photomicrograph of specimen showing large, empty vacuoles, which had contained silicone. Note the giant inflammatory cells and infiltrate cells typical of free silicone in tissue. **(E)** Patient after subcutaneous mastectomy. **(F)** Patient following subpectoral placement of gel prostheses for reconstruction.

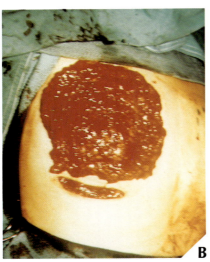
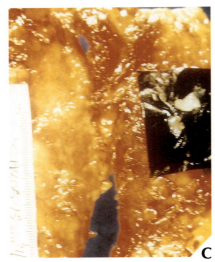
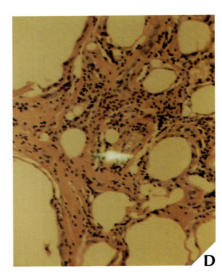
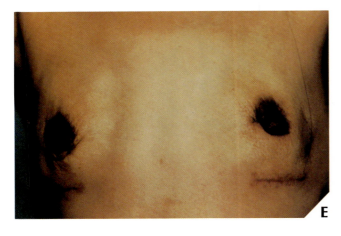
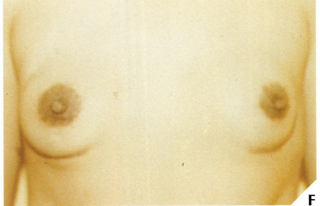

neous nodularity was noted throughout the area. Mammograms demonstrate the dense, diffuse volume of the silicone throughout the subcutaneous tissue (Fig. 9.6).

PATIENT HISTORY AND EXAMINATION

Although complications may occur from any surgery, the complication of the dissatisfied patient postoperatively can frequently be prevented by careful preoperative screening and thorough explanation of the patient's anatomical limi- tations. Due to variations in body configuration, the patient's expectations cannot always be achieved through breast augmentation.

Physical examination of the back will demonstrate scoliosis and misalignment of shoulders (Fig. 9.7). It will be projected on the ventral surface as an alteration in thoracic wall symmetry and, frequently, nipple alignment (Fig. 9.8). In this patient the nipple height is asymmetric, the thoracic wall is more prominent on the left side (which creates a different projection of the breast), and tight cleavage is impossible to attain, due to the convexity of the sternum. This should

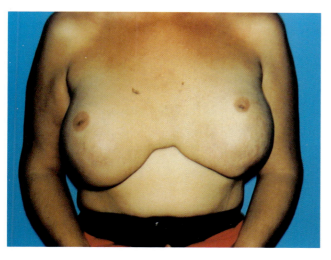

Figure 9.5. Male transsexual who underwent massive injection of silicone by non-physician for breast enlargement.

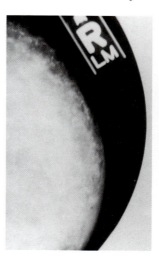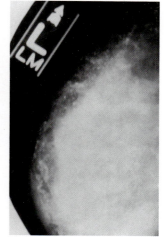

Figure 9.6. Mammogram illustrating mass dispersion of free silicone throughout the subcutaneous tissue.

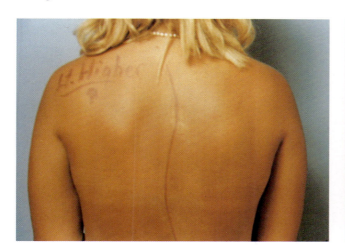

Figure 9.7. View of the patient's back indicating a degree of scoliosis and shoulder misalignment.

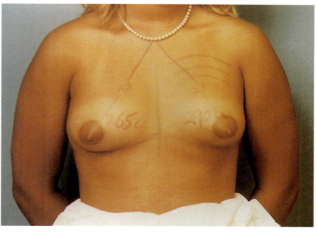

Figure 9.8. Anterior view of patient with alterations in chest anatomy. Note the more prominent left thoracic wall. Estimated implant size has been written on breast.

be pointed out to the patient during the initial consultation. In the patient in Figure 9.9, the left nipple is located laterally on the breast, near the anterior axillary line and the midclavicular line; this will be the postoperative condition as well (Fig. 9.10). Neither of these patients was disappointed with the postoperative result since they understood that, while breast enlargement was possible, their anatomy would dictate nipple projection, position, and slight asymmetries, which were present preoperatively.

Measurements and notes of anatomical variations should be recorded on a diagram and attached to the patient's chart (Fig. 9.11). An informed consent is mandatory when undertaking any aesthetic procedure (Fig. 9.12).

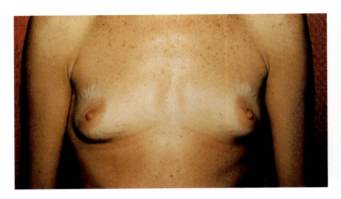

Figure 9.9. Marked lateralization of the left nipple preoperatively.

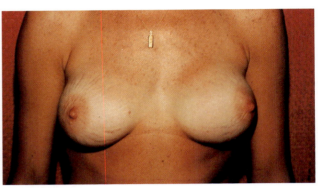

Figure 9.10. Postoperatively, nipple will remain in lateral position. This result should be discussed with the patient preoperatively.

Figure 9.11. Diagram for recording surgical plan and discrepancies of chest wall.

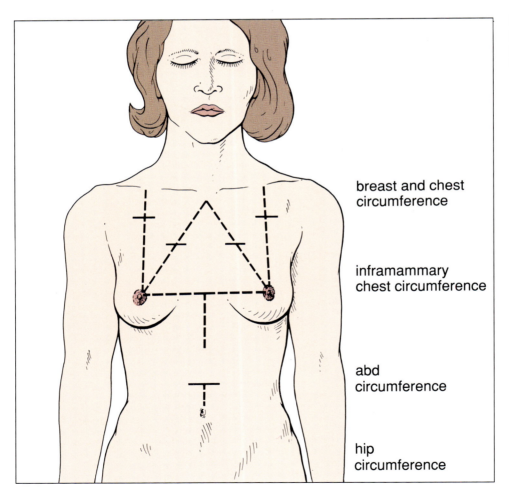

breast and chest circumference

inframammary chest circumference

abd circumference

hip circumference

INFORMED CONSENT TO OPERATION

PATIENT:_____

DATE:_____TIME:_____

I hereby authorize Dr. James L. Baker, Jr., and/or associates to perform the following procedures on myself:

_____

_____

_____

1. I recognize that, during the course of the operation, unforeseen conditions may necessitate additional or different procedures than those set forth above. I therefore further authorize and request that the above-named surgeon, his assistants, or his designees perform such procedures as are, in his professional judgement, necessary and desirable, including, but not limited to, procedures involving pathology and radiology. The authority granted under this paragraph shall extend to remedying conditions that are not known to the above doctors at the time the operation is commenced.

2. I consent to the administration of local anesthesia to be applied by or under the direction and supervision of the above doctors, with the exception of

_____
(None or a particular one)

3. I recognize that when general anesthesia is used it presents additional risks over which the above doctors have no control and I agree to discuss the risks of general anesthesia with the anesthesiologist before surgery is performed.

4. I am aware that the practice of medicine and surgery is not an exact science, and I acknowledge that no guarantees have been made to me as to the results of the operation or procedure.

5. I consent to be photographed before, during and after the treatment; that these photographs shall be the property of the above doctors and may be published in scientific journals and/or shown for scientific reasons.

6. I agree to keep the above doctors informed of any change of address so that they can notify me of any late findings, and I agree to cooperate with the above doctors in my care after surgery until completely discharged.

7. I am not known to be allergic to anything except. (list) _____

_____

_____

Figure 9.12. (A) Generic informed consent form.

AUGMENTATION MAMMAPLASTY:
(An operation for increasing the size of the breasts)

8. This procedure has been personally explained to me by the above doctors, and I completely understand the nature and consequences of the procedure. The following points, among others, have been specifically made clear:

a. The operation has been done for several years, but the end results are not, and cannot be determined for a number of years yet to come.

b. Research indicates that the material implanted in the body does not cause malignancy in human subjects.

c. There is a possibility that my body may not tolerate these implants, making it necessary to remove the implants. This occurs in a small percentage of cases.

d. A cyst may form in the area adjacent to the implants, causing fluid accumulation which may require drainage by needle or removal of the implants.

e. The breasts can become firm (capsule formation and contraction). This condition can be permanent and can cause pain and discomfort.

f. No guarantee has been given as to size and shape of the breasts. Good results are expected but not guaranteed.

g. In some patients the margin of the implants can be felt.

h. The incision will heal with a scar which will be permanent.

i. Postoperative bleeding may occur around the implant requiring a second operation for its removal.

j. After being exposed to cold temperatures (i.e., swimming in cold water), the breasts may feel cooler than surrounding body tissues.

k. Pregnancy is not recommended for at least six (6) months after the surgery.

l. Numbness or hypersensitivity of the nipple may be experienced following surgery.

m. The procedure is subject to the same postoperative complications as other surgical procedures.

n. The implant shell theoretically could be broken at some point in the life of the implant or during the duration it is implanted. The gel contained within is medical grade and the same as the shell design and would in all probability be confined to the space behind the breast where the implant was implanted. This should not cause any serious side-effect. However, removal and replacement with a new implant will be required.

I have read the above consent and received a copy of it. I fully understand the contents of the consent and authorize and request the above doctors to perform this surgical procedure on me.

Witness	Date	Patient or Legal Guardian

Figure 9.12. (B) Informed consent form specific to breast augmentation.

POSTOPERATIVE COMPLICATIONS

The common complications of breast augmentation may be summarized as follows:

1. Hypertrophic scars
2. Mondor's syndrome
3. Sensory changes to the nipple/areolar complex
4. Infection
5. Implant extrusion
6. Hematoma
7. Displacement of the prosthesis
8. Implant rupture and/or deflation of inflatable prosthesis
9. Capsular contracture and related complications, including implant rupture
10. Steroids and other complications
11. Pneumothorax

Hypertrophic Scarring

While true keloid formation is uncommon, hypertrophic or unsightly scars can be expected in 2 to 5% of patients (Figs. 9.13 and 9.14). The inframammary approach provides the best camouflage for an unsightly scar, as long as the incision is placed just above the inframammary crease, allowing the breast to fold over and conceal the scar. Preoperative planning should include developing symmetrical placement of the incision by using a standard means of incision positioning, placing the scar in the middle of the breast approximately 1 cm above the new inframam-mary crease (Fig. 9.15). When the scar is placed too high on the breast (Fig. 9.16), it will be unsightly, even when it is not hypertrophic.

When two different prostheses are being used for correction of breast asymmetry, it is wise to

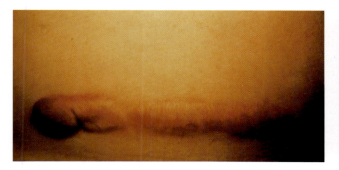

Figure 9.13. Keloid scar of inframammary incision.

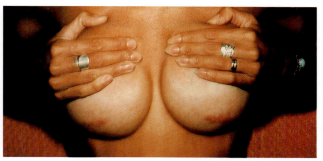

Figure 9.14. Hypertrophic scarring from inframammary incision.

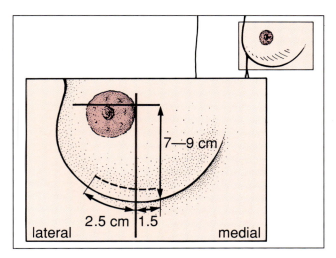

Figure 9.15. Markings for positioning inframammary incision just above inframammary crease. A line is drawn vertically on the medial side of the nipple from 7 to 9 cm, depending on implant size to be used. This should place the incision approximately 1 cm above the inframammary crease. The incision line is then drawn approximately 1.5 cm medially and 2.5 cm laterally, which will place the incision in the best position for later concealment.

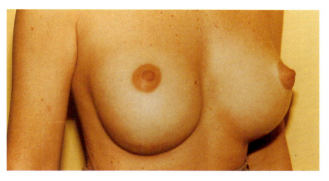

Figure 9.16. An inframammary incision placed too high on the breast.

mark the size planned for insertion on each breast when the incision areas are drawn to avoid inserting the implants in the wrong sides (Fig. 9.17). There is nothing more embarrassing to the surgeon than to have a left side smaller than the right preoperatively, only to find the left side even smaller than the right postoperatively. This mistake can occur during surgery and produce a very dissatisfied patient postoperatively.

When the transaxillary approach is used and results in unsightly scarring, the patient will have to be careful in selecting clothing that shows the axilla, especially in choosing her evening wear (Fig. 9.18).

While periareolar incisions tend to carry a slightly lower incidence of hypertrophy, it has a significant disadvantage: when the pocket has to be re-entered for additional procedures, such as hematoma evacuation or release of capsular contracture, scarring in the subareolar area can occur. The scar can create marked distortion and indentation of the nipple/areola complex, which is extremely unsightly and even more difficult to correct (Fig. 9.19). Unsightly scarring is treated on an individual basis by steroid injection and/or revision. While revision is usually successful in improving the appearance of the scar, the patient must be warned that a scar as unpleasing, or even worse, may occur with any secondary procedure.

When nonabsorbable suture is used for subdermal approximation, it can result in later migration of the suture material through the scar, requiring its removal (Fig. 9.20). This complication can be avoided by using absorbable suture material for this closure.

Mondor's Syndrome

Mondor's syndrome is an uncommon condition manifested by painful cord-like "banjo strings" subcutaneously, just below the inframammary crease. These cords are thrombosed veins, and the condition is benign (Fig. 9.21). The etiology is not known, with the syndrome usually presenting itself within the first several weeks after surgery and subsiding spontaneously several weeks thereafter. No treatment is indicated; however, the discomfort is usually alleviated by the use of anti-inflammatory drugs, such as ibuprofen and/or warm compresses. Steroid injection or surgical intervention is contraindicated. The patient should be reassured that the condition is of no consequence and will regress spontaneously.

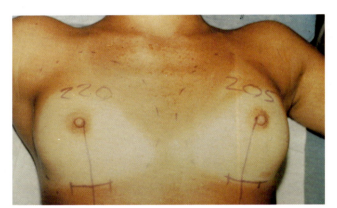

Figure 9.17. Implant size marked on the patient prior to surgery to avoid any intraoperative confusion of implant placement.

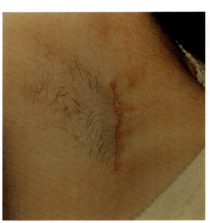
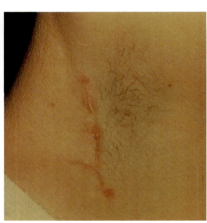

Figure 9.18. Hypertrophic axillary scars following transaxillary approach.

Sensory Changes to the Nipple/Areola Complex

Permanent alteration of nipple sensation will occur in approximately 15% of patients undergoing breast augmentation. It is imperative to discuss and find out the importance of nipple sensation to the patient preoperatively to avoid postoperative disappointment of both patient and spouse should this complication occur. In my preoperative interview, I ask each patient to rate the importance of nipple stimulation in her sex life on a scale of 1 to 10, with 10 being the ultimate in sexual pleasure. The most common response is between 4 and 5. It does not appear to play a large role in the majority of patients with breast hypoplasia; a small percentage of the patients can have orgasm from nipple stimulation with no genital play. It is of prime importance to stress to all patients that 15% of women undergoing this procedure will have permanent alteration of sensation, which can be manifested as bilateral total numbness, and that removal of the implant, should this phenomenon occur, will *not* result in restoration of sensation. Those patients who rate nipple stimulation highly are encouraged to consider the operation carefully, discuss it with their loved one, and make their decision to undergo the operation only if they feel that improved breast contour is of greater importance than the pleasure derived from nipple stimulation.

Fortunately, in most cases sensation does return over a period of time, although years may be required for reinnervation. While diminished

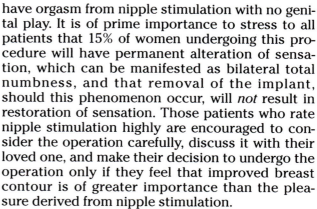

Figure 9.19. Inversion and distortion of the nipple/areola complex following periareolar augmentation. The left pocket had to be re-entered for hematoma.

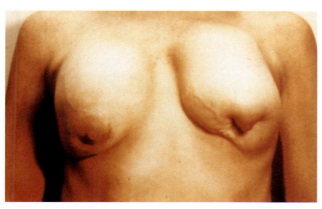

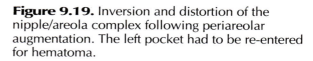

Figure 9.20. Nonabsorbable suture migrating through inframammary incision.

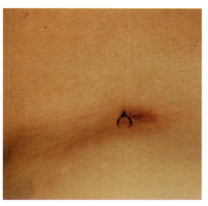 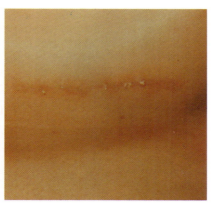

Figure 9.21. Cord-like banjo strings pathognomonic of Mondor's syndrome.

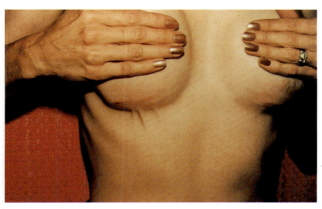

sensation occurs from all surgical approaches, it is least common with the transaxillary approach and slightly more common with the periareolar approach. The lateral cutaneous branch of the fourth intercostal nerve is thought to provide the majority of sensation to the nipple/areola complex. The nerve usually penetrates into the posterior aspect of the breast at the intersection of the lateral border of the pectoralis major muscle with the fourth intercostal space (Fig. 9.22). (This corresponds to 4 o'clock on the left breast and 8 o'clock on the right.) Midway en route to the nipple/areola complex, the nerve divides into five fasciculi, with one central branch to the nipple and two upper and two lower branches. Since the lower-most branch pierces the areola consistently at 5 o'clock on the left and 7 o'clock on the right, postoperative sensation may be preserved in part by planning the periareolar incision more medial from 10 o'clock to a few millimeters medial to 5 o'clock on the left breast, and a few millimeters medial from 7 o'clock to 2 o'clock on the right breast, instead of the usual 9- to 3-o'clock incision.

With the inframammary approach, the large nerve trunk is usually identifiable at the lateral extent of the pocket, as described above, and care should be taken to dissect it free and preserve it, when it is at all possible. In some patients, stretching the nerve over the prosthesis while preserving it may result in hypesthesia in the nipple/areola complex, which usually diminishes over a period of weeks or months.

If the nerve enters too far medially and the correct pocket dimensions cannot be dissected, it is better to sacrifice the nerve than to produce asymmetry or indentation of the lateral border of the breast contour. Resection of this nerve will not always result in numbness of the nipple;

hence, it is presumed that there is additional innervation to the nipple/areola complex by another route.

Infection

Fortunately, postoperative infection of the augmented breast is rare, occurring in approximately 1% of patients. The infection is usually unilateral, and, when caused by common bacterial pathogens, it occurs within several weeks of the operative procedure. While *Staphylococcus epidermidis* has been implicated in the cause of capsular contracture, it rarely is a causative agent of postoperative infection of a clinical nature. It can frequently be cultured from ductal secretion at the nipple and is of questionable importance if the glandular tissue is violated in the duct center, as in concomitant biopsy with augmentation.

Staphylococcus aureus is the most common pathogen in the instances when infection does occur (Fig. 9.23). The onset is usually insidious, with a rise in temperature, swelling, and discomfort. If contamination occurs with pseudomonas, the patient will experience extreme discomfort, far beyond the symptoms found upon examination. A pseudomonas appears to irritate the nerve endings to a great extent, causing severe pain that is disproportionate to the amount of swelling noted. The breast is frequently nonoutstanding upon examination. When the patient has a minimal to moderate amount of postoperative unilateral swelling with extreme pain, pseudomonas should be suspected as the contaminant.

The occurrence of *Mycobacterium fortuitum* is fortunately rare, but it was noted in 17 patients in 3 states between March 1975 and October 1978. Periprosthetic infection with no evidence of systemic disease occurred from 1 to 2 weeks to over

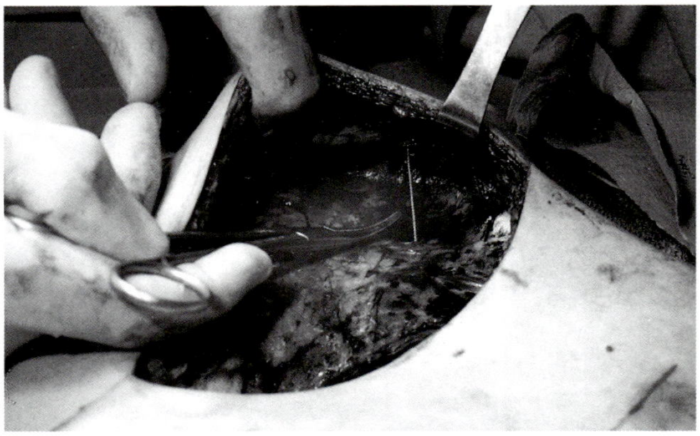

Figure 9.22. Dissection showing the lateral thoracic nerve branch as it courses from the pectoralis muscle border into the breast parenchyma. (Courtesy of Dow Corning)

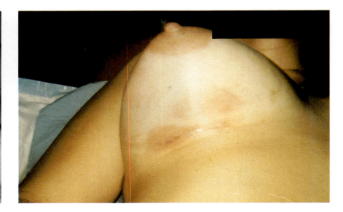

Figure 9.23. Breast with postoperative infection. Note areas of hyperemia and enlargement of breast without evidence of ecchymosis.

2 years after breast augmentation with silicone prostheses. The mycobacterium complex is an unusual pathogen and is difficult to culture. None of the patients had a temperature elevation above 100°F. The presenting symptoms included breast swelling in all patients, some tenderness to palpation, and erythema at the incision or the area overlying the implant.

Spontaneous drainage through the incision site was noted in 33% of the patients having this pathogen. This discharge and the fluid present in the pocket around the prosthesis were nonodorous and either serosanguineous or purulent. Gram stain of the fluid usually revealed many polymorphonuclear leukocytes with few, if any, organisms. Initial cultures of this fluid were often reported to be sterile, with occasional growth of "diphtheroids" or possible *Nocardia*. While the onset of infection occurred 1 week to 2 years following surgery, the median time from implantation of the prosthesis to the onset of symptoms was 1 month. All but one patient had unilateral infections. The organism is poorly receptive to standard antibiotic therapy (nor will pre- and postoperative antibiotic therapy prevent the occurrence). Treatment consists of triple sulfa QID for 2 to 3 weeks. If there is no evidence of infection, the patient is again placed on triple sulfa for several days preoperatively, continuing this regimen through the postoperative period for 1 to 2 weeks.

While mycobacterium will always necessitate the removal of the prosthesis for a period of weeks to months, augmented breasts with infections caused by routine bacteriological organisms have been successfully reimplanted after performing a capsulectomy with profuse Betadine irrigation. Then reinsertion of a new prosthesis can be performed with appropriate antibiotic therapy. I place all patients undergoing breast augmentation on a broad-spectrum antibiotic for 9 days, beginning 2 days preoperatively. My experience with postoperative infection has been 0.1%. Of the seven patients afflicted, all have been unilateral infections consisting of one *Mycobacterium fortuitum*, two pseudomonas, and the remainder staphylococcus infections.

Extrusion of the Implant

In the 1960's and early 1970's, extrusion of the prosthesis was a not too unusual phenomenon when Dacron coating was used on the posterior wall of the implant. The Dacron increased the amount of capsular contracture present. In a very thin patient with minimal breast tissue, the amount of contracture could actually erode the implant through a weakened area in the overlying tissue (usually at the incision site).

In the 1970's, when the use of steroids became popular, occasional erosion due to overlying atrophy compounded by contracture was noted, either in the pocket or intraluminal in the prosthesis itself (Fig. 9.24). Treatment consisted of removal of the prosthesis, repair of the defect, capsulotomy or capsulectomy, and replacement of the prosthesis (beneath the pectoralis muscle in the most severe cases).

Hematoma

Postoperative hematoma will occur in approximately 1% of all breast augmentations. The onset is most commonly seen within 48 hours; however, very late cases (up to 3 weeks postoperatively) have been reported (Fig. 9.25).

In large hematomas, treatment consists of surgical evacuation of the hematoma with irrigation of

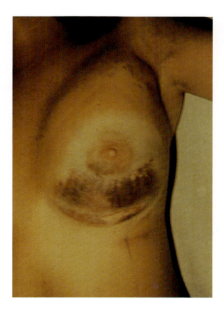

Figure 9.25. Postoperative hematoma.

Figure 9.24. Erosion of the prosthesis following postoperative use of steroids. Note bluish area above obvious erosion site, indicating impending erosion at that site as well.

the pocket and reinsertion of the prosthesis. While a considerable amount of blood can be lost into a large pocket, the need for transfusion is extremely rare. Alternatives, such as postoperative oral iron replacement therapy and adequate IV infusion to replace blood volume are usually adequate treatment.

Displacement of the Prosthesis

The dislocation of the prosthesis, usually downward, is most commonly found when the inframammary incision is used and is due to ptosis of the flap (Fig. 9.26). This can result from suture breakdown or the pooling of steroids placed in the pocket. Implant displacement is far less commonly seen in the periareolar or transaxillary approaches.

Treatment consists of opening the incision, dissecting the subcutaneous flap free, and reapproxi-

mating it to the fascia of the chest wall with a nonabsorbable suture. During the primary surgery, it may be advisable to use nonabsorbable suture for reapproximation of this flap to diminish the incidence of this minor complication.

Implant Rupture and/or Deflation of the Inflatable Prosthesis

While proponents of the inflatable prostheses frequently claim lower capsular contracture rates, with the added benefit of a nonsilicone gel-containing prosthesis, the problem with these protheses has always been occasional spontaneous deflation, either due to leakage at the valve or a hole in the prosthesis at a point of wear (Fig. 9.27). The implant is designed to be maximally inflated to avoid the capsular contracture from compressing the implant and creating a fold in the shell. Compression produces weaken-

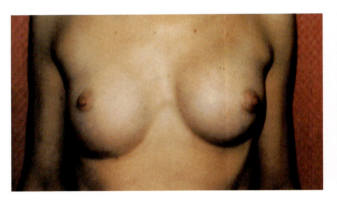

Figure 9.26. Implant ptosis (right side). Correction is achieved by reopening the incision and reapproximating the flap with nonabsorbable suture.

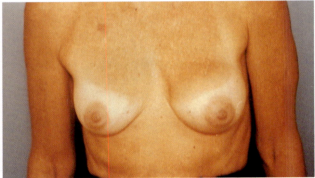

Figure 9.27. Spontaneous deflation of the right breast following attempted needle aspiration of cyst by a general surgeon, which punctured the prosthesis.

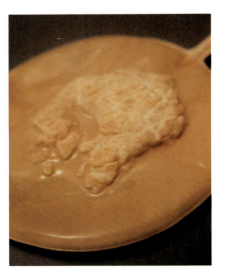

Figure 9.28. Salt crystals noted intraluminally in prosthesis.

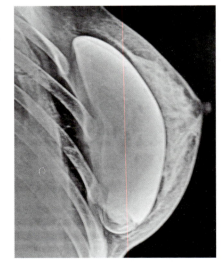

Figure 9.29. Xerogram showing implant rupture in the inferior pole. Note irregularity of shell integrity with gel extrusion at 6 o'clock.

ing along the fold and molecular movement of the silicone, creating what is known as a fold-flow phenomenon. It is usually along one of these folds that a pinpoint leak occurs. Deflation can also be caused by accidental damage to the implant during attempted needle aspiration of a breast cyst. It is not uncommon to find the salt crystallized within the deflated prosthesis after absorption of the saline (Fig. 9.28). The condition is treated by reoperating with replacement of the prosthesis.

Rupture of the Gel Prosthesis

Gel implants have come under scrutiny during the past year because of the potential complications caused by silicone gel in soft tissue. The silicone gel may "bleed" or the prosthesis may rupture, with dispersion of the gel into the breast or surrounding tissues. It is imperative that the surgeon discuss the pros and cons of silicone implants with their patients preoperatively and help them understand the scientific data known at this in time. In June 1988, the FDA classified breast implants as Class III devices; under this classification manufacturers must demonstrate the safety and efficacy of their devices through scientific studies. Many scientific studies have been done, and silicone, including liquid silicone for injection, is probably one of most studied "drugs" in history.

It is well known that minute quantities of silicone can travel through the implant shell and will often be picked up by the body's white cells and/or isolated in the surrounding tissues. However, at the present time there is no evidence that this small amount of silicone is harmful to the body. All needles and syringes are coated with silicone to minimize pain on injection; hence,

patients receiving an IM or IV injection will have minute quantities of silicone introduced into their bodies. Also, minuscule quantities of silicone can be found in many patients since it is a frequent ingredient of many over-the-counter drugs, including antacids. Silicone is also found in clothing, furniture, and cosmetics.

Some have wondered whether silicone has any possible cause and effect on connective tissue diseases. While several published studies have questioned the possible relationship between breast implants and scleroderma or other collagen diseases, including rheumatoid arthritis, none have been substantiated to date. Given the very small number of patients who have developed these diseases in the general population and the large number of patients with breast implants, it is a logical conclusion that inevitably some patients with breast implants will develop these diseases in the same ratio as the general population. However, should a woman express concern about the development of such a disease after augmentation has been performed, the implant can easily be removed. If the patient still desires correction of breast contour, either saline inflatable prostheses or the new Misti "Gold"-textured silicone prostheses (produced by Bioplasty) can be inserted. The latter contains no silicone gel and was approved for implantation by the FDA in October 1990.

Should rupture of the prosthesis occur, it is usually diagnosed by mammography (Fig. 9.29). In such instances, it is advisable to exchange the prosthesis and remove any free gel from the pocket. Should traumatic rupture of the prosthesis occur with extreme force, extrusion and propulsion of the gel through the capsular wall into the breast tissue may result (Fig. 9.30). Removal of the extruded gel resulted in a subtotal mastecto-

Figure 9.30. Dispersion of silicone gel through lower pole of breast.

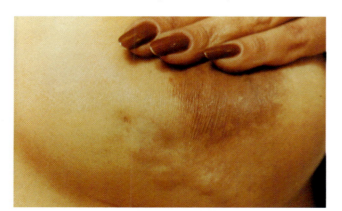

my to remove siliconomata throughout the lower portion of the breast (Figs. 9.31 and 9.32). It should be noted that siliconomata within the breast tissue will limit the effectiveness of mammography.

While breast prostheses do complicate mammography, research has shown that compensatory measures by an experienced radiologist can overcome this obstacle. Multiple views should be taken in all patients having undergone breast augmentation with silicone prostheses. One-view mammography is ineffective. In the Eklund technique, which is another method of choice, the breast is positioned so that the implant is pushed against the chest wall and the glandular tissue is pulled forward for radiologic examination. It is helpful for the surgeon to establish a working relationship with a competent local radiologist and to refer patients with breast augmentation to him or her for mammographic studies.

Capsular Contracture and Related Complications

Capsular contracture following breast augmentation most commonly occurs within 6 to 12 months following surgery. All implantable devices will develop a scar tissue layer, or capsule, around the foreign body. When this capsule contracts, distortion of the implant can occur. Since the soft prosthesis is usually compressed into a spherical shape, the term *spherical contracture* is used when discussing breast firmness. The Baker classification has been devised to categorize the degree of contracture (Fig. 9.33).

Myofibroblasts appear to have a role in initiating and/or producing scar contracture. Since the drug papaverine sometimes produces cell relaxation, the contracture may be minimized with 150 mg BID of the agent for several months (or until improvement occurs). The regimen will be most

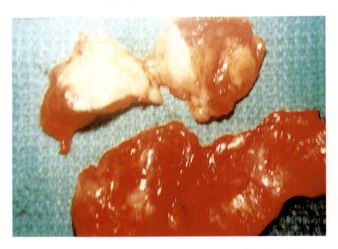

Figure 9.31. Postoperative specimen of subtotal mastectomy showing massive siliconomata.

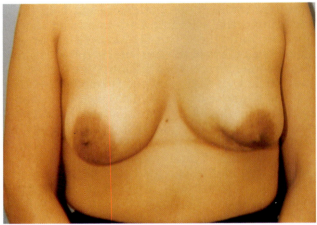

Figure 9.32. Appearance following subtotal mastectomy. Reconstruction of the breast was performed later.

Figure 9.33. Baker Classification of Implant Contracture

Class	Condition
I	Normal—no contracture
II	Mildly firm—rarely problematic
III	Moderately firm—patient is aware of firmness
IV	Severe—patient requires treatment

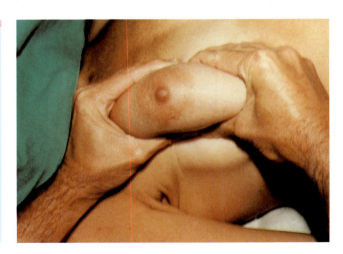

Figure 9.34. Common closed "squeeze" capsulotomy technique.

effective at the earliest onset of the contracture, when the myofibroblasts are greatest in number and are most active.

Various modalities for the treatment of this condition have been proposed. A closed "squeeze" capsulotomy may rupture the membrane (Fig. 9.34) and produce the desired softness. However, as with any procedure, it is not without potential complication. All patients should be aware of the possible complications resulting from closed capsulotomy; it is recommended that a written consent form be completed prior to performing this procedure (Fig. 9.35). Incomplete rupture of the capsule may result in abnormal distortion and

CLOSED CAPSULOTOMY CONSENT

PATIENT:_____

DATE:_____ TIME:_____

1. I hereby authorize James L. Baker, Jr., M.D. and/or his associates to perform a procedure to attempt to rupture the scar capsules surrounding my breast implants by squeezing the breasts, known as Closed Capsulotomy, on myself.

2. The procedure listed in Paragraph 1 has been explained to me by the doctor and/or his nurse and I completely understand the nature and consequences of the procedure. The following points have been made specifically clear:

    a. There is a possibility that a blood clot may form in the area adjacent to the implants which might require surgical correction, which may have to be performed under general anesthesia.

    b. The procedure is not always successful and/or bizarre shape of the breast can occur which could necessitate surgery for correction.

    c. Recurrence of the contracture (hard breast) can occur even if the capsulotomy is successful.

    d. Breakage of the implant can occur which would necessitate surgical correction.

    e. Thinning of an area of the tissue over the prosthesis may occur which could necessitate surgical correction or removal of the implant.

    f. If surgery is necessary following the capsulotomy it may be necessary to make an incision in an area other than where the previous scar is located.

    g. Surgical fees would be charged if surgery should become necessary as a result of this procedure.

    h. No guarantee has been given as to the expected result.

3. I am aware that the practice of medicine and surgery is not an exact science, and I acknowledge that no guarantees have been made to me as to the results of the operation or procedure.

4. I agree to keep the doctor informed of any change of address so he can notify me of any late findings, and I agree to cooperate with the doctor in my care after surgery until completely discharged.

5. I have read the above consent and fully understand same and do authorize the doctor to perform this procedure on me.

6. I am not known to be allergic to anything except: (List) _____

_____

(Witness)_____ (Patient)_____

Figure 9.35. Consent form for closed capsulotomy.

shape of the breast, commonly known as the *dumbbell effect* (Fig. 9.36). This outcome may require surgical revision with open capsulotomy/capsulectomy for correction. While superficial ecchymosis may occur (Fig. 9.37), it is self-limiting and of no consequence. However, a hematoma may result from a tear of a vessel within the capsular wall, which would then necessitate surgical evacuation. The patient should be made aware of the potential costs of the procedures prior to consenting to the closed capsulotomy in order to avoid later disagreement between surgeon and patient.

Capsular contracture following the transaxillary approach may produce migration of the prostheses toward the axilla (Fig. 9.38). Capsulectomy in the axillary area and tissue approximation with capsulotomy of the remaining pocket are necessary if the patient desires correction. Closed capsulotomy has been very ineffective with a transaxillary approach, either performed subpectorally or superpectorally.

To avoid damage to the implant prior to its removal in open capsulotomy, it is recommended that the electrosurgical scalpel be used for final penetration of the capsular wall to the surface of the implant (Fig. 9.39). As long as the cutting tip is free of carbon particles, the implant will not be damaged and can easily be removed intact (Fig. 9.40). Surgical capsulotomy at the base, with scoring of the dome (if a smooth-walled implant is to be replaced), is usually adequate. It is best to

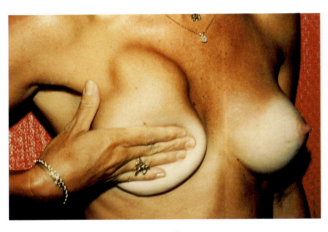

Figure 9.36. A dumbbell irregularity following closed "squeeze" capsulotomy.

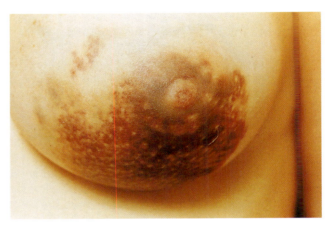

Figure 9.37. Subcutaneous ecchymosis following closed capsulotomy. The condition is of no pathologic significance and is self-limiting.

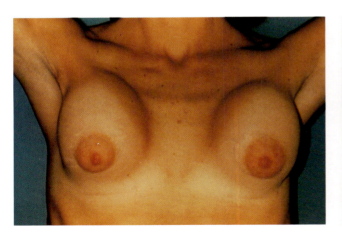

Figure 9.38. Migration of prostheses toward axilla following transaxillary approach with postoperative capsular contracture.

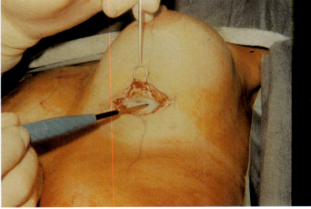

Figure 9.39. Use of the electrosurgical scalpel to split the capsule wall, avoiding damage to the prosthesis.

place "checkerboard" cuts into the dome capsule, if it is to be left intact, to release the overlying breast tissue and improve contour.

When severe calcification of the capsule is noted (Fig. 9.41), capsulectomy is required. Leaving these fragments of calcium imbedded in the capsule wall can result in damage to the surface of the prosthesis.

A total capsulectomy is necessary when the new textured surface implants are used for replacement (Fig. 9.42) since, due to their design, they must be in contact with the soft tissue to allow the capsule to form within the irregularities of the surface. While the use of these implants is increasing in the hope of diminishing capsular contracture, it is too early to determine their effectiveness in this regard.

Steroids and Subpectoral Placement of Implants

Steroids have been used intraluminally, in the pocket, or by injection in an attempt to control scar contracture, either before the scarring has begun or after it has occurred. It should be understood that steroids are not without their inherent complications, and it is probably best to avoid their use in breast augmentation.

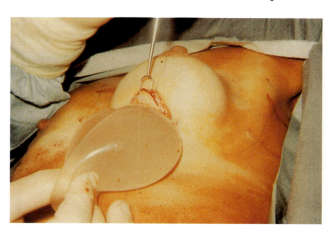

Figure 9.40. Removal of the intact prosthesis.

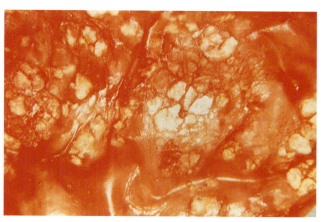

Figure 9.41. Massive calcification throughout the capsule wall. The capsule must be removed when this is found since the fragments of calcium have extremely sharp edges and can damage a new prosthesis.

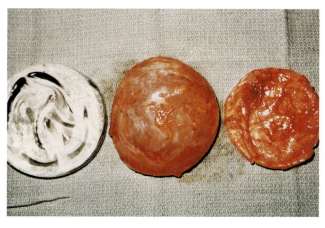

Figure 9.42. Specimen with total capsulotomy. Note the implant is contained within capsule. (Courtesy of Dow Corning)

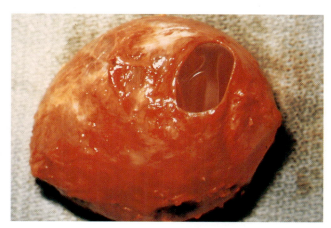

When soluble steroids are placed intraluminally, they can create massive soft tissue atrophy with marked diminution of breast tissue volume and ptosis of the prostheses, as noted in the patient in Figure 9.43. This patient had a unilateral, severe contracture, which was operated on several times before this attempt. In this procedure, 120 mg of Solu-Medrol was placed intraluminally in an inflatable prosthesis; the results were massive atrophy and ptosis of the breast. Treatment consisted of removal of the source of the diffusing steroid, allowing the soft tissue to recover, and replacement with a prosthesis *without* steroids.

Steroid injection has also been attempted in the pericapsular subcutaneous tissue. The use of Kenalog or Depomedrol is common in this attempt to soften scar tissue. However, localization of the long-acting steroid may produce severe localized atrophy, resulting in implant herniation (Figs. 9.44 and 9.45). Treatment may mandate removal of the prosthesis, with rotation of capsular or soft tissue flaps from the posterior wall of the breast to cover the defect (if localized advancement suturing of the tissue is not adequate), and immediate implant replacement.

Another attempt to minimize capsular contracture is the placement of the prosthesis in the subpectoral space. Studies have shown, however, that this method is ineffective in preventing capsular contracture. If contracture occurs with subpectoral placement, distortion of the prostheses is common and the rim of the muscle may be seen overlying the implant. When the pectoralis muscle is tensed (e.g., during exercise), elevation with distortion of the implant can occur (this phenomenon can occur even without capsular contracture), producing an effect known as the "dancing breast". To correct this undesirable result the prosthesis is replaced in the suprapectoral space (Figs. 9.46 and 9.47).

Coagulation of bleeding points in a patient with minimal breast tissue or in the medial aspect

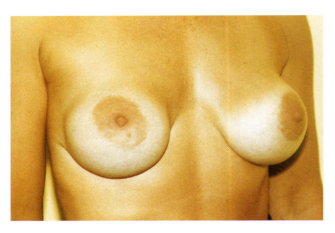

Figure 9.43. Severe atrophy and ptosis of right breast following intraluminal use of steroids.

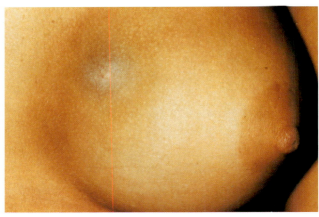

Figure 9.44. Localized, severe subcutaneous and dermal atrophy following injection of Kenalog.

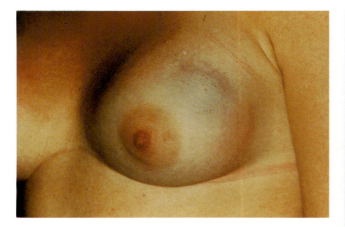

Figure 9.45. Tissue that has undergone extreme atrophy following subcutaneous injection of Kenalog for capsular contracture. Note the "blue dome" appearance.

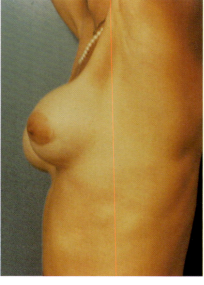

Figure 9.46. Subpectoral position of prostheses, which elevate irregularly and tend to rotate laterally when arms are raised.

where the tissue is especially thin may result in a full-thickness burn, creating an overlying defect, which requires primary closure after eschar separation (Figs. 9.48 and 9.49).

Pneumothorax

Pneumothorax following augmentation has been reported, but fortunately it is a very uncommon complication. The risk is much greater when an intracostal block is used for anesthesia. However, since most surgeons use a spinal needle for infiltration of the submammary space with local anesthesia, it is imperative to be cognizant of where the needle is tracking at all times, i.e., in relationship to the ribs and intercostal spaces. A wide-bore needle, which will not deflect when a rib is accidently encountered and penetrate the intercostal space into the thoracic cavity, is recommended (18- to 20-gauge, as opposed to a 25-gauge spinal needle). The surgeon should perform the injection perpendicular to the ribs to diminish the chance of producing iatrogenic pneumothorax (Fig. 9.50).

To create very tight cleavage, it is possible to traverse the midline in the subcutaneous space,

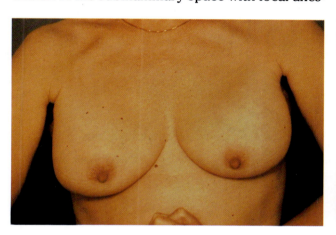

Figure 9.47. With subpectoral placement, elevation and distortion of prosthesis on the left side are marked when the pectoralis muscle is tightened. On the right, implant was placed above the muscle.

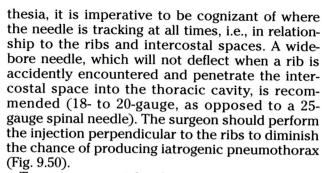
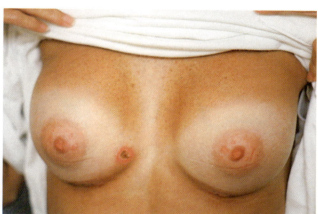

Figure 9.48. Full-thickness overlying tissue loss secondary to electrocoagulation of subdermal vessels for hemostasis.

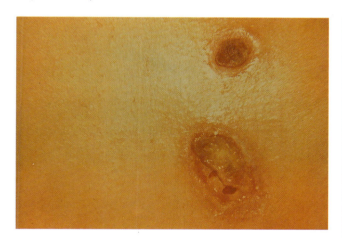

Figure 9.49. Electrocautery damage to overlying skin following hemostasis.

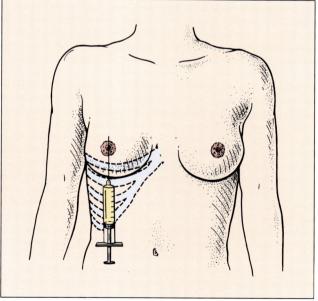

Figure 9.50. Needle should be kept perpendicular to the ribs to avoid inadvertent intercostal penetration and pneumothorax during local anesthesia injection.

creating union of the two pockets. This will produce distortion over the sternum, with communication of the implants across the midline (Fig. 9.51).

While transaxillary augmentation does not produce scar tissue on the breast, it may be difficult to obtain symmetrical pockets at the inframammary crease. When performed subpectorally, there is a danger of producing severe distortion, due to irregular pocket development. Therefore, the surgeon should be skilled in this procedure prior to attempting it (Fig. 9.52).

Sensitivity to Betadine may produce an acneoid eruption when the material is in contact with the skin for a period of time (Fig. 9.53). Excess Betadine should be washed from the skin following surgery. Oral steroid therapy may be required to treat severe eruptions.

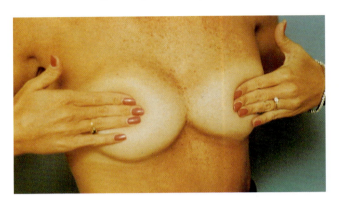 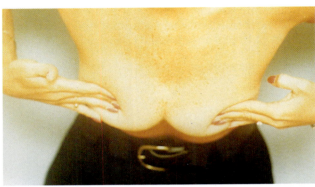

Figure 9.51. Dissection across the midline, creating communication between the pockets. Care should be taken to avoid crossing the midline.

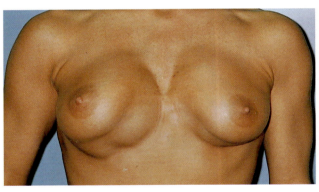 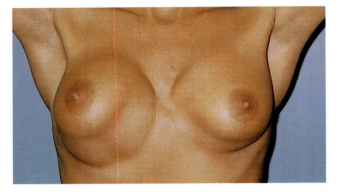

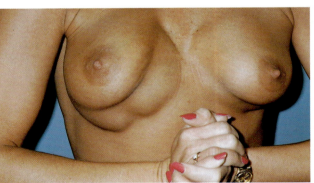

Figure 9.52. Severe deformity following transaxillary subpectoral placement of the prostheses. Note the marked irregularity of the pockets, as well as disruption of the pectoralis muscle. This deformity is extremely difficult to correct.

CONCLUSION

Breast augmentation is one of the most satisfying surgical procedures performed. Studies of large groups of women have reported 90+% acceptance rate, with only 2% to 4% of patients stating they would not have the procedure repeated. Care should be taken to fully inform the patient of the possible complications, to impress upon her the importance of maintaining contact with the surgeon, and to request annual office visits (at least) so that any new data on implant safety and efficacy can be discussed. The importance of mammography by a competent radiologist familiar with breast implants should also be discussed, and informed consent specifically for breast augmentation should be reviewed and signed by the patient. Allow the patient to take home a copy of the consent. She and/or her spouse may then review it at leisure and contact you should any questions need to be answered prior to surgery. Finally, the various types of prostheses should be discussed with the patient so that she can make a reasonable decision.

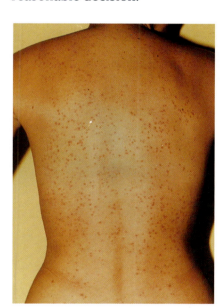

Figure 9.53. Severe acneoid eruption of back following Betadine sensitivity.

BIBLIOGRAPHY

Baker JL Jr: Augmentation mammoplasty. In Grabb C, Smith JW, (eds): Plastic Surgery, 3rd ed. Little, Brown, Boston, 1979.

Baker JL Jr: Augmentation mammoplasty. In Owsley JQ Jr, Peterson RA, (eds): Symposium on Aesthetic Surgery of the Breast, Scottsdale, Arizona 1975. St. Louis, CV Mosby, 1978.

Baker JL Jr: Breast augmentation and capsular contractures. In Barrett BM, Jr, (ed): Manual for Patient Care in Plastic Surgery. Little, Brown, Boston, 1982.

Baker JL Jr: The effectiveness of alpha-tocopherol (vitamin E) in reducing the incidence of sperical contracture around breast implants. Plast Reconstr Surg 65:696, 1981.

Baker JL Jr, Bartels RJ, Douglas WM: Closed compression technique for rupturing a contracted capsule around a breast implant. Plast Reconstr Surg 58:137, 1976.

Baker JL Jr, Chandler ML, LeVier RR: Occurrence and activity of myofibroblasts in human capsular contracture tissue surrounding mammary implants. Plast Reconstr Surg 68:905, 1981.

Baker JL Jr, Donis R: Genesis and management of the hard augmented breast. In Habal M, (ed): Advances in Plastic and Reconstructive Surgery, Vol 6. Year Book Medical, Chicago, 1990.

Baker JL Jr, Kolin IS, Bartlett ES: The psychosexual dynamics of patients undergoing mammary augmentation. Plast Reconstr Surg 53:652, 1974.

Baker JL Jr, Mara JE, Linville J: Diagnosis and treatment of masses in the augmented breast. Rocky Mt Med J, 74:255, 1978.

Baker JL Jr, LeVier RR, Speilvogel DE: Positive identification of silicone in human mammary capsular tissue. Plast Reconstr Surg 69:56, 1982.

Baker JL Jr, Penn JG: Augmentation mammoplasty. In Goldwyn RM, (ed): The Unfavorable Result in Plastic Surgery, Avoidance and Treatment, 2nd ed. Little, Brown, Boston, 1984.

Courtiss EH, Goldwyn RM: Breast sensation before and after plastic surgery. Plast Reconstr Surg 58:1, 1976.

Farina MA, Newby BG, Alani HM: Innervation of the nipple-areola complex. Plast Reconstr Surg 66:497, 1980.

Little GA, Baker JL Jr: Results of closed compression capsulotomy for treatment of contracted breast implant capsules. Plast Reconstr Surg 65:30, 1980.

Morbidity and Mortality Weekly Report Center for Disease Control, Dec 22, 1978. Vol 27, No. 51, Pg. 513.

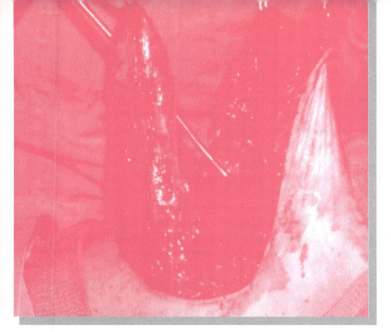

REDUCTION
MAMMAPLASTY

Eugene H. Courtiss
Robert M. Goldwyn

CHAPTER 10

PREOPERATIVE PROBLEMS

Realistic Expectations

Although realistic expectations on the part of both the patient and surgeon cannot guarantee a happy outcome after aesthetic surgical procedures, particularly following reduction mammaplasty, they are a vital element preoperatively. Thus, if the patient's expectations are appropriate, she may be a candidate for reduction mammaplasty. If her expectations are unrealistic, surgery should be denied or at least delayed. Operating on patients who have unrealistic expectations of how their lives or appearance will change after surgery may be catastrophic.

Aesthetic Result

Techniques for measuring breast volume have been suggested; however, they are imprecise. Bra-cup sizes may be used as references, but the patient should not be guaranteed a specific size bra.

Medical Risks

If the patient is in good health and does not have contravening medical disease, she is probably a

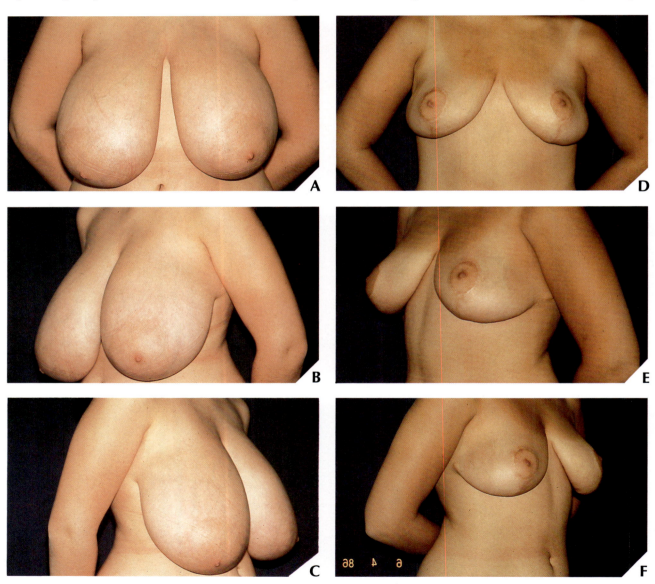

Figure 10.1. Good result following inferior pedicle procedure. **(A-C)** Before surgery. **(D-F)** One year after surgery.

good candidate for reduction mammaplasty. Those with medical conditions should be properly evaluated.

Obesity

As in all surgery, patients who are overweight are not as good candidates for reduction mammaplasty as those who are thin. Overweight patients have a greater tendency for fat necrosis and infection. In addition the aesthetic result in patients who are overweight is not as favorable as in those who are thin.

Tendency for Thickened Scars

Patients who have a tendency to develop thickened scars, often called a keloid tendency, may be more likely than others to scar severely, paticularly at the ends of the horizontal, inframammary scar. These patients should be forewarned accordingly.

Medications

Patients who are taking aspirin or any other medication that alters blood coagulation should stop taking such medication 2 weeks prior to surgery.

Technique

There are many techniques for performing reduction mammaplasties. For most patients, the authors prefer using the inferior pedicle technique (Fig.10.1). However, we recognize that other surgeons may favor other techniques. Regardless of the technique the surgeon employs, the limitations of the technique should be understood and the surgeon should be prepared to use another technique when indicated. Thus, when the distance of the nipple/areola transpostion is minimal, the superior pedicle method may be preferable (Fig. 10.2). At the other extreme, when the breasts are massively

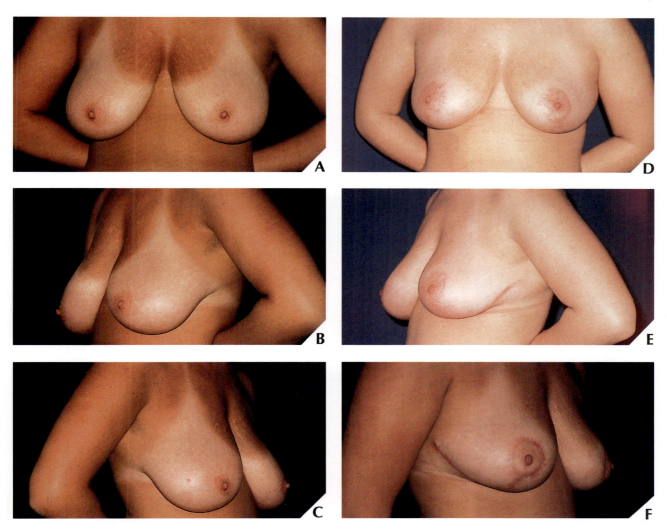

Figure 10.2. Good result using superior pedicle procedure. **(A-C)** Before surgery. **(D-F)** Eight months after surgery.

enlarged, transplantation of the nipple and areola as a free graft may be the method of choice (Fig. 10.3).

Preoperative Marking

Because the breasts shift significantly when patients are supine, the breasts should be marked preoperatively while the patient is either sitting or standing. This should be done before the patient is anesthetized since it allows the patient another opportunity to discuss her objectives with the surgeon.

Whether the marking is complete or partial depends on the surgeon. However, the most important marking are transference of the level of the inframammary fold onto the anterior surface of the breast and identification of the central meridian of the breast. These lines form the basis for the location of the nipple/areola complex,

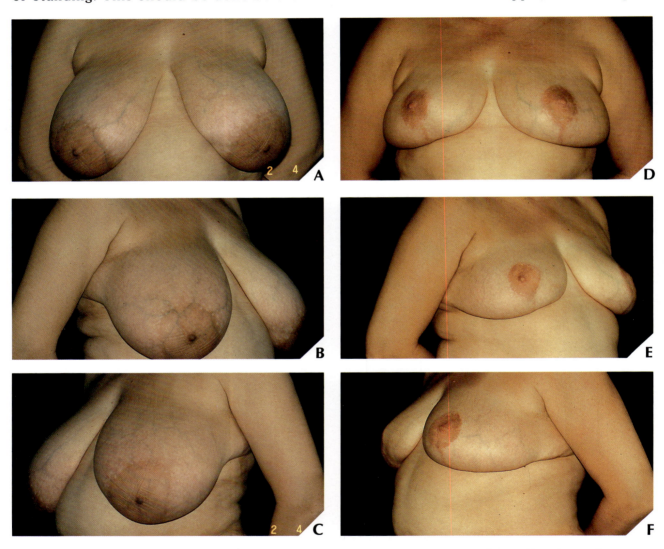

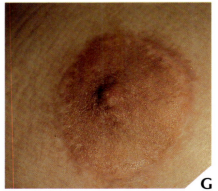

Figure 10.3. Good result using transplantation. **(A-C)** Before surgery. **(D-F)** One year after surgery. **(G)** Close-up of nipple at 1 year postoperatively.

which should be kept on the low side. It is easy to raise the nipple and areola in a secondary procedure but impossible to lower it without leaving a superior scar.

Patients who have giant areolae should be treated as if the condition does not exist. They should be informed that it may be necessary to leave some areola and later, after the skin has stretched, excise it.

Patients who have webbing between their breasts present special problem. Excision across the midline may result in a thick web scar. As a result, we avoid incisions that cross the midline connecting the two breasts. Instead we rotate our excision pattern laterally and use liposuction to remove fat under the skin (Fig. 10.4).

Asymmetry

Patients who are asymmetric should have their breasts marked to treat the problem. In addition, the condition should be discussed with the patient and recorded in the medical record.

INTRAOPERATIVE PROBLEMS

Blood Loss

Because blood loss during reduction mammaplasty may be significant, efforts should be made to minimize the amount lost. We employ hemostasis, pressure, electrocoagulation, and epinephrine-containing solutions.

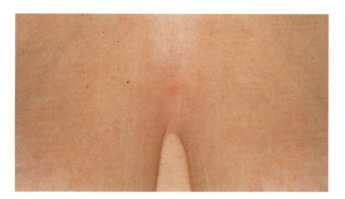

Whether patients should provide their own blood prior to surgery is debatable. Because of the blood-saving measures mentioned above, blood loss during reduction mammaplasty infrequently requires transfusion. We do not routinely prepare autologous or homologous transfustion. However, in large-breasted women, particularly those who bruise easily or have bled during other operations, despite normal bleeding studies, the use of autologous blood may be indicated.

Vascular Compromise of Nipple/Areola Complex

Vascular compromise of the nipple/areola complex may be due to epinephrine drift, compression of the pedicle, or transection of the blood supply of the pedicle.

Epinephrine drift can be prevented by not injecting the area with the drug; it is self-limiting. Vascular compromise secondary to compression of the pedicle can be distinguished from that secondary to transection of the blood supply by removing all sutures and evaluating the color of the nipple/areola complex. If it is still questionable (or if the areolar skin is normally very dark), fluorescein should be injected intravenously and the nipple and areola evaluated using a Wood's light. If the areola fluoresces, careful closure, without kinking the pedicle, may begin. If this causes tension and the color turns dusky, thinning the flaps or pedicle, which may be done with a suction cannula, should be per-

Figure 10.4. Webbed breasts. (Same patient as in Fig. 10.6).

formed (Fig. 10.5). Another alternative is to leave the wound partially open. It will heal or may be closed secondarily.

If the nipple/areola complex does not fluoresce, it should be removed and placed on a dermal bed as a free graft without coring out the nipple. The distal nipple may slough but muscle will remain and surprisingly good nipple projection may result.

Difficult Closure

If the skin closure is too tight, poor scars or wound breakdown may occur. To prevent this, the surgeon has several options: 1) additional fat and breast parenchyma under the medial or lateral flaps may be removed; 2) if the tight closure is due to lack of skin (rather than tension), some of the skin removed in the specimen can be replaced as a split-thickness skin graft, provided the surgeon has not passed the skin off with the specimen; or 3) the wound can be closed partially, allowing it to heal secondarily with contraction and revising the scar later if necessary.

Dog Ears

If dog ears remain at the ends of the flaps, advancing the medial and lateral flaps toward them-

selves will minimize them. This maneuver also helps decrease tension on the vertical suture line. Dog ears due to fat can be excised sharply or removed by suction. Small dog ears usually disappear with time or can be excised in 3 to 6 months postoperatively.

Asymmetry

Asymmetry first noted intraoperatively should be addressed by whatever surgical measures are required to obtain the best possible symmetry. When this is done, care should be taken to keep the nipple/areola complex properly located, particularly vertically. It is important to have the patient symmetrically positioned on the operating table and sitting upright.

EARLY POSTOPERATIVE PROBLEMS

Hematoma

Large collections of fluid or blood may cause vascular compromise. Thus, if a large hematoma is detected, the patient should be returned to the operating room, the hematoma evacuated, bleeding vessels coagulated, and antibiotics (if not given previously) administered (Fig. 10.6).

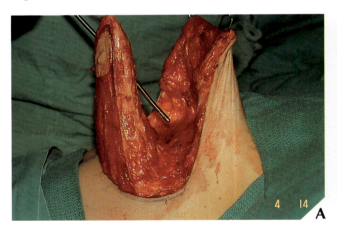

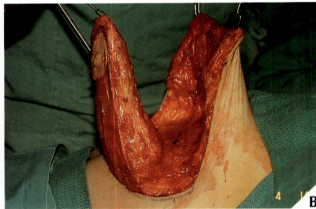

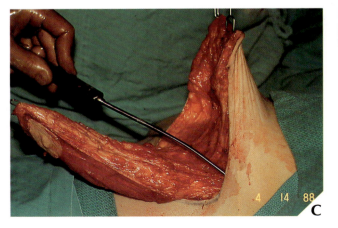

Figure 10.5. Cannula used to remove fat. **(A)** Inferior pedicle showing cannula. **(B)** Pedicle being thinned. **(C)** Cannula thinning axillary fat.

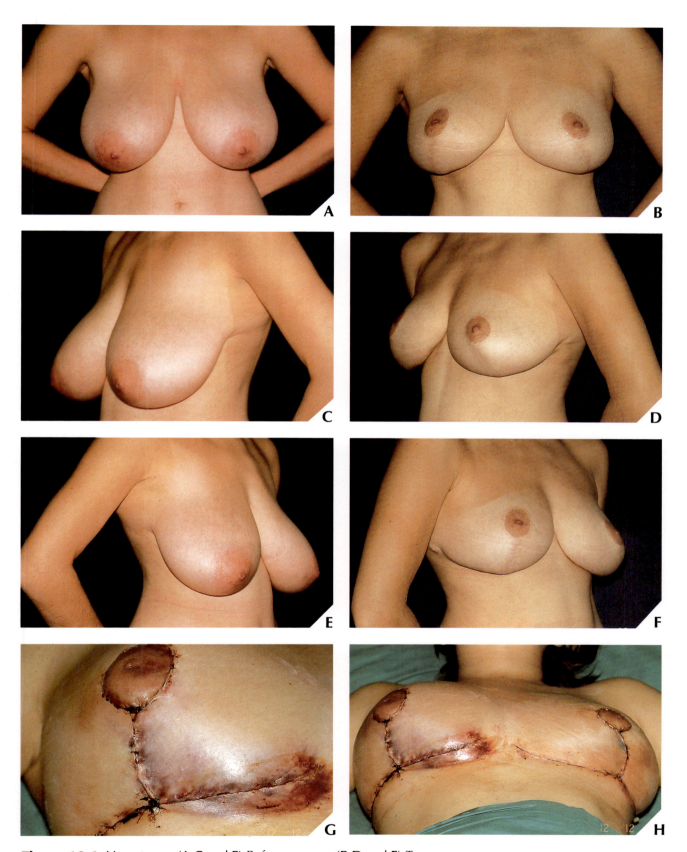

Figure 10.6. Hematoma. (**A,C** and **E**) Before surgery. (**B,D** and **F**) Two years postoperatively. (**G** and **H**) Evening of surgery.

Although drains do not prevent hematomas, they may be indicated after one has been evacuated. Small hematomas are usually detected a week or so after surgery when there is swelling or spontaneous drainage.

Dark Nipple/Areola Complex

If the nipple/areola complex appears dusky, the cause must be diagnosed and treated. Failure to do so may result in at least partial necrosis of the nipple/areola complex.

The entire dressing should be removed and the breast examined. If edema has compromised the venous outflow, removal of a few sutures may be sufficient. However, if the breast is very firm and engorged, a hematoma is probably present. In such instances, or if no apparent cause exists, the patient should be returned to the operating room and the sutures removed. Any hematoma present should be evacuated and any kinking of the pedicle treated. If, despite all efforts, the blood supply of the nipple/areola complex remains compromised, the nipple and areola should be excised and replaced on a well-vascularized dermal bed as a full-thickness skin graft.

If the nipple/areola complex is first noted to be dusky at 24 hours, medicinal leeches may be helpful (Fig. 10.7). Regardless of the cause, failure to treat the problem will result in at least partial necrosis of the nipple/areola complex (Fig. 10.8).

Decreased Sensation of the Nipple/Areola Complex

If, in the immediate postoperative interval, the patient has decreased sensation of the nipple/areola complex nothing should be done. In all probability the patient has a neuropraxia that will resolve within 3 weeks.

LATE POSTOPERATIVE PROBLEMS

Unexpected Malignancy

Prior to undergoing reduction mammaplasty, women over 35 years old should have a mammogram if their family history is positive for breast cancer in women over 30. If, in spite of a negative preoperative mammogram, the patient is found to have a malignancy, a surgeon who treats carcinoma of the breast should be consulted.

Obviously during surgery and in processing, the specimens should be carefully separated to avoid confusion about which side contained the malignancy.

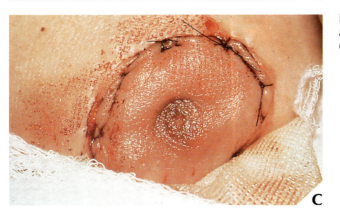
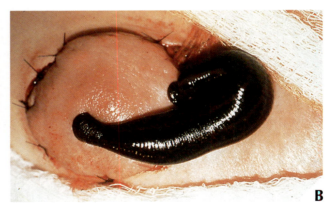

Figure 10.7. Use of leeches. **(A)** Dusky nipple and areola. **(B)** Leech on nipple/areola complex. **(C)** Result.

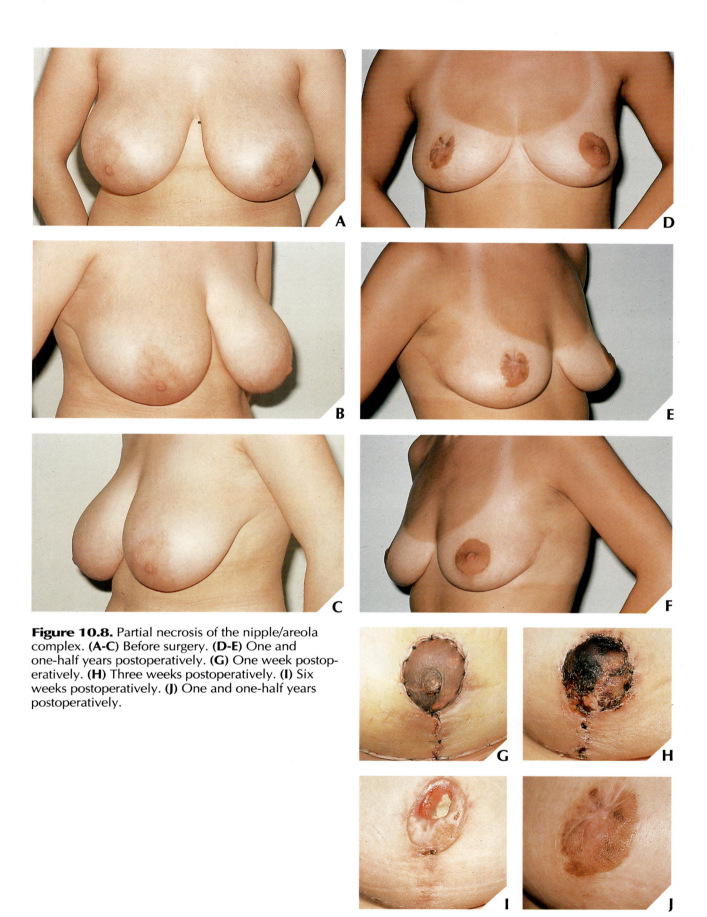

Figure 10.8. Partial necrosis of the nipple/areola complex. **(A-C)** Before surgery. **(D-E)** One and one-half years postoperatively. **(G)** One week postoperatively. **(H)** Three weeks postoperatively. **(I)** Six weeks postoperatively. **(J)** One and one-half years postoperatively.

Infection

If the breast is warm and tender, or the patient has a fever, an infection is probably present. Suture removal, drainage, and antibiotics should be instituted.

Fat Necrosis

Fat necrosis usually presents as spontaneous draining of oily fluid. It is self-limiting and requires no treatment. On occasion fat necrosis will present as a mass. In such cases, the diagnosis

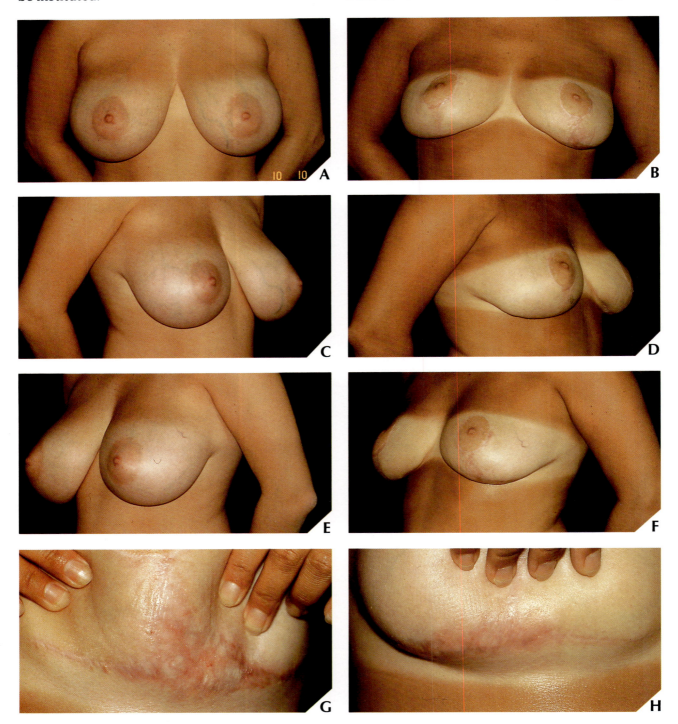

Figure 10.9. Poor healing at inverted "T." (**A, C** and **E**) Before surgery. (**B, D** and **F**) Nine months postoperatively. (**G** and **H**) Close-up demonstrating poor healing.

should be made by biopsy and treatment by drainage should be instituted. Debridement with saline gauze packing is occasionally necessary.

Poor Healing
Poor healing either from tension or no apparent cause may occur. Most commonly it develops at the inverted "T," but may occur at any location (Fig. 10.9). Measures such as suture removal, debridment, and dressing changes should be employed. Even if the defect is large, healing is by secondary intention and contracture may be preferable to skin grafting.

Loss of Nipple/Areola Sensation
Most patients have decreased nipple sensation after a reduction mammaplasty. As an aside, large-breasted women tend to have less breast sensa-

tion in general. Sensation of the breasts should be evaluated preoperatively. Usually the condition improves significantly with time although several years may be required. In any event, there is no known treatment for lost or impaired sensation.

Location of Nipple/Areola Complex
If the nipple/areola complex is located too low, elevation is not difficult to achieve.

If the nipple and areola are too high, lowering them by excision of a pie shape of tissue above the inframammary fold may be attempted (Fig. 10.10). However, usually this maneuver results in only temporary improvement. To obtain a permanent correction, a direct V-Y maneuver may be used, but this leaves a scar above the areola. Since the treatment options for a low nipple/areola complex are unsatisfactory, prevention is critical.

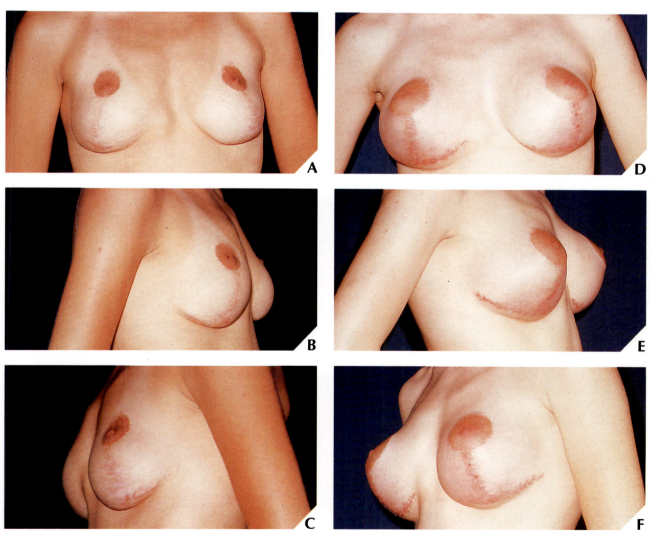

Figure 10.10. Treatment of high nipple/areola complex. Two years previously, patient had a mastopexy by another surgeon. **(A-C)** Post-mastopexy. A bilateral aug- mention mammaplasty and excision of skin horizontally were performed to pull down nipple/areola complex. **(D-F)** One month after surgery. (continued on next page)

Areolar Deformities and Color Changes

If the areola is deformed, revision may be indicated after sufficient time has elapsed to permit full scar maturation. Correction may necessitate treating an inverted nipple or an asymmetric areola. If the color of the areola is poor, tattooing may be helpful.

Poor Scarring

Obtaining fine, hairline scars in breast reduction may be difficult. Usually the circumareolar scar heals kindly, as does the vertical scar. However, the horizontal component may not heal well, especially at the lateral and medial ends (Fig. 10.11). Occasionally, steriod injections, silicone gel sheeting, and scar revision may be beneficial.

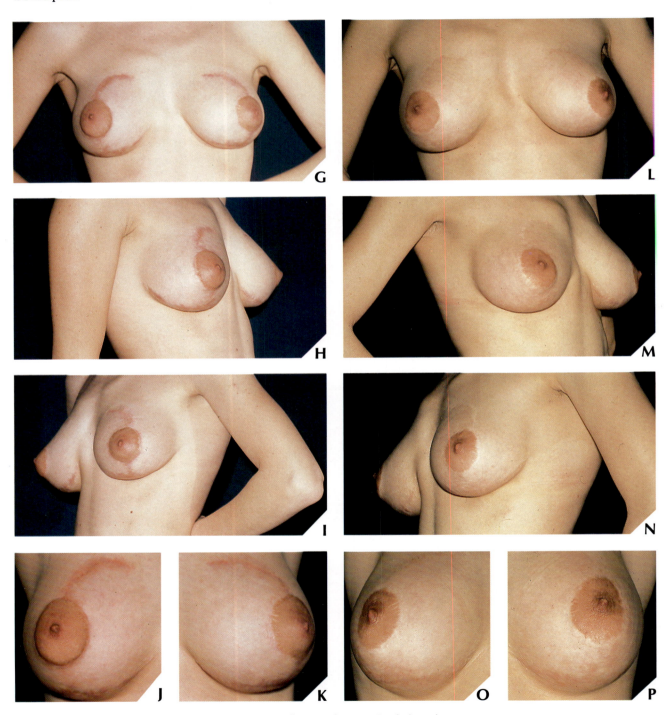

Figure 10.10.(cont'd) A V-Y maneuver was done to lower nipple/areola complex. **(G-K)** Four months after V-Y procedure. **(L-P)** Five years after last surgery.

Asymmetry

If the patient's breast are asymmetric, a secondary procedure may be beneficial after sufficient time has elapsed to permit final healing. If the asymmetry is due to loss of fat, contouring with suction may be helpful. If it is not, then additional techniques, such as local excision and local flaps, may be necessary.

BIBLIOGRAPHY

Courtiss EH, Goldwyn RM: Breast sensation before and after plastic surgery. Plast Reconstr Surg 58:1, 1976.

Courtiss EH, Goldwyn RM: Reduction mammaplasty by the inferior pedicle technique. Plast Reconstr Surg 59:500, 1977.

Courtiss EH, Goldwyn RM: Update. A reduction

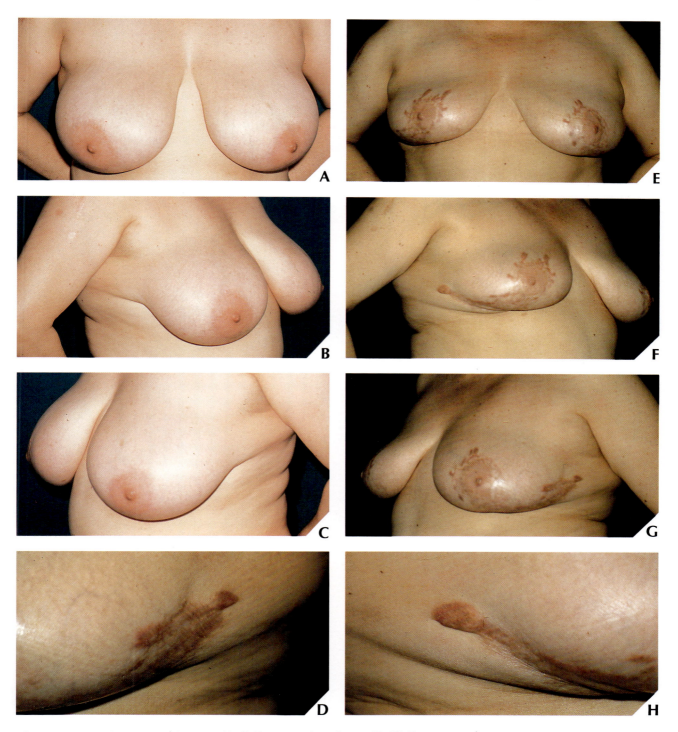

Figure 10.11. Hypertrophic scar. **(A-C)** Preoperative views. **(D-H)** Ten years after surgery.

mammaplasty by the inferior pedicle technique. Plast Reconstr Surg 66:646, 1980.

Georgiade NG, Georgiade GS, Riefkol R: Aesthetic Surgery of the Breast, WB Saunders, Philadelphia, 1990.

Goldwyn RM, Courtiss EH: Reduction mammaplasty using inferior pedicle technique. In Regnault P, Daniel R (eds): Aesthetic Plastic Surgery. Little, Brown, Boston, 1984.

Goldwyn RM (ed): Reduction Mammaplasty. Little, Brown, Boston, 1990.

Goldwyn RM, Courtiss EH: Inferior pedicle technique. In Goldwyn RM (ed): Reduction Mammaplasty. Little, Brown, Boston, 1990.

McKissock PK: Reduction mammaplasty. In Courtiss EH (ed): Aesthetic Surgery: How to Avoid it and How to Treat it. CV Mosby, St. Louis, 1978.

McKissock P: Complications and undesirabel results with reduction mammaplasty. In RM Goldwyn (ed): The Unfavorable Result in Plastic Surgery, Little, Brown, Boston, 1984.

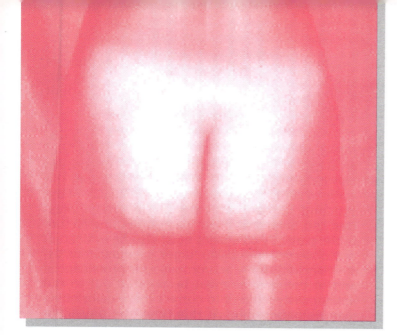

BODY CONTOUR SURGERY

W. Graham Wood

Fredrick M. Grazer

CHAPTER 11

The most distressing aspect of a plastic surgeon's professional life is the development of a postoperative complication. The best way to minimize this peril is to do everything possible to prevent complications from occurring. Risk prevention begins with the clinical competency of the operating surgeon. Core surgical training, as well as body contour training, are mandatory parts of the training curriculum. These are the basics on which innate ability and experience merge to form clinical competency.

Assuming the surgeon is clinically competent, the next major criterion in complication prevention is patient selection. The motivation and expected goals of the patient must be critically analyzed by the surgeon. The psychological status of the patient and the physical state of the patient from a surgical/anesthetic point of view should also be analyzed. Family/genetic history that might give clues to surgical and/or anesthetic risks must be determined.

Every patient requesting body contour surgery has a motivating reason. Body contour surgeons must closely examine the motivations and expectations of the patient, using their experience, skill, and thorough understanding of the patient's desires. The astute surgeon should be able to advise the patient of the percent improvement that can be expected from a proposed procedure. If the patient is aware of and accepts the motivating stimuli, the gamut of possible complications, and the percentage of improvement that can be expected, that patient can then be considered a potential candidate for surgery.

The surgeon should be fully aware of the enlightened attitudes of our changing society and the motivational needs of the patient, without being judgmental and reliant on outdated notions of teachings in the past. As long as the patient has a thorough understanding of the percent improvement that can be realistically expected, minor body contour defects may be corrected even though the improvement might be relatively slight. If the patient is well informed and accepting of all of the above-mentioned parameters, he can be extremely gratified and appreciative of even a small percentage of improvement.

THE PREOPERATIVE CONSULTATION

There is only a certain amount of time available for the surgeon to interview the patient. Even if multiple interviews are a part of the preoperative planning, it is impossible to analyze all of the facets of a patient's psychological make-up. Sometimes the person we initially judge to be stable turns out to be emotionally inept. If signs of emotional problems are noticed at the time of consultation or preoperative evaluation, the surgeon must decide whether or not the patient needs preoperative psychological evaluation.

Examination and evaluation of the patient's chief complaints should be conducted on a disrobed patient. This is necessary so that the surgeon can evaluate the anatomical area of concern and its adjacent areas. In the examination, the surgeon should note the texture and quality of the skin and subcutaneous tissue. Underlying muscles and bone that might be contributing factors to the patient's complaint must also be evaluated. Any observations of skin turgor, subcutaneous tissue flaccidity, bony and/or muscular prominences and/or concavities must be pointed out to the patient since surgery to correct these deformities may be impossible. At this time, the physician must be careful to examine for umbilical hernias, inguinal hernias, abdominal wall hernias, and incisional hernias and inform the patient of these abnormalities. The patient must be informed if autologous fat grafting will be necessary to fill in existing depressions that cannot be corrected by other surgical measures. It is also appropriate at this time to point out any surgical maneuvers that would be necessary to modify underlying muscle or bony prominences.

To better demonstrate the nature of the proposed surgery, it is helpful to take polaroid photographs of the areas of chief complaint. Anterior, posterior, left lateral, and right lateral photographs should be taken and placed in clear polyethylene folders so that both the patient and the surgeon can mark on the transparent overlay. The patient can identify those areas that are of chief concern. As an adjunct to describing the proposed procedure, the surgeon can mark on the overlay with a different colored pen. Alcohol on a cottonball can be used to easily erase any lines on the sketches that do not meet with approval. Using this pictorial method of communication, it is easier for each of the parties to grasp what the other has in mind. Evaluating the photographs also affords an excellent opportunity for the patient's wants and desires to be expressed and for the surgeon to indicate whether or not the patient's desires are realistic.

There are few body contour surgeries performed in which a change on the frontal or posterior plane does not produce a secondary change on the lateral plane and vice versa. It is very important for the patient to understand that changing one anatomical area can produce a secondary change in another area. Once this concept is understood, the patient will be better prepared to accept the postoperative results. The right and left sides of the human body are, by nature, slightly unequal, therefore achieving exact left/right volumetric equality and left/right horizontal and vertical symmetry is extremely difficult. Pre-existing asymmetries must be pointed out to the patient in the preoperative planning stage.

During the patient education process, the use of photographs of pre- and postoperative results of the surgeon's past surgeries will give the patient an opportunity to evaluate preoperative body types and defects similar to his or her own. This better enables the patient to ask pertinent questions about his or her deformity. This method of education also gives the patient an opportunity to note and compare the aesthetic preference of the surgeon with his or her own. The up-front-and-honest patient may express displeasure with the postoperative results of previous patients' surgeries. Admittedly, this is not flattering to the surgeon's ego; however, the emotionally mature surgeon should realize the benefits derived from a patient who can express both delight and displeasure while viewing the surgeon's past surgeries. Through this process, the basis for rejection can be decided upon by both parties involved. Had this awareness not been cultivated, postoperative differences of opinion of the patient and surgeon might result. The patient with a passive personality does not openly communicate differences in aesthetic preference to the surgeon at the time of consultation. This type of patient, if not pleased with the surgeon's aesthetic taste, at least has the opportunity to seek consultation elsewhere. Likewise, the surgeon has the opportunity to decline to do the proposed surgery if the patient's expectations exceed the realm of capability of the surgeon.

Finally, postoperative photographs can also be used to demonstrate placement of incisions so that the patient can judge whether or not the postoperative scars would be acceptable.

By far the most frequent postoperative complication is an undesirable result. An undesirable result may not only be caused by complication or sequelae, but by the inability of the doctor and patient to communicate and understand what reasonable improvement can be expected. For a patient to be pleased with a postoperative result, it is absolutely necessary that the limitations that must be exercised to ensure patient safety are understood. It is also paramount that the surgeon be able to deliver the improvement expected by the patient. Should the surgeon or patient feel uneasy about their communication at the first consultation, a second consultation at a later time could provide both parties an opportunity to thoughtfully address the issues raised at the original consultation. At the second consultation, if either the surgeon or the patient has an uneasy feeling about the appropriateness of the procedure or the expectation of the results, the probable course of action should be to postpone the proposed procedure until there is a better meeting of minds.

PREOPERATIVE CONSIDERATIONS

With the increased number of facilities for collecting autologous blood, its use is now the rule rather than the exception. The replacement of blood should be considered for any operation where there is a probable blood loss of more than 1 unit. The economy and safety of autologous blood replacement is well established. Postoperative recovery has been greatly improved in patients with a unit replaced for a unit lost. The patients not only look and feel better in the recovery room, they also return to their daily physical activities and their professional pursuits much more rapidly than those patients who were not given autologous blood replacement. The ultimate decision for autologous blood replacement rests in the hands of the surgeon. Today, many well-informed patients are requesting autologous blood replacement because of public awareness of its salutary effect.

The family history is a very important aspect of the presurgical work-up. The classical family history should be taken, with particular emphasis on relatives who might have had malignant hyperthermia or familial coagulopathies. History of coronary artery disease and diabetes should be noted. If there is a family history of malignant hyperthermia, the anesthesiologist or anesthetist will need to be appraised of this finding. If there is a family history of coagulopathies, a work-up by a hematologist may prove to be beneficial. The patient's past history, with emphasis on surgical and anesthetic history, should be obtained. The history of both over-the-counter and prescription medications must be reviewed and a written list of contraindicated medications prior to surgery should be given to the patient. The patient must also be instructed on which maintenance medications that they might already be taking should be continued up to and after the day of surgery.

Routine laboratory and diagnostic procedures should be performed preoperatively to rule out any pre-existing medical problems that might be detrimental to the patient if the proposed surgery is performed. If red flags go up in the family history, personal medical history, physical examination, or laboratory and/or diagnostic procedures, the appropriate specialist should be consulted and clearances received before the surgery is done.

Many hospitals and institutions require that laboratory work and other diagnostic procedures be performed not more than 72 hours prior to surgery. We disagree with this practice and feel that preoperative laboratory data and other diagnostic tests and procedures should be performed at least 1 week before surgery so that any abnormalities would be noted in time for the appropriate specialists to be consulted and a plan of action initiated to remedy the problem. Receiving findings indicating abnormalities in laboratory and diagnostic work-ups at the eleventh hour causes confusion and errors in judgment as to whether or not the proposed surgery should be performed or cancelled.

In excisional body contour surgery, pre- and postoperative smoking can produce catastrophic results in tissue undermining procedures. Patients *must* be made aware of all probable complications should they elect to continue to use tobacco products. They must be given a written statement warning them of the hazards to the surgical flaps and the cardiovascular and pulmonary hazards that smoking could cause during the intra- and postanasthesia periods. If excisional body contour surgery is to be performed and the patient will not agree to stop smoking for 2 weeks before and 2 weeks after surgery, the surgeon should seriously consider not performing the surgery. The patient must be reminded that drugs that prolong the bleeding mechanism must be avoided. The patient should be given appropriate warnings on direct sun exposure immediately postoperatively. The photochemical reaction of the sun with the hemoglobin pigment may prolong bruising. Patients sun bathing after excisional flap surgery, such as an abdominoplasty, should be instructed not to wear dark-colored swim suits since clothing of dark colors attract heat, which has been reported to result in tissue ischemia. Sun screens should always be used liberally when sun exposure is anticipated.

It is recommended that all patients be placed on a balanced diet preoperatively and understand the necessity of maintaining it for optimum postoperative healing. Female patients should be informed that future pregnancy might impose deleterious effect on their breast and abdominal surgery. Personal hygiene should be stressed in the preoperative and immediately postoperative phase of recovery. Patients also need to be given some idea of the amount of postoperative pain to expect. They should be alerted to the duration of time required for postoperative recovery.

A decision must be made on whether or not the surgery will require hospitalization or be performed in an out-patient setting. It must be decided in advance if a recuperation facility is needed or if the patient can recover at home. If a halfway house is needed, reservations should be made well in advance to accommodate the patient.

If there is a probability of using surgical drains, the patient should be advised preoperatively. If patients are not advised preoperatively, when they awaken and find out they have drains, oftentimes they feel that something might have gone wrong during the surgery. This may cause a great deal of unnecessary anxiety.

The patient should always be advised of the surgeon's fee. The assistant surgeon's fee should also be quoted, when applicable. The patient should be made aware of all operating room costs, the anesthesia costs, and the expenses for preoperative diagnostic studies and postoperative prescription. Depending upon the policy of the operating surgeon, the patient should be advised about possible expenses if a complication were to arise postoperatively. Misunderstandings about the financial arrangements of surgery can precipitate disagreements after surgery that can turn into a complication for the surgeon.

INTRAOPERATIVE CONSIDERATIONS

The operating room personnel must be competent in the prep and drape of the patient in order to minimize the risk of infection. The surgeon should supervise these maneuvers to assure quality control. It is especially important that the inner depth of the umbilicus be properly prepped if it is to be used as an entrance for the suction cannula.

Prevention of systemic complications during the intra- and postoperative period focuses on adequate autologous blood replacement and crystalloid and colloid IV fluid volume replacement. The patient should be preloaded with crystalloid in the presurgical holding area. It is mandatory that the anesthetist not get behind on fluid replacement during the intraoperative period. The general guidelines for crystalloid minimal replacement is 2 l per 1 l of loss if no blood transfusion is given, and 1.5 l per 1 l of loss if autologous blood is given. If more than 1.5 l are lost, 1 unit of colloid or whole autologous blood should be transfused in addition to the fluid replacement. If more than 2000 ml are lost, 1 unit of whole autologous blood should be given for each additional 500 ml lost.

We recommend using intraoperative corticosteroids with 500 mg of Solu-Medrol or the equivalent given intravenously. An IV alcohol for prophylaxis of pulmonary fat emboli syndrome is also routinely given. The IV alcohol administered intraoperatively has provided an additional margin of safety in our opinion, but the primary treatment for postoperative, full-blown fat emboli syndrome is megadoses of IV corticosteroids. Intraoperatively, IV steroids, IV alcohol, and IV antibiotics are given routinely. The regimen consists of 500 mg of IV Solu-Medrol, 5% alcohol and 5% dextrose; they are started before surgery begins and are administered during the entire course of surgery. Each 100 ml contains 5 ml of dehydrated alcohol and 5 gm of dextrose administered as follows: 150 ml per 50 lb body weight up to 150 lb; thereafter, 250 ml per 50 lb body weight, not to exceed 1000 ml per 4-hour period.

With alcohol administration, anesthetic gas flows may be reduced slightly. When IV alcohol is used there might be some mild hypotension during the immediate postoperative recovery period. This is handled with appropriate fluid replacement and has not been a problem in our practice. Alcohol may also contribute to some additional postoperative nausea. We have found that the intraoperative use of IV Inapsine, 0.625 mg, may help prevent some postoperative nausea.

POSTOPERATIVE CONSIDERATIONS

An additional intravenous injection of the appropriate antibiotic is given in the recovery room, and the patient is continued on oral antibiotics for a 7-day period postoperatively.

Age, obesity, smoking, and a history of thrombophlebitis and pulmonary embolism all increase the incidence of deep-vein thrombosis in the patient postoperatively. The use of oral contraceptives and the existence of varicose veins are additional risk factors that may present in patients undergoing body contour surgery. Elastic stockings during and after surgery and/or alternating inflating/deflating anti-embolism stockings may be used. Patients are encouraged to plantar flex their feet while laying in bed, and usually they begin ambulation the day of surgery. Progressive ambulation is encouraged and mandatory the day after surgery and thereafter.

If there are signs and symptoms of deep-vein thrombosis and/or thromboembolism, a multidisciplinary team comprised of a vascular surgeon, radiological sub-specialist, internist, and the operating plastic surgeon must convene. First, the clear-cut diagnosis and/or probability factors must be balanced against the risk factors of treatment, if indeed the probability of such is uncertain.

Intraoperatively, if the surgeon suspects that there are circulatory problems developing, the appropriate measures must be taken to determine the etiology of the ischemia and corrective measures must follow. The cause of any postoperative flap ischemia must be determined, and, if not surgically correctable, the immediate use of hyperbaric oxygenation should be considered. It is very important to remember that excessive pressure from an abdominal binder may cause compromise of circulation. Excessive pressure from abdominal binders may also inhibit the excursions of the diaphragm and give rise to postoperative pulmonary complications.

The commitment of the surgeon and his staff does not end once successful surgery has been performed. It is very important that the surgeon and his staff be aware of the high incidence of psychological depression that often complicates recovery of the aesthetic surgery patient. All staff members must be alerted to the signs and symptoms of postoperative depression. Depression sometimes may be precipitated by the use of steroids. The surgeon has the responsibility to determine when postoperative depression cannot be treated by the tincture of time and reassurance alone. It is his responsibility to direct the patient to the appropriate health care specialist for treatment should the need arise.

No matter how pleasing the aesthetic result, thee is often a period of psychological adjustment to the change in the patient's appearance. The surgeon and his staff must be aware of this and not be offended if the patient is uncomplimentary, even if the surgical result is excellent. Occasionally, the surgeon's critical eye may make him dissatisfied with some small detail in the patient's postoperative result. If the patient is pleased with the results, the surgeon's voiced observations of slight imperfection can generate unnecessary patient dissatisfaction.

When the patient is ready to be picked up from the recovery room, the responsible party is reminded of the "dos and don'ts" of postoperative care before the patient is discharged. Written orders are given to the responsible party, including instructions for wound care, dressing changes, drain care, personal hygiene, and prescribed drugs. The responsible party is given verbal and written descriptions of symptoms of vascular compromise, hematoma, and wound infection. The patient is cautioned on driving an automobile or performing hazardous tasks during the immediately postoperative period and anytime while pain medications are being taken. The responsible party is given the surgeon's emergency telephone number in case problems or questions should arise. An appointment card is also given, stating when the patient should return for postoperative follow-up care.

It is the surgeon's responsibility to be available to respond to an emergency or to provide coverage for another clinically competent plastic surgeon should an emergency arise during the postoperative period.

CHRONIC POSTOPERATIVE COMPLICATIONS

Chronic infection and sinus drainage are treated according to standard surgical principles. These consist of incision, drainage, and debridement. Gram stain, culture, and sensitivity, including a search for occult pathogens such as acid-fast bacilli/mycobacterium and fungi, are mandatory. It is wise for the surgeon to work in concert with an infectious disease specialist who would conduct the regimen of antibiotic therapy.

Chronic induration generally improves with time; however, the use of dilute depository corticosteroid injections may produce some salutary response. The use of ultrasound has also been helpful.

The seldom-encountered complication of postoperative chronic pain is apt to be associated with improper surgical contouring technique in which the incisions have been placed over pressure point areas and/or keltoid formation has taken place over pressure point areas. Proper positioning of surgical scar sites is important in prevention of pressure point pain. Careful use of dilute steroid injections along the scar line where the pain persists is sometimes beneficial. In cases of severe, chronic pain resulting from improperly placed incisions, repositioning of the scars may be necessary. Systemic anti-inflammatory non-steroidal medications may prove to be helpful in certain cases of chronic pain. Occasionally, chronic pain patients who do not respond to the conventional measures must be sent to pain specialists for consultation.

Rarely, cases of postoperative hyperpigmentation develop and are usually a result of temporarily impaired circulation. This mechanism is quite similar to the hyperpigmentation seen in stasis ulcer problems. A hyperpigmentation condition will generally disappear as the injured tissue repairs itself. Avoidance of sun exposure is indicated and perhaps a dermatological evaluation should be done. The use of skin bleaching creams such as Eldoquin Forte (4% hydroquinone USP) has been effective in selected cases.

Hypopigmentation is even rarer than hyperpigmentation and the treatment consists of a specific duration of sunlight exposure. This regimen in some cases has stimulated the pigment to return. Sun exposure, combined with the use of Trisoralen (trioxsalen), under the direction of a dermatologist has also been helpful in select cases.

Permanently altered sensation as a complication is very rare; usually any decrease in sensation is transitory. Permanently altered sensation usually only occurs in cases where skin reduction is involved. Sensation generally improves over time. If a deficit is persistent, the patient usually learns to live with the deficit without letting it interfere with quality of life.

BODY CONTOUR COMPLICATIONS

Regardless of the care in planning and execution of the surgery, complications will arise. The following atlas of cases demonstrates classical body contour complications and the methods used to correct the problems.

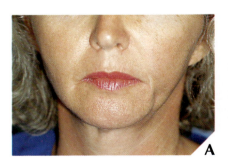 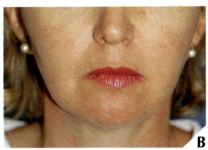

Figure 11.1. (A) Iatrogenic defect in the face of an over-suctioned patient. **(B)** This type of defect can be treated by autologous fat grafting and/or unilateral integument tightening. The same principles of correction apply to other areas of the face, including the mandibular line and submental areas.

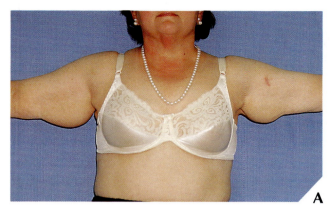 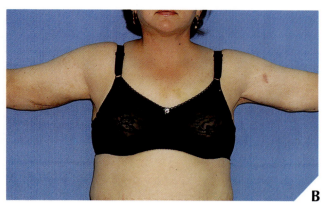

Figure 11.2. (A) Over-reduction of adipose tissue in the brachial area in which the integument did not conform properly during the postoperative period.

(B) Brachioplasty with excision of excess skin was necessary to correct this deformity.

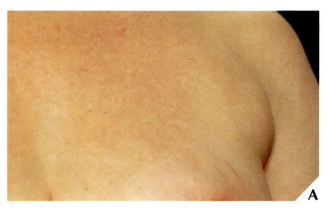 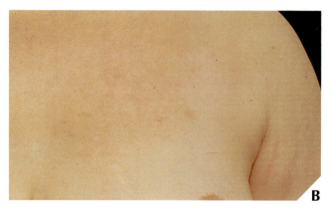

Figure 11.3. (A) Excess adipose tissue in the axillary area of a patient following breast reduction. **(B)** Cor-

rection of this defect was achieved using a 2.8-mm suction cannula to evacuate the excess adipose tissue.

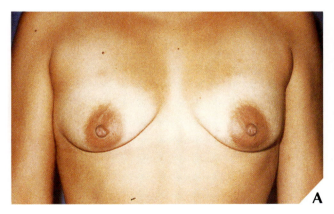 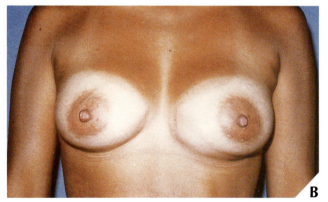

Figure 11.4. In an attempt to perform a suction aspiration breast reduction, excess flaccid integument and loss of the soft tissue breast mound with downward pointing nipples resulted **(A)**. **(B)** Reconstruction was

achieved by transaxillary breast augmentation, keeping in mind that a mastopexy might also be necessary if proper elevation of the nipple/areola complex was one of the surgical goals.

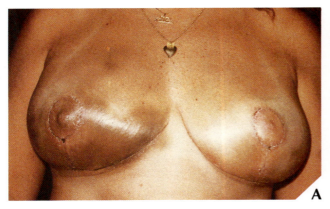

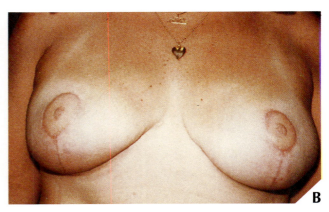

Figure 11.5. (A) Hematoma formation on the first day following breast reduction. **(B)** Suction aspiration of a 225-ml hematoma without any recollection of

blood worked very nicely to speed this patient's recovery.

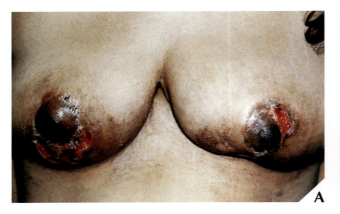

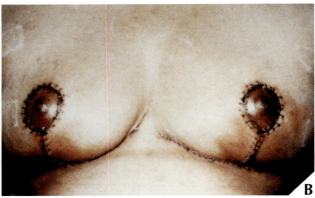

Figure 11.6. (A) Postoperative integument and soft tissue necrosis secondary to vascular embarrassment with necrosis and subsequent infection following a breast reduction. Correction of this defect required a

secondary inferior pedicle breast reduction. **(B)** The reconstruction produced acceptable left/right volumetric equality with vertical/horizontal symmetry of the nipple/areola complexes.

Figure 11.7. Postoperative accumulation of hematoma in the abdomen following abdominoplasty. This problem can be corrected by suction aspiration without reformation of hematoma.

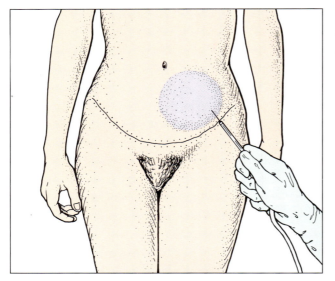

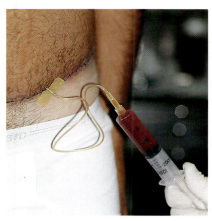

Figure 11.8. Aspiration of a seroma in a patient with abdominal wall reconstruction. A standard 16-gauge scalp vein set, with standard 20-ml hypodermic syringe, was used to evacuate the seroma. Aspirations on this patient were repeated at periodic intervals. The rare occurrence of a postoperative lymphocele in the lower extremity would be aspirated in the same manner.

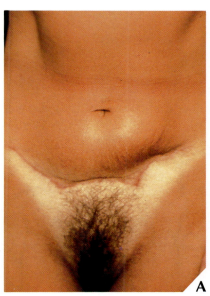

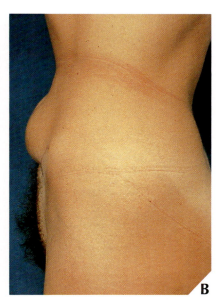

Figure 11.9. (A,B) Pseudocyst that formed during the postoperative period following an abdominal wall reconstruction. Repeated needle and syringe drainages failed to correct this deformity. **(C,D)** Surgical excision of the pseudocyst was necessary with recontouring of the skin flap on the left side of the abdomen.

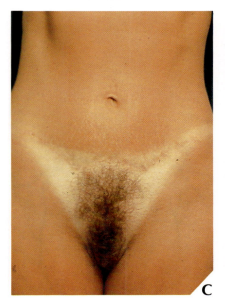

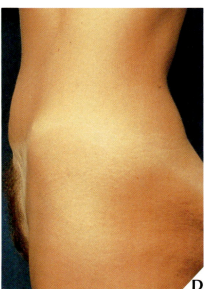

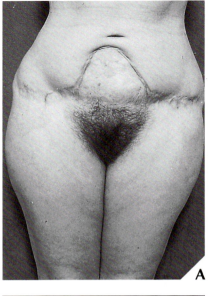

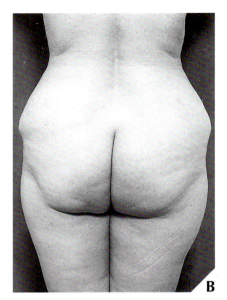

Figure 11.10. (A,B) Tissue necrosis in an abdominal wall reconstruction was treated initially with a split-thickness skin graft to cover the exposed rectus abdominus muscle. (C) Stage I reconstruction required vigorous suction of the adipose tissue in the posterior and lateral flanks. This removal of subcutaneous fat was necessary to provide excess integument that could later be rotated medially to cover the ventral abdominal wall defect. Suctioning adipose tissue in the upper pole of the buttocks and flank areas resulted in a pronounced protuberant and unaesthetic appearance of the trochanteric area of the buttocks and flanks. Therefore, camouflage suctioning of the trochanteric area was necessary to create an aesthetic balance. (D) The Stage II procedure was performed 3 months later with transpositional advancement of the excess skin gained from wide undermining laterally. The split-thickness graft was excised and covered with the medially advanced flap. (E) The inverted "T" closure of the medial advancement of the two lateral abdominal/flank flaps, and (F) the lateral extent of flap dissection into the lateral and posterior areas. The latter was necessary to gain the length needed for the closure.

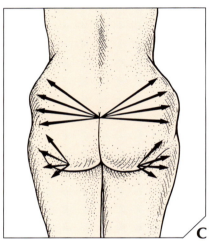

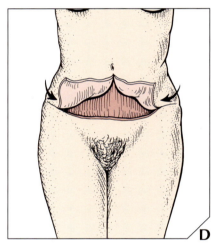

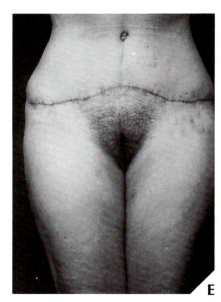

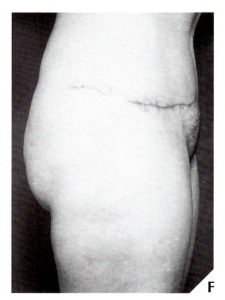

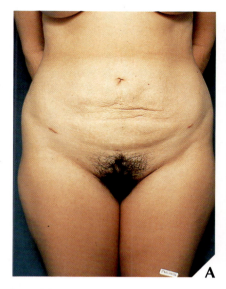 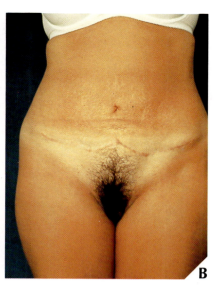

Figure 11.11. **(A)** Over-reduction in the lower abdomen due to overly aggressive aspiration of subcutaneous fat, which resulted in redundancy of the integument. **(B)** This condition was corrected by the standard procedure for lower abdominal integument reduction.

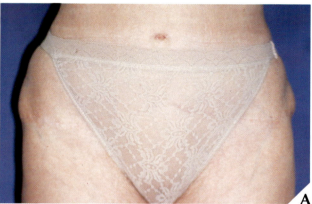 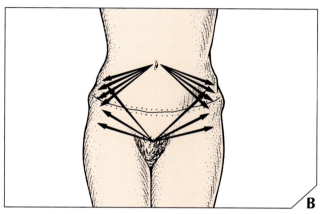

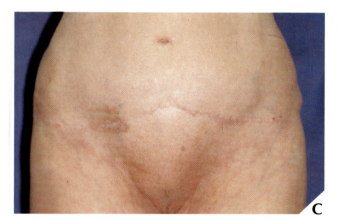

Figure 11.12. **(A)** Postoperative appearance of an abdominoplasty with undue fullness in the lateral flanks. **(B,C)** This was corrected by suction-assisted lipectomy using a 3.7-mm cannula introduced through small stab incisions in the umbilicus and in the hair-bearing area of the pubis.

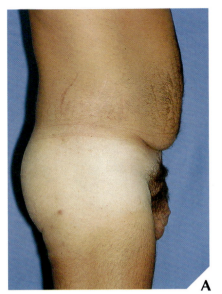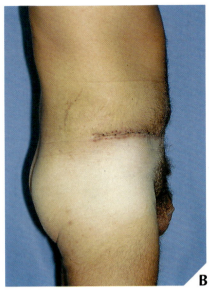

Figure 11.13. (A) A misguided attempt at abdominal contouring using suction alone without removal of redundant integument. The surgeon did not assess preoperatively that some percentage of the abdominal contour defect was caused by intra-abdominal fat in the omentum and mesentery. Reconstruction of this deformity involved two procedures: (1) plication of the rectus abdominus fascia of the abdominal wall to correct the overdistended abdomen secondary to the intra-abdominal fat and (2) traditional procedure for lower abdominal integument reduction. (B) Postoperative appearance.

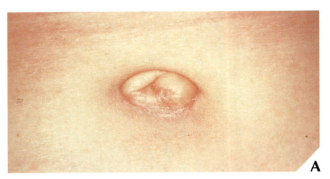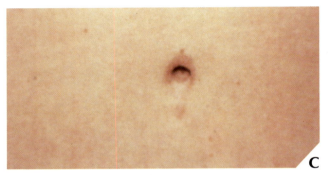

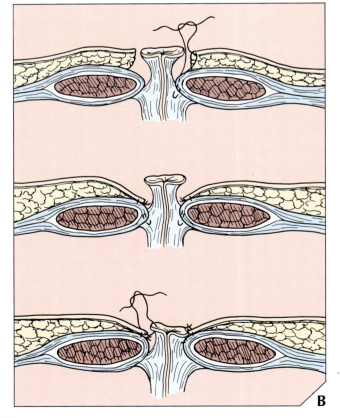

Figure 11.14. (A) An unaesthetic, large, protuberant umbilicus in a patient following abdominoplasty. (B) Correction consisted of an umbilicalplasty that decreased the circumference of the umbilical stalk. Employment of a single suture to tie down both the abdominal circumferential skin and the skin on the circumference of the umbilicus to the rectus abdominous sheath below produced a smaller invaginated umbilicus, which was more aesthetically pleasing (C).

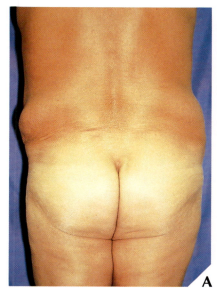

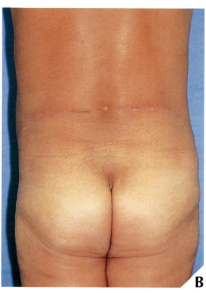

Figure 11.15. (A) A bilateral flank deformity in a male patient that had failed to improve on two previous suction aspiration procedures. **(B)** Correction consisted of a belt lipectomy with excision of the excess flaccid integument.

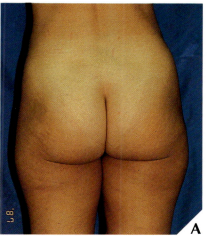

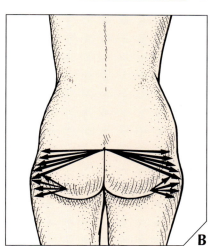

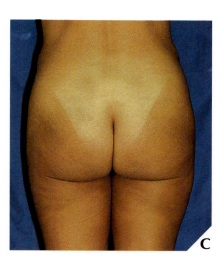

Figure 11.16. The patient had suggested that the surgeon only suction the waist and upper hip area and the surgeon obediently complied. **(A)** It was only after the surgery had been performed that both the patient and surgeon realized that this maneuver alone, without proportionately reducing the lower trochanteric area, would accentuate a heretofore non-problematic trochanteric area. **(B,C)** Correction of this deformity simply involved using a 3.7-mm cannula to reduce the contour of the trochanteric area. Small stab wound incisions were concealed in the vertical and the horizontal creases of the buttocks.

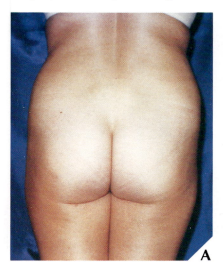

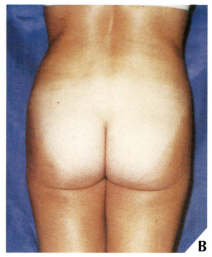

Figure 11.17. (A) The same error as described in Figure 11.16, except the patient directed the surgeon to reduce lower trochanteric area without giving thought to decreasing the projection of the waist and upper hips proportionately. **(B)** Correction consisted of a 3.7-mm cannula aspiration using two small stab incisions concealed in the vertical crease of the buttocks.

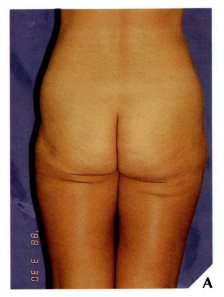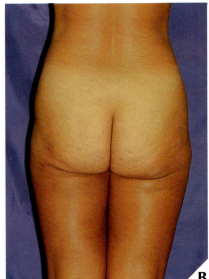

Figure 11.18. (A) common deformity produced by over-reduction of adipose tissue in the subgluteal area, which creates an unaesthetic horizontal fold when the patient is standing. This deformity is not detectable on the operating table where the effect of gravity is 45° out of phase; therefore, the potential for this deformity must be accounted for in the preoperative marking. **(B)** Correction consists of suction contouring with a 3.7-mm cannula.

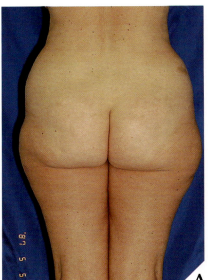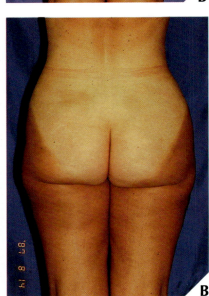

Figure 11.19. (A) Suction contouring that failed to create left/right volumetric equality, with much greater volume on the right side. Correction consisted of aspiration with a 3.7-mm cannula of the excess volume on the right side. **(B)** Stab incisions were concealed in the vertical and horizontal creases of the buttocks.

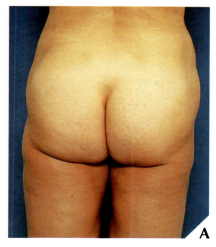

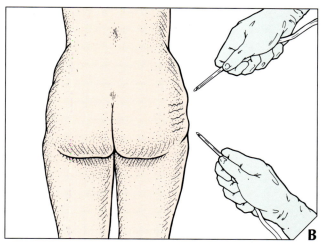

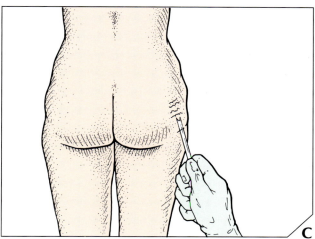

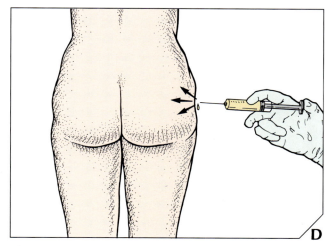

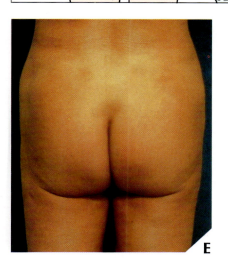

Figure 11.20. **(A)** Common iatrogenic deformity. **(B)** Correction of this depression consisted of suction with a 2.8-mm cannula introduced through two small stab incisions several inches above and below the deformity to feather out the rim between the high ridge and the low concavity. **(C)** Following this procedure, a V-tipped, 3-mm cannula was introduced through one of the stab incisions and the fibrous septi that caused the skin to adhere down to the lower subcutaneous tissue were cut. Lysis of fibrous septi is a preliminary step before injection of autologous fat **(D)**, which is used to fill the remaining defect of the concavity. Overfilling of the defect to allow for fat absorption is at the discretion of the experienced surgeon. **(E)** Postoperative appearance.

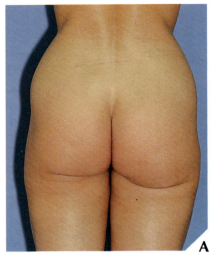

Figure 11.21. (A) Iatrogenic contour deformity with horizontal asymmetry of the subgluteal fold. **(B)** Correction consisted of suctioning the lower horizontal fold with a 3.7-mm cannula.

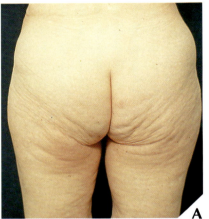

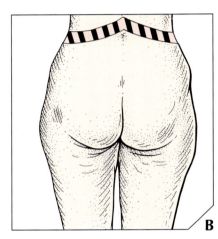

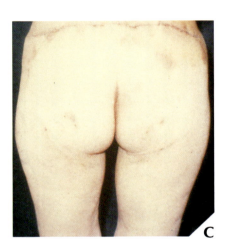

Figure 11.22. (A) Over-reduction of subcutaneous adipose tissue in the buttocks and subgluteal area, resulting in excessive subgluteal redundancy. **(B,C)**

Correction consisted of skin reduction to elevate and tighten the redundant integument of the buttocks and subgluteal area.

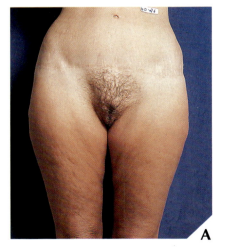

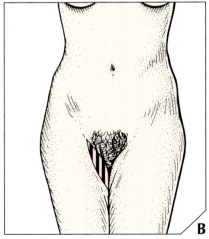

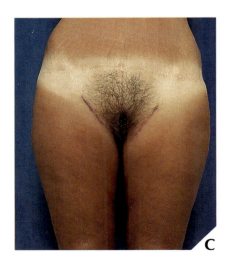

Figure 11.23. (A) One of the most unforgiving anatomic areas for over-reduction of adipose tissue, namely the medial thigh and inguinal area. **(B,C)**

Correction consisted of a unilateral medial thighplasty, which was designed to tighten the redundant integument in the medial thigh area.

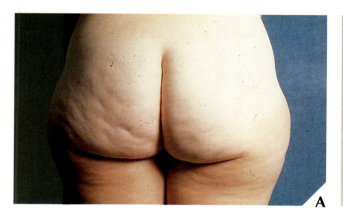
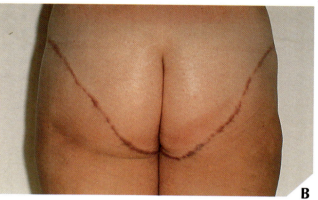

Figure 11.24. (A) Iatrogenic defect secondary to removal of too-much subcutaneous adipose tissue, resulting in redundancy of the integument in the trochanteric area. **(B)** Correction of this defect consisted of excision of integument and subcutaneous tissue to lift and tighten the redundant skin.

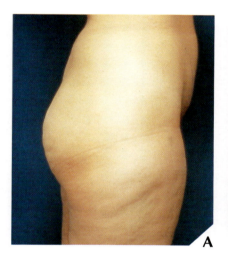
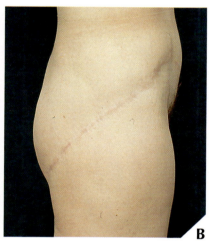
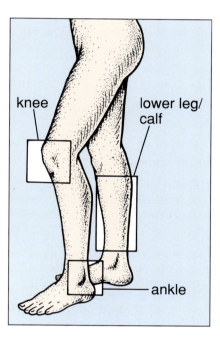

Figure 11.25. (A) Over-reduction of subcutaneous adipose tissue that resulted in an unaesthetic ptosis of the buttocks. **(B)** Correction consisted of excision of skin and subcutaneous tissue to restore contour. This procedure may be performed unilaterally and/or bilaterally, depending upon the nature of the defect.

Figure 11.26. Other anatomic areas where over-reduction of subcutaneous adipose tissue can cause contour irregularities. Unfortunately, integument reduction in these areas leads to unsightly visible scarring. Deformities are best handled by autologous fat grafting of any contour defects that produce a concavity and suction contouring of any high spots. Iatrogenic contour defects in these areas are extremely hard to correct.

BIBLIOGRAPHY

Grazer FM, Wood WG: Abdominal contouring. In Curtis EH (ed): Male Aesthetic Surgery. CV Mosby, St. Louis, 1990.

Grazer FM, Wood WG: Atlas of Body Contouring and Suction Assisted Lipectomy. Churchill Livingstone, New York, 1992.

Grazer FM, Wood WG: Body contour surgery. In Barrett BM (ed): Patient Care in Plastic Surgery. Blackwell Scientific, Cambridge, in press.

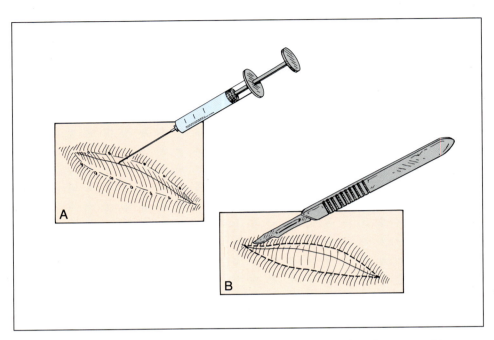

Figure 11.27. The two basic means of addressing hypertrophic scarring. **(A)** The procedure of choice for hypertrophic scarring is injection of dilute solutions of depository corticosteroids, such as Kenalog 10, into the scar. Serial injections are used at approximately 1-month intervals until the desired decrease in scar tissue is reached. Maintenance injections at periodic intervals may be necessary in order to prevent further development of hypertrophicity. **(B)** Unacceptable scars having an unsightly appearance due to width and concavity are best addressed by scar revision. The use of intercuticular sutures can help prevent widening if there is tension on the wound edges. The use of pressure dressings is also beneficial in the treatment of hypertrophic scarring.

Index

O

Obesity, in mammaplasty, 10.3
Obstruction, lacrimal duct, 2.5
Ophthalmopathy, thyroid, 5.10, 5.18, **5.12**
Optic
  chiasm injury, 2.7
  nerve, 5.18, 5.19
Otoplasty, 8.2–8.13, **8.1–8.19**
  allergic reaction, 8.5, **8.5**
  antihelix modification, 8.7–8.8, **8.11,
    8.12, 8.14**
  auditory canal distortion, 8.10
  bleeding, 8.3–8.4, **8.2**
  cartilage
    floppy, 8.8, 8.9, **8.13–8.15**
    irregularity, 8.12–8.13, **8.11, 8.12**
  complications
    general, 8.3–8.6, **8.2–8.8**
    specific, 8.6–8.8, 8.10–8.13, **8.9–8.19**
    surgical, 8.6–8.8, 8.10, **8.9–8.15**
  conchal
    reduction, 8.6–8.7, **8.9, 8.10**
    setback, 8.10
  earlobes, prominent, 8.10
  helix, hidden, 8.11
  hematoma, 8.4
  infection, 8.4–8.5, **8.3, 8.4**
  keloids, 8.5, **8.6, 8.7**
  pain, 8.3
  psychological considerations, 8.6, **8.8**
  relapse, 8.11–8.12, **8.17**
  scarring, 8.3, 8.5, **8.6, 8.7**
  shape changes, 8.10–8.11, **8.15, 8.16**
  suture erosion, 8.10, **8.18**
  suture exposure, 8.12, **8.18**
  telephone deformity, 8.13, **8.19**
Oximeter, 2.2

P

Paresis
  blepharoplasty, 5.19
  eyelid, 5.20
  facelift surgery, 3.5, **3.6**
  nasolabial, 6.19, **6.37, 6.38**
Paresthesia
  brow lift surgery, 4.2
  chin augmentation, 6.30
  facelift surgery, 3.4
  forehead lift surgery, 4.2
Parrot beak deformity, 1.7–1.9, **1.6–1.8**
  See Rhinoplasty, complications
Pinocchio tip deformity, 1.14–1.15, **1.15**
Pneumocephalus, 2.7
Pneumothorax, mammaplasty, 9.21, **9.50**
Port-wine stain, 7.4
Premandible, anatomic zones, 6.5–6.6, **6.7, 6.8**
Psychological considerations
  body contour surgery, 11.2, 11.5
  facelift surgery, 3.7–3.8
  face peel, 7.15
  otoplasty, 8.6, **8.8**

  rhinoplasty, 2.21, **2.37**
Ptosis
  acquired, 5.10, 5.12, **5.14**
  congenital, 5.10, 5.13
  eyelid, 5.9, 5.10, 5.21, 5.22–5.23, **5.5, 5.6,
    5.29, 5.30**
Pustules, 2.7, **2.12**

R

Raynaud's disease, 3.6, 3.7
Rhinoplasty
  augmentation, 1.2, 1.7, 1.8, 2.13, 2.16, **1.1, 1.2**
  bacteremia, 2.5
  bleeding, 2.4, **2.4, 2.5**
  bone
    infracturing, 1.3, 1.4, 1.10, 1.14, 1.15, 1.16, **1.9, 1.14,
      1.15, 1.17**
    rasping, 1.3, 1.4, 1.8, 1.10
    reduction, 1.14
  complications
    allograft rejection, 2.17
    breathing difficulties, 2.17–2.19, **2.30–2.33**
    columella, 1.20, **1.17, 1.18**
    columella, hanging, 1.5–1.8, 1.12, **1.5, 1.6, 1.12**
    columella, retracted, 1.10, **1.10**
    donor site, 2.12–2.13, **2.23, 2.24**
    flap necrosis, 2.27–2.29, **2.47–2.49**
    grafts, 1.16, 1.18
    intracranial, 2.7
    nasal tip, broad, 1.9–1.10
    nose, crippled, 2.12, **2.22**
    nose, crooked, 2.10, 2.12
    nose, long, 1.10–1.12, **1.9, 1.11, 1.12**
    nose, short, 1.12–1.13
    Pinocchio tip deformity, 1.14–1.15, **1.15**
    saddle nose deformity, 1.4–1.6, 1.8, 1.10, 1.12, 1.18,
      1.20, 2.8–2.9, **1.4, 1.5, 1.8, 1.12, 1.16, 1.18, 1.20,
      1.21, 2.15, 2.18**
    skin perforation, 2.23, **2.38**
    supratip deformity, 1.7–1.9, **1.7, 1.8**
    tip projection, 1.2–1.4, 1.6, 1.10, 1.14, 1.20, **1.1–1.3,
      1.8–1.11, 1.14, 1.16, 1.21**
  ecchymosis, 2.2
  edema, 2.2, 2.5–2.7, 2.26–2.27, **2.2, 2.9–2.11**
  effect of alcohol, 2.20
  erythema, 2.19, 2.20
  hematoma, 2.4–2.5, **2.3**
  hemostasis, 2.3, 2.4, 2.26, **2.6**
  hypertension in, 2.2
  infection, 2.5, 2.7, **2.8**
  open, 2.2–2.29, **2.1–2.49**
  primary, 1.2, 1.3, 1.9, 1.10, 1.15, 1.16, **1.1, 1.2,
    1.9, 1.11**
  psychological considerations, 2.21, **2.37**
  reduction, 1.2, 1.3, 1.7, 1.12, 1.14, 1.15
    hump, 1.2, 1.3 1.5, **1.1, 1.2**
  scarring, 2.25–2.26
  secondary, 1.4, 1.7, 1.8, 1.10, 1.12, 1.14, 1.16, **1.3,
    1.5–1.7, 1.12, 1.14, 1.18, 1.20, 1.21, 2.11**
  steroid atrophy, 2.5, 2.7, **2.11**
  telangiectasia, 2.19, 2.20 **2.34**
Rhytides, face peel, 7.3, 7.10, 7.13